The Drama of DNA

THE DRAMA OF DNA

Narrative Genomics

Karen H. Rothenberg

and

Lynn Wein Bush

OXFORD
UNIVERSITY PRESS

OXFORD
UNIVERSITY PRESS

Oxford University Press is a department of the University of Oxford.
It furthers the University's objective of excellence in research, scholarship,
and education by publishing worldwide.

Oxford   New York
Auckland   Cape Town   Dar es Salaam   Hong Kong   Karachi
Kuala Lumpur   Madrid   Melbourne   Mexico City   Nairobi
New Delhi   Shanghai   Taipei   Toronto

With offices in
Argentina   Austria   Brazil   Chile   Czech Republic   France   Greece
Guatemala   Hungary   Italy   Japan   Poland   Portugal   Singapore
South Korea   Switzerland   Thailand   Turkey   Ukraine   Vietnam

Published in the United States of America by
Oxford University Press
198 Madison Avenue, New York, NY 10016

Library of Congress Cataloging-in-Publication Data
Rothenberg, Karen H., 1952– author.
The drama of DNA : narrative genomics / Karen H. Rothenberg and Lynn W. Bush.
    p. ; cm.
Includes bibliographical references.
ISBN 978-0-19-930935-1 (alk. paper)
I. Bush, Lynn W., author.   II. Title.
[DNLM: 1. Genomics.   2. Drama.   3. Teaching—methods. QU 460]
QH431
611'.018166—dc23
2013037248

9 8 7 6 5 4 3 2 1
Printed in the United States of America
on acid-free paper

To our families, with enduring love

CONTENTS

PART THREE: Narrative Genomics on Stage: DNA, Society, and Theatre

Online Links to Original Genomic Plays
Chapter 2 "Imagining a Genomic Crystal Ball"
Chapter 3 "It's Not That Simple!" and "It's So Complicated!!" (sequel)
Chapter 4 "The Paradoxes in Pandora's Box" and "Paradoxes Within Pandora's
   Box" (fuller version)
Chapter 5 "What's Next?!"

Note: Six full-length plays, adapted to varying degrees for the narratives
in these chapters, can be accessed at the companion website for this book,
http://global.oup.com/us/companion.websites/9780199309351/.

FOREWORD

The past decade has brought spectacular advances in technologies for analyzing genomes, in particular methods for "reading out" the sequence of DNA. These advances have catalyzed the spread of genomic approaches for studying human disease across the biomedical research landscape, which in turn has brought an impressive acceleration in the acquisition of fundamental knowledge about the genome's role in health and disease. To capitalize on these successes and to facilitate the use of genomics in medical care (i.e., genomic medicine), we need a better understanding of the professional and societal implications of routinely acquiring and using human genomic information.

Among the many things to consider is the need for healthcare professionals to interpret and communicate genomic information to their patients; yet that information is often associated with immediate uncertainty and its predictive value will almost certainly evolve over time. And yet that very genomic data have great potential to redefine our conceptualization of health, disease, and identity.

Effectively examining the implications of genomic advances requires interdisciplinary collaborations. Toward that end, narrative genomics developed by Karen Rothenberg and Lynn Bush offers a novel path to enhance the understanding and dialogue among clinical geneticists, genetic counselors, bench scientists, primary care physicians, bioethicists, policy makers, other researchers and healthcare professionals, patients, and patient advocates. Many of their papers and plays have been posted on the National Human Genome Research Institute (NHGRI) website—www.genome.gov—for widespread access. Their narratives extend beyond the provision of genomic information, and illustrate what they call "the dialogues and dilemmas" of genomic research and its application to medicine.

Having a compilation of Rothenberg and Bush vignettes in book form also facilitates using the narratives and accompanying questions in the medical education setting. Interest in their creative approach has been expressed by members of the scientific community following exposure to their initial publications and presentations at professional meetings (e.g., the annual meetings of the American College of Medical Genetics and Genomics and the American

Society of Human Genetics) and at a number of academic medical centers in the United States and abroad.

Personally, I have had the opportunity to participate and "act" (very liberally defined!) in several sessions at the National Institutes of Health and elsewhere involving Rothenberg and Bush's original plays as well as scenes from existing theatre. My experiences confirm that their novel approach successfully generates a constructive dialogue about the ethical, psychological, and societal challenges that develop with the infusion of genomics into real-world situations. Understanding these important transitional challenges is a key component of the mission of NHGRI, as we aim to chart the course from genomic research to genomic medicine.

As Director of NHGRI, I have also supported the use of Rothenberg and Bush's vignettes and existing theatrical excerpts at policy meetings, training sessions, and trans-NIH bioethics programs—and most recently, as part of a multiyear collaboration with the Smithsonian Institution's National Museum of Natural History's exhibition *Genome: Unlocking Life's Code*, which commemorates the 10th anniversary of completing the Human Genome Project.

It is with the spirit of providing a valuable resource for enhancing teaching and an interdisciplinary dialogue in genomics that I welcome Rothenberg and Bush's contribution represented by this book. From my perspective, these pages provide an innovative vehicle to illuminate the human element and to facilitate insight into the challenges facing individuals, families, professionals, and society as we move into a future of genomics-based health care.

Eric D. Green, MD, PhD
Director, National Human Genome Research Institute
National Institutes of Health
Bethesda, Maryland

PREFACE

We share an appreciation for the power of dramatic narratives to bring to life the complex challenges posed by emerging genomic technologies. Narrative genomics developed from our belief in this creative pedagogical approach to illuminate issues to the genomics community. And so this book evolved.

As fate would have it, our paths crossed while we were both at Columbia University five years ago at interdisciplinary seminars on health law, bioethics, science policy, and narrative medicine. Neither of us is shy, and it soon became apparent that we both had a strong interest in enhancing dialogue and understanding about the ethical, psychological, and policy challenges raised by generating and sharing vast amounts of genomic information. With diverse backgrounds in psychology, genetics, law, and bioethics, we both had woven dramatic narratives into our teaching and scholarship to enhance the educational experiences within our varied professional contexts. Once we met, we were a team.

We initially collaborated on the creation of a short vignette play in the context of genomic research and the informed consent process that was performed at the NHGRI-ELSI Congress by a geneticist, genetic counselor, and other conference attendees. The response by "actors" and audience fueled us to write many more plays of varying lengths on different genomic issues, as well as to explore the dialogues of existing theatre with genetic and genomic themes—all to be presented and reflected upon by interdisciplinary professionals in the genomics community at conferences and academic institutions across the globe.

This book would not have been possible without the support and generous feedback of so many colleagues. Nancy King first introduced us to the concept of "readers' theater" and inspired and encouraged us to develop narrative genomics. Jim Evans guided us with his insights and watchful genomics eye throughout our endeavor, and enthusiastically acted in most of our plays, beginning with our first performance in which he brilliantly played a snarky 19-year-old.

A very special thank you to Eric Green, Director of NHGRI, for embracing from day one the benefits of narrative genomics as a creative technique to facilitate understanding of the implications of genomic technologies on professionals and society—not to mention his many starring performances!!! We want to express our deep appreciation to other colleagues at NHGRI and the NIH Department of Bioethics, especially Ben Berkman, Barbara Biesecker, Christine Grady, and Sara Hull, for their reviews, commentaries, the sharing of our work with faculty and fellows, and acting roles from pilots at the NIH to final scripts on stage. A special thank-you for the encouragement of the Division of Genomics and Society—Joy Boyer, Larry Brody, Jean McEwen, and Nicole Lockhart, and the support of the Division of Policy, Communications, and Education, including Vence Bonham, Christina Daulton, Carla Easter, Raymond MacDougall, Jeannine Mjoseth, Laura Rodriguez, and Larry Thompson—not to mention so many of these folks and others at NHGRI who have participated in our play readings over the last few years. We are also so grateful for the artistic talent of Darryl Leja, who created the image for this cover, and Annette Sante for her outstanding technical assistance and enduring patience.

Our gratitude extends to all the members of the genomics community who so generously "volunteered" to be actors and discussants at numerous conferences over the years, especially Jeff Botkin, Carlos Bustamante, Malia Fullerton, Steve Joffe, Eric Juengst, Barbara Koenig, Michelle Lewis, Amy McGuire, Bob Nussbaum, Pearl O'Rourke, Heidi Rehm, Ginna Sybert, Wendy Uhlmann, Ben Wilfond, and Susan Wolf. We want to thank Elisa Hurley and Joe McInerney for their support in sharing this pedagogical method broadly with their interdisciplinary membership through videotaping of our plays. And for giving us a global presence, we thank David Weisbrot and his colleagues in Australia, Tim Caulfield in Canada, Hub Zwart in the Netherlands, and colleagues at the Wellcome Trust in the United Kingdom. In addition, we are greatly appreciative of our diverse audiences for their important role in actively participating in the performance discussions.

We wish to thank our colleagues at Columbia for their advice and support throughout the years, and are particularly grateful to Ruth Fischbach and George Hardart at the Center for Bioethics for so generously embracing narrative genomics as an educational method to use with colleagues and medical students; Wendy Chung, Brynn Levy, Jacinda Sampson, and Kwame Anyane Yeboa for contributing their expertise in clinical genetics and neurogenetics; James Colgrove for his mentorship on public heath ethics and the historical underpinnings of bioethics; Rita Charon for sharing her scholarly interest and enthusiasm for narrative medicine; and Kendall Thomas for his academic leadership on the study of law and culture. And at Maryland Law, we thank our colleagues with the Linking Law and the Arts initiative, including Taunya Banks and the late Katherine Vaughns, and Diane Hoffmann of the Law and Health Care Program—with a very extra special thanks to Sue McCarty for her expertise and patience in helping us format our extensive references and her thorough review of this book manuscript. Our appreciation also extends to the faculty of the Berman Institute of Bioethics at Johns Hopkins, especially Ruth Faden, Gail Geller, Jeff Kahn, Nancy Kass, and Jeremy Sugarman for their interest and experience in integrating narratives into bioethics teaching and scholarship.

We are indebted to Chad Zimmerman, our outstanding editor at Oxford University Press, for his unwavering support and thoughtful guidance in making this book become a reality—having faith in the value of narrative genomics as a creative educational technique for the genomics community. Our thanks also extend to Meredith Keller, Emily Perry, and others on the editorial staff at Oxford for their valuable contributions to this book project.

Finally, we want to express to our husbands, Jeff and Paul, our love and appreciation for enduring years of listening to us morning, noon, and night on the phone creating plays and drafting, editing, and re-editing this book long distance. As we reflect on the creative process, we dedicate this book to our children—who have enriched our lives beyond our imagination.

A NOTE FROM THE AUTHORS

The Drama of DNA is meant to provide an analytical foundation and pedagogical approach to the many complex challenges surrounding clinical genetics, genomic medicine, and its related disciplines. Because we hope to facilitate interdisciplinary discourse and reflection on the complexity of the scientific, ethical, psychological, societal, legal, and policy issues discussed within the chapters and online plays, we have provided an extensive reference section at the end of this book that gathers multiple sources together under numeric headings. These reference groups are referred to by number throughout the text, and are often re-cited in different chapters to reflect that these complex issues arise in multiple contexts. We consider each reference entry important individually, and together the numbered groupings highlight the breadth of scholarship on these multidisciplinary and interrelated issues as a resource to enhance teaching.

CHAPTER 1

Setting the Genomic Stage

Why Genomics, Why Narratives, Why Now?

Genomics has the potential to be transformative, raising ethical dilemmas for professionals and our society that call forth novel ways to enhance understanding of these challenges. We have developed *narrative genomics*, using characters and dramatic dialogue, as an pedagogical technique to bring to life the diverse voices, varied contexts, and complex processes that encompass the nascent field of genomics as it evolves "from base pairs to bedside."[1,2] This creative approach focuses on inherent challenges currently posed by the comprehensive interrogation and analysis of DNA through sequencing the human genome with next generation technologies—extending far beyond the scope and implications of a single gene in the context of genetics and its narratives.[3] These chapters capture the drama of DNA in genomic narratives that can be imagined and shared to illuminate our gaze on the people, the helices, and the future within.

Narrative genomics can juxtapose both complementary and disparate views,[4] engraving images[5] of often conflicting experiences and perspectives when encountering new genomic technology and information. Dramatic vignettes offer a unique analytical stage for imagining the bioethical and scientific past, present, and future, and the dramatization of relationships surrounding genomics creates the potential to stimulate self-reflection and new perceptions, sparking *the moral imagination*[6] through the lens of others. By casting light on all "the storytellers" and the complexity of interactions inherent with this powerful technology, narrative genomics can create vivid scenarios through which to imagine the challenges faced by individuals, families, and professionals on the genomic path ahead.

We build upon the legacy of using case vignettes as a clinical teaching modality, and our experience suggests similar value within the research and public policy domains in illustrating potential psychosocial risks and benefits as witnessed through narrative genomics. We are also inspired by "readers' theater"[7] and "narrative medicine"[8] as approaches[9] that helped us to expand our analyses of the implications of genomic technologies. While film, plays, television, literature, and narrative prose have often been utilized in academic and medical settings to facilitate empathy and spotlight ethical and legal controversies such as end-of-life issues, organ donations, and health law,[10] to date there appears to be few dramatizations focusing on next-generation sequencing (NGS) in genomic research and medicine.[11]

This book was written with the belief that creative interdisciplinary approaches need to be encouraged to foster a greater appreciation for how society evaluates, processes, and shares genomic information that may implicate future generations.[i, 12-14] Narrative genomics highlights the breadth of individuals affected by next-gen technologies—the conversations among professionals and families—while bringing to life the spectrum of emotions and challenges that envelop genomics. The selection of dialogue in this book encompasses abbreviated excerpts adapted from our original genomic plays (linked online in their entirety) and existing theatre, some of each that we have presented nationally and internationally, including at professional society meetings and academic medical institutions. Varying iterations of the dramatic narratives have been experienced (read, enacted, witnessed) by geneticists, genetic counselors, other healthcare professionals, basic scientists, bioethicists, policy makers, lawyers, patient advocates, and students to enhance insight and facilitate interdisciplinary dialogue.[ii]

Our exploration of the drama of DNA begins by focusing the imagination on whole-exome and whole-genome sequencing (WES and WGS, respectively). Contemporary issues are brought to life through a variety of fictionalized characters and their dramatic narratives, illustrating potential benefits and dilemmas facing individuals, families, and professionals with comprehensive genome technology and the information it generates.[iii, 15-18] Presently there is considerable variation and debate in the literature and among professionals over the terminology to best describe information generated through genome sequencing, and while we prefer the terms "genomic information" and "genomic findings," this book also includes the phrases "incidental findings," "secondary findings," and "research results" interchangeably to reflect current patterns of usage.[19,20]

Part I, "Narrative Genomics: Exploring Process in Context," revolves around three narratives that place the issues in differing contexts and build upon each other. The three chapters evolve from an institutional review board (IRB) and advisory committees considering an aggregated WGS research protocol with participants who are unknown to the investigators (Chapter 2); to a pediatric clinical geneticist who has a long relationship with a family recruited for WES clinical research as they all experience the informed consent process and disclosure of findings (Chapter 3); to an expert public health policy committee analyzing the philosophical and practical implications of implementing new-born genomic sequencing (NBSeq) as a pilot statewide initiative (Chapter 4).

Part II, "Integrating Narrative Genomics: A Case Study Drama," presents a fuller fictionalized genomic *case* that integrates most of the seminal issues and themes we explored in the preceding chapters with several significant contextual variations. This narrative involves a family known to the genetic counselor, with some members engaged in both clinical research with NGS and diagnostic targeted genetic testing. The four scenes move from an IRB deliberation, to the informed consent process, to a clinical ethics consultation, and then to the return of genomic findings (Chapter 5).

Dramatizations are brought to life through another avenue in Part III, "Narrative Genomics on Stage: DNA, Society, and Theatre," in which excerpts from some existing theatrical narratives illuminate the historical path to the genomics revolution, beginning with Rosalind Franklin's crystallographic image of the double helix to the molecular genetics of Alzheimer's disease (Chapter 6).

The Drama of DNA has been structured to provide an analytical foundation that builds from Part I through Part III to reinforce the fact that many complex issues surface repeatedly in varying contexts.[21] Because narrative genomics is a pedagogical approach intended to facilitate discourse as well as provide reflective reading on the interrelatedness of the cross-disciplinary issues posed, we have included an extensive references section at the end of this book that groups multiple citations together numerically delineated by themes, most of which are cited in more than one chapter.

We reflect on the reality that as the evolution of next-gen sequencing progresses exponentially into clinical research, medicine, and screening, so too will the discovery of incidental findings and ethical complexities.[22-24,76] Many challenges surround the promise of genomic technology and the power of genomic information, as they alter conceptions of identity and dynamics within personal, familial, and professional relationships.[25-30] Controversial issues abound—such as determining whether, what, to whom, when, and how genomic information should be disclosed to individuals and their families[31,32]—and whose voices matter in making these determinations.[33-39]

Unlike some diagnostic or screening methods, comprehensive genomic sequencing can reveal a vast amount of potent information that extends beyond the individuals to include blood relatives and ancestral groups, and thus, anticipation of the ethical, legal, social, psychological, and policy implications necessitates additional forethought.[40-46] Therefore, when WGS is involved in either the research or clinical setting, it is particularly important that plans and policies be formulated early on and clearly elucidated throughout the informed consent process,[47-50] including any duty to recontact or ancillary care obligation issues.[51-53] Although the lengthy consent form language may allude to the possibility of learning secondary results, many individuals consider the potential for discovering incidentals with WGS/WES to be highly remote. Further complicating the discovery of incidental findings, it often is the case that the original question for which genomic study was indicated will go unanswered.

The element of surprise can be emotionally unsettling, particularly when neither families nor professionals fully anticipate the range of findings that will be routinely discovered upon the application of this powerful technology, and the impact that information will yield.[54,55] Neither the clinician-researcher nor the individual can always predict whether their preferences for the return of results will change or who will bear the burden and distress from the return of unanticipated findings.[56] Moreover, there is little consensus regarding under what circumstances, if any, a consent form's request "not to know" may go unhonored.

The judgment regarding the disclosure of secondary results attained in genomic research and medicine remains controversial,[57-59] and the need to clarify definitions such as variable penetrance and susceptibility is essential.[60,61] There is great debate as to what revelations constitute urgency for disclosure and who should decide, as well as what findings are deemed clinically relevant, actionable, or predictable.[62-64] Caution is also advised to avoid misinterpretation of susceptibility with a diagnosis of disease, especially when it is low-risk or represents a broad range of phenotypes.[65,66]

Implications need to be considered for individuals who previously identified themselves as healthy as well as those defined by their genetic condition.[67-70] Next-generation sequencing raises challenges when children, especially otherwise "unaffected" children, are faced with findings that threaten their identity and raise novel concerns about their future.[71-78] As investigations involving minors engender even more complex ethical and psychological challenges, the need for heightened sensitivity by professionals becomes magnified, as does the unsettling nature for researchers and clinicians.[79-86] Differential approaches must be weighed not only to consider whether, but to whom and when, results may be disclosed.[87-89]

Even when there is "ideal" genetic counseling preceding and following genomic sequencing,[90-91] the psychological stress regarding expectations and anticipations may often impede individuals from adequately hearing and integrating the information. Moreover, genomics professionals and other healthcare providers face potential distress in light of serious incidental findings to report, or those with uncertainty regarding the consequences.[92]

With these debates and dilemmas as our backdrop, the scenario for Chapter 2's dramatic narrative, "Anticipating the Future," spotlights WGS and the need for ethics consultations in a variety of contexts, including IRBs and genomics advisory committees. The drama particularly highlights the roles professionals should play within each group to minimize psychosocial harm, ideally in advance of genomic testing. This dialogue brings to life significant challenges with the process and systemic questions raised when "a plan" does not adequately consider potential risks,[93–96] especially with children.[102–105] Along with exploring reactions toward planning protocols in anticipation of results generated from the genomic study, the narratives adapted from *Imagining a Genomic Crystal Ball* illustrate inherent tensions among professionals and the need for guidance from institutional boards, advisory committees, and professional societies.[97–101]

Chapter 3, "Informing the Future," showcases the practical application of the issues highlighted in Chapter 2, with distinctions that are context-driven and relationship-oriented. This new cast of characters sheds light on the complexity of emotions, reactions, and implications throughout the informed consent process and during disclosure of genomic information. The vignette illuminates some of the challenges that may arise from the multidimensional role of the clinical geneticist-researcher when recruiting a long-standing patient and family for participation in a genomic study. The narrative commences by illustrating *It's Not That Simple!*,[4] with dialogue that focuses on dilemmas often facing family members during the informed consent process for genomic research and medicine, and concludes with some of the professional, personal, and familial dilemmas surrounding the reporting of genomic findings to illuminate that *It's So Complicated!*[4] Such issues considered in the chapter include the blurring of boundaries between genomic research and clinical practice,[106] the therapeutic misconception,[107] privacy and confidentiality,[108–112] biobanking,[113–115] reporting incidental findings to *unaffected* children, the role of assent,[116,117] and broader implications for blood relatives and ethnic communities.

The genomic narratives in Chapter 4, "Reframing an 'Open Future,'" finds another group of interdisciplinary professionals situated in a different advisory role, this time public health policy, examining many of the ethical, legal, and psychosocial issues previously raised in the earlier chapters. This dramatization highlights a very contemporary debate—the future of a shifting landscape from NBS to NBSeq.[118–123] Set in a government conference room, an expert committee has been convened to advise a state agency on whether to pilot newborn whole-genome sequencing as a population-based screening program.[124–127] As they consider some of the implications of WGS involving all infants statewide, the committee moves from the philosophical sphere of generating paradoxes to brainstorming a list of salient challenges of a more practical nature.[128–134,154] Of paramount concern expressed by many of the experts is the impact on a child's "right to an open future."[136] Many other issues are raised by the committee including informed consent,[137–142] social justice,[143–145] incidental findings,[154] and implications on parental stress-infant attachment,[146–153] as this narrative explores *The Paradoxes in Pandora's Box*.

The drama of DNA in Chapter 5, "Reconceptualizing the Past, Present, & Future," is a four-scene fictionalized genomics case study that integrates most of the issues and implications highlighted in previous chapters. To emphasize just how much context matters, themes explored in Part I (Chapters 2–4) are interwoven into a fuller dramatic narrative that evolves from an IRB meeting through the informed consent process and a clinical ethics consultation to the disclosure of incidental findings. Based on an original, full-length genomic play, *What's Next?!*, Part II (Chapter 5) illuminates the ethical, psychological, social, legal, and policy concerns surrounding the attaining and sharing of massive amounts of information generated by next-generation sequencing, particularly when involving *unaffected* children and pregnant women.

Some enduring concerns also represented in earlier genomic narratives (and explored in some existing plays that follow) include difficulty adequately anticipating challenges and minimizing potential risks from the planning stages to the return of findings, the implications of the graying of boundaries between research and clinical medicine, and the perceived blurred distinction between diagnostic capabilities and genomic screening technologies. To delve further into controversial issues brought to life in this case narrative, we have included a *focus question* to ponder between each scene regarding the sharing of genomic information and the institutional processes that are needed to anticipate challenging scenarios before the promise of genomic technology can be realized.

Narrative genomics is presented in a different format as Chapter 6, "Dramatizing the Past, Present, & Future," illuminates key moments in genetic and genomic history with existing theatrical narratives. By situating theatrical dialogue in historical context beginning with the search for the structure of DNA, Part III (Chapter 6) highlights varying perspectives on the evolution of the ethical, legal, social, psychological, and policy implications of genetics and genomics. Although the scientific landscape shifts, the hopes and fears expressed in theatre from long ago parallel many contemporary issues, including the ongoing struggle to appreciate the impact of emerging genomic technologies on relationships and identity. Therefore, to enhance our current discourse on these enduring concerns as we translate genomic innovations from the lab to the clinic, we reflect on their constancy by exploring how perceptions and relationships have shaped—and been shaped by—genetics and genomics as portrayed through dramatic vignettes from existing theatrical productions spanning generations.

Weaving in historical events that have colored the public's imagination surrounding genetics and genomics, we selected narratives that illuminate affective responses within personal and professional relationships to genomic technology with contrasting contextual subtleties. This last chapter encompasses three sections moving through time.[251–262] "The Theatrical Double Helix and 'Chromozones'" explores the late 1940s through the early 1960s—the nascent years of trying to understand the basic structure of DNA and its subsequent application to society—in Ziegler's *Photograph 51* and Albee's *Who's Afraid of Virginia Woolf?*

The second section, "Mapping and Manipulating Fate," moves to the 1990s—from the initiation to the completion of sequencing the human genome—with narratives from Tolins' *The Twilight of the Golds*, Stephenson's *An Experiment with an Air Pump*, Mullin's *The Sequence*, Djerrassi's *An Immaculate Misconception*, and Churchill's *A Number*. The final section, "A Genomic Crystal Ball in the Post-Mapping Decade," explores theatrical narratives with themes reflecting our recent attempts to understand ancestry and control heritable disorders in Medley's *Relativity*, Atkins' *Lucy*, Loomer's *Distracted*, Fortenberry's *The Good Egg*, and White's *The Other Place*. Narrative excerpts from these playwrights' dialogue dramatize the persistence of aspirations and concerns we still face today—the promises and perils of genomic innovations transforming human relationships and individual, familial, and cultural identities.

While contemporary ethical, social, psychological, and legal issues echo debates of an earlier time as society continues to search for biological explanations and solutions, these persistent challenges emerge with increasing frequency as genomic advances generate more and more information. The risks of revealing genomic information that is even suggestive of disease or a stigmatizing disorder to healthy participants or family members must be carefully weighed against medical benefits, especially when involving children. We believe that the genomic research, clinical, policy, and bioethics communities can benefit from engaging in further dialogue together, reflecting on these unresolved dilemmas to enrich health care and the policy process.

Our dramatic narratives generate many questions about the implications of genomic research and medicine on a multitude of dimensions, including familial and professional relationships, personal and group identities, and practical concerns such as privacy issues. Therefore, to enhance discourse and synthesize some key "teachable moments" for further analysis, we have provided a list of discussion questions at the end of each chapter, as well as one or two *focus questions* at the end of each scene within the narratives of Parts I and II and the online linked original plays.

The complexity of these contemporary issues is brought to life through narrative, "just because it is not our life, [it] places us in a moral position that is favorable for perception and it shows us what it would be like to take up that position in life."[276] Since the potential exists for genomics to dramatically transform society, educational techniques should be encouraged to promote a better understanding of the ethical challenges facing individuals and professionals in the present and future. Dramatizations embedded in genomic narratives illuminate the human dimensions and complexity of interactions among family members, medical professionals, and others in the scientific community. By facilitating discourse and raising more questions than answers on difficult issues, narrative genomics links the promise and concerns of next-gen technologies with a creative pedagogical approach for learning from one another.

NOTES

i. A small segment of this book is adapted from the authors' prior body of work in this field, including Rothenberg and Bush, "Manipulating Fate: Medical Innovations, Ethical Implications, Theatrical Illuminations"; Bush and Rothenberg, "Dialogues, Dilemmas, and Disclosures: The Return of Results and Incidental Findings"; Rothenberg and Bush, "Genes and Plays: Bringing ELSI Issues to Life"; and Rothenberg, "From Eugenics to the 'New' Genetics: The Play's the Thing."

ii. Although memorization and rehearsals are not necessary, the dramatic narratives are intended to be read in advance by the volunteer "actors" to gain familiarity with the characters and issues. Following performance of the vignettes, as well as between acts in the lengthier original plays, we encourage discussion among panelists/professors, actors, and the audience.

iii. While the characters in these narratives are fictitious, as are some diseases noted, italicized consent form language excerpts are based on composites of actual consent documents. The referenced community, names, and designated disorders are modifiable, and, depending on cultural and other demographic variables, the way in which the genomic information is received and shared will differ, as will expectations.

Moreover, cognizant that perspectives can dramatically shift depending on the nuances and context presented, most genders are not specified and the age ranges highlight the additional responsibility required when considering sharing genomic information attained from families that include pregnant women and fetuses, newborns and children.

PART ONE

Narrative Genomics

Exploring Process in Context

CHAPTER 2

Anticipating the Future

Genomic Protocols & Ethics Consultations

The complexities and processes of integrating genomic research and medicine are brought to life in a variety of contexts in the narratives of "Anticipating the Future with WGS," an adaptation of our play *Imagining a Genomic Crystal Ball*. This dramatic narrative provides the opportunity to imagine, contemplate, and debate complex ethical and psychosocial dilemmas posed by research protocols[94,98] that increasingly propose the application of cutting-edge genomic technologies[15] in ways that challenge the boundaries of current ethical norms—especially when whole-genome sequencing involves pregnant women and their fetuses,[99,155,156] newborns, and children, including *unaffected* siblings.[72,83–86]

Autism spectrum disorder (ASD) was selected as the condition under study for this hypothetical vignette (although several other disorders are equally applicable) to explore shifting perspectives of *normal* in the context of genomic findings as well as phenotypic expression, and illuminate how genetic variations, behavioral manifestations, and their categorizations are subject to modification over time. The provocative research protocol is intended to help us grapple with personal, professional, and societal implications that may ensue when reconceptualizing boundaries of *normal* as discoveries are made using whole-genome sequencing on vulnerable populations.[43,67–71,93,136]

SCENE I: THE IRB MEETING

The fictionalized drama begins at West Coastal Children's Hospital, part of Pacific University Medical Center, where an IRB meeting is in progress. The second protocol, titled "Investigating Genotype-Phenotype Variations in Autism Spectrum Disorders Using Whole-Genome Sequencing," is about to be reviewed by IRB committee members including:

> Dr. Pedonc, a pediatric oncologist and the IRB chair
>
> Dr. Neurow, a pediatric neurologist and the primary reviewer
>
> Dr. Psychlaw, a clinical child psychologist with JD degree
>
> Dr. Farmeth, a pharmacologist and ethicist
>
> Mr./Ms. Comparent, community member and parent of an adult child with autism

The site Primary Investigator (co-PI), Dr. Pigene (pronounced "PIE-gene"), Chief of Neurodevelopmental Genetic Pathology, is outside in the hallway, waiting to be called in to respond to queries.

As Chair, Dr. Pedonc initially expresses concern that "several aspects of this research design will likely be controversial," and notes the limited time for discussion due to the day's full agenda. Without further ado, Dr. Neurow provides the requisite details for the IRB, cognizant that some members typically do not read their files in advance beyond a quick glance, and not everyone seated will have ample understanding of the potential implications of the comprehensive genomic technology proposed.[157-160]

More specifically, Dr. Neurow explains that this protocol is a multisite aggregate study in which neurogeneticist Dr. Pigene is serving as co-primary investigator (co-PI) and builds upon the research team's earlier international research project[161-163] investigating copy number variation (CNV) on children already diagnosed with autism spectrum disorder (ASD).[164] The protocol under review today uses these investigators again to study the same group of kids with ASD—this time utilizing whole-genome sequencing (WGS). In addition, this new project will include their biologically related siblings below the age of 18 without an ASD diagnosis and their undiagnosed parents—including pregnant moms—with all participants getting WGS.[173]

When Dr. Neuro mentions that family members will be recruited by the Autism Spectrum Parent Advocacy Network ("Autism Network"), a "yellow flag" is raised for Dr. Farmeth, who interrupts: "Are they funding this?" Somewhat defensively, Mr./Ms. Comparent quickly responds: "I should make clear, up front, that I have no conflict of interest to report—I don't belong to the Autism Network." Potential conflict of interest[165] can take many forms beyond the financial, including, at times, balancing the benefits of hearing the voices of advocacy groups[166] and professional organizations in evaluating new research with the potential risk of loss of objectivity.

As is often the arrangement between advocacy groups and researchers,[95] the Autism Network is giving Dr. Pigene access to the stored blood specimens[102,113] used in the initial collaborative study from the children diagnosed on the autism spectrum. The researchers now propose to employ WGS on the *affected* kids who participated in the original study, and for whom Dr. Pigene's team determined through targeted sequencing to have deletions and duplications on chromosomes highly associated with ASD. Dr. Farmeth advises that "we have to be mindful" of the multitude of genetic variants and epigenetic factors that have been reported to potentially influence the phenotypic expression of this complex disorder—such as variations in the severity across the spectrum, including within families.[167-169,175]

Dr. Neurow also highlights that research results from the original study were not returned to the families,[45,76,170] as stated in the consent.[47,84,87] Because these children, now ages 4 through 18, have biobanked specimens available to the researchers,[105] the new protocol suggests there is no need to collect blood from them again. Eyebrows are raised after hearing that the co-PI "just" wants to collect samples for WGS from their *unaffected* sibs under 18 years of age[43] and their parents:

DR. PEDONC: This seems to be a very ethically complex expansion of Dr. Pigene's previous study from my perspective.

DR. FARMETH: I agree with that. And I don't understand why they involve *normal* children with getting sequencing of their *whole* genomes? The sibs are all reported to be *unaffected* if I understand correctly?

MR./MS. COMPARENT: The protocol specifies that the sibs are reported by parents to be *neurotypical* . . . like their parents' report of themselves.

DR. PSYCHLAW: But *reported unaffected* doesn't always equate with *being unaffected* . . . and I am not just referring to the psychosocial impact of living with a sibling or child who has autism.

When an IRB is evaluating a protocol involving children, Subpart D requires a risk/benefit analysis for all the children participating in the study[83]—both *affected* and *neurotypical*.[86] This is a big challenge, particularly when a protocol includes *unaffected* children in genomics research.[85] For example, the sibs perceived as *unaffected* may turn out to have deletions or duplications or other variants that are found to be a risk factor for autism, and risk factors may be identified now or in the future.[159]

Dr. Farmeth expresses concern about whether having that genomic information "then makes them *affected* and considered any less *normal* in their eyes or others', including their parents'."[177] Pondering the significance of this question, Dr. Psychlaw cautions that this can fuel an identity crisis in adolescents who already are tackling issues of identity formation.

Easing the intensity of the moment, Dr. Neurow interjects, "I'm not sure *any* teenager acts *normal.*"

Although it is unclear from the protocol whether siblings will ever learn this information, IRBs should require investigators to further elaborate about the plan to return results,[18] both related to autism as well as to the incidental findings that will arise with WGS.[19,22,77,78]

To further complicate matters, Dr. Farmeth wonders aloud, "What if WGS uncovers a genetic mutation on an infant that is similar to the *affected* kid with autism?"[178] Mr./Ms. Comparent replies without hesitation, "I'd certainly want to know that information, and I think so would most parents in the autism community."[188] Troubled by this, Dr. Farmeth looks directly at Dr. Pedonc and stresses, "We don't even know what most of this information means yet."[179]

"And while the importance of getting parent input is invaluable, I urge us all to be a bit cautious when speaking on behalf of many others," suggests Dr. Pedonc, "as there is not likely to be one representative, unified 'parent perspective' even within a selected group, and particularly not when there is such a broad spectrum of experiences and needs as with the autism community."[176]

Dr. Psychlaw returns to probing whether that preference[28,33] would be the same if parents who viewed themselves as "neurotypical" found out from whole-genome sequencing that they had the same mutation as their child *affected* with autism. Mr./Ms. Comparent considers this: "Hmmm... I'm not certain if I'd want to know that information about myself now that I'm older. Just things about my kids... Could I have autism?" Dr. Farmeth tries to explain, "Well, from my research on pharmacogenetics, having those variants could mean several things, including potentially nothing. *All* of us have *many* mutations with differing degrees of penetrance.[61,64,66] Some variants found in such testing have no known significance, and the vast majority are of unknown significance."[62,92] After listening carefully, Mr./Ms. Comparent deduces, "So this means I could have a deletion and it might not have anything to do with autism."

Dr. Neurow confirms the reality: "Potentially, yes." To add to the complexity, some genotypes, phenotypes, and diagnostic labels that are characterized as *abnormal* today may be recategorized over time as *normal*. And vice versa. Even now, there is no agreement on how to categorize Autism Spectrum Disorder in this country and around the world.[180]

Further adding to the complexity posed by this research protocol is an option for prenatal whole-genome sequencing. The Chair feels compelled to discuss in closed session this "provocative add-on" to the main study. "So potentially a mom who has a kid with ASD is not only agreeing to participate for herself but also for her fetus?" asks Dr. Farmeth. To which the primary reviewer confirms and comments, "Dr. Pigene justifies that this fetal add-on has the potential to expand our knowledge of variations in genotype-phenotype expression with its longitudinal, natural history study design."

As the conversation moves forward, so too does the tension on the most controversial issue:

DR. PSYCHLAW: Fetal research? How do they envision that could possibly be ethical?

MR./MS. COMPARENT: Don't you think it borders on being unethical *not* to do something? There is so much that needs to be learned about autism, and Dr. Pigene has devoted his whole career working to help the autism community.

DR. PSYCHLAW: But it's so much more complex than that—sometimes boundaries get blurred and limits are needed, especially for those most vulnerable.

DR. FARMETH: Are parents going to decide to terminate the pregnancy based on one of these "variants of unknown significance"?

Clearly the investigator and the IRB have to adequately consider Subpart B of 45 CFR 46, which specifically addresses human subject protection for research involving fetuses and pregnant women.[99] Reiterating that there is no way to get through all the salient issues they want to raise today, Dr. Pedonc outlines for the IRB their next steps. Once the co-PI is invited in, they will ask a few pressing questions regarding the *main* project, and then try to get to the *optional* fetal study so Dr. Pigene and colleagues "will have a clue" where this entire study stands with respect to the IRB's determination.[181]

Focus Question: What would you want to ask the co-investigator, Dr. Pigene, if you were on this IRB?

There are certainly many challenges to be addressed when collecting and sharing genomic information on adults, and even more so with children—particularly those who participate without having either the symptoms or condition under study, and are unable to consent for themselves.[116–117,195] Furthermore, these issues are played out in the context of a larger reality in which there is little consensus on what constitutes a *normal* genome—and there may never be consensus. With this perspective in mind, the dramatic narrative continues.

Dr. Pedonc calls in Dr. Pigene to respond to the IRB members' queries while respectful of their time constraints given the day's full agenda. When Dr. Farmeth asks Dr. Pigene to explain why this protocol using blood samples previously collected and stored from the *Autism Network* on ASD kids does not have a "provision to re-consent" for the new study, the researcher looked puzzled and a bit annoyed. Dr. Pigene's rationale was that because the informed consent document for the previous project studying copy variants specified "will be used for further research," why would there be *any problem* with just stating in the protocol "no re-consent is needed"?[172]

Recognizing the need to *inform* the participants that whole-genome sequencing has the potential to reveal a vastly different amount and type of information than what the original study provided,[23,49,103,104] Dr. Pedonc sternly advises the co-PI, "You have to *plan* for that" in the protocol and informed consent document and process.[48] Assuring the IRB that there was "a *plan*," Dr. Pigene confirms that "decisions related to returning results on children will, *of course*, be decided by the parents."[76–80] This "*plan*," however, raises more questions than answers.

DR. PSYCHLAW: Don't the sibs and adolescents have a right—independent of their parents—to know, or not to know, their genomic information when they are older?

MR./MS. COMPARENT: [*quickly interjects*] The autism community wants Dr. Pigene to learn everything possible about autism. And most of the parents want to know everything they know about our children.

DR. PIGENE: Parents can tell their children *if* something turns up that is *abnormal*.

Children traditionally are given the opportunity for an *open future*, and there is a vast amount of genomic information that can be discovered on every participant—including findings that have nothing to do with autism. Incidental findings that fall outside the boundaries of *normal* can be especially troubling and need to be considered in the context of the IRBs risk-benefit analysis.[136,177]

DR. PSYCHLAW: And what about those parents who thought their adolescent was functioning just fine and perhaps was just a little quirky? Now they learn their *non-ASD* kid they thought was *neurotypical* turns out to have the same variant associated with autism as their *affected* kid. Does this genomic information make the kid less functional and *not normal*?

DR. PEDONC: [*quickly adds*] Well, let's make sure to consider the risk to "neurotypical" sibs of WGS and possibly revealing incidental findings that carry mutations suggestive of other neurodevelopmental or psychiatric disorders.

DR. NEUROW: And take a look at the benefits—Dr. Pigene describes new opportunities to better understand the spectrum of neurodevelopmental and neuropsychiatric disorders.

Actually, to date, we know of very few mutations that are even associated with 1% of individuals with ASD. Putting this statistic in context, when Dr. Farmeth asks, "Do we presently know with any certainty the combination of deletions or duplications that represents falling out of the range of genetically *normal*?," Dr. Pigene pauses, then counters: "Well...we have some evidence...but that's why we are doing the research and why it's so important to do this study." As is often the case, researchers and IRBs struggle to find the right balance between pushing forward on the promise of emerging genomic technologies while being mindful of the potential perils of having a limited scientific foundation to build upon.[182]

Regardless of the value of the study, Dr. Neurow reminds us we need to better understand the logistics, asking, "Will you disclose to the parents that some of the mutations we are examining have also been seen in schizophrenia, for example,... as well as in a group of *neurotypical* controls?"

MR./MS. COMPARENT: Wait a second, I'm confused. You're asking the parents to enroll in a study about autism. Why are you talking about schizophrenia? That sounds even worse than autism...I'm not comfortable opening up that can of worms...

DR. PEDONC: [*interrupts*] Frankly, we don't necessarily know what any of those variants would mean for anyone.

Recently, a number of empirical genomic studies have reported the prevalence of a single variant being associated with so many psychiatric and neurologic phenotypes and hence challenging specific diagnoses for such conditions as schizophrenia, autism, and bipolar disorder,[183] each with varying degrees of stigma attached.[30] Dr. Pigene responds with a bit of exasperation: "But I hope you agree this is really worthwhile research—we hope to learn about the variable severity of ASD and other genetically related disorders." In support of the research endeavor, Dr. Neurow addresses his IRB colleagues: "I believe it's an important study," noting that this is particularly so given the recent revisions to the "official label" in DSM-V, used to access many educational and health services,[186] which always evokes passionate debate regarding the inclusion and exclusion of milder criteria. So, too, do the different perspectives on the power of genomics given varying phenotypic expression.[44]

DR. NEUROW: The more we can interrogate the genome to hone in on variations that delineate conditions, the better.

DR. FARMETH: With all due respect, do you really think this research protocol is going to provide the answers to resolve that debate?

DR. PEDONC: We all can be hopeful. Changes in how we define a disorder can have a positive impact on public policy and perceptions of stigma.

DR. PIGENE: This project not only has the potential to identify *rare* variants, but we're expecting that they may act in *combination* with additional variants—to allow us to better categorize distinct diseases that have otherwise been associated with their shared variants.

Dr. Psychlaw attempts to return to the protocol to get some clarity of the details. "So any sib not diagnosed with ASD to date you are categorizing as an *unaffected* sibling?" Dr. Pigene confirms that siblings are included whether or not they have ever received a diagnosis of, or are symptomatic with, any other neurodevelopmental disorder, a psychiatric condition, or other disorders.

DR. FARMETH: Let me ask you, Dr. Pigene. In trying to understand the genetics of autism, you get all these siblings to participate—is all this inclusion worth the risk?

DR. NEUROW: Let's look at it another way. Wouldn't it be a greater risk not to have the complete picture of variants from the kids and parents?

This short dialogue between IRB members reflects the challenges of having to balance benefits and risks in new areas of genomic research in which medical and psychosocial implications are yet to be understood and difficult to quantify. A starting point may often be an evaluation of inclusion criteria. In this context, when Mr./Ms. Comparent questions what criteria for inclusion will be used for parents, Dr. Pigene responds that both *affected* and *neurotypical* would meet the criteria for inclusion. "We want to have cross analysis in the study, to investigate both what may be heritable versus de novo as well as genotype-phenotype expression. We'll try to see what the variants mean and if we can determine which are typically within *normal* limits."

Afterward, Dr. Pedonc expresses significant concerns to Dr. Pigene regarding the *added optional* study design, commenting that it "seems like it is tacked on and may in fact be an independent study, requiring its own protocol." Dr. Neurow clarifies that the main protocol includes mothers of the ASD probands, including mothers who are currently pregnant, with an *option*, under separate consent form, as it should be, for additional research using noninvasive prenatal whole-genome sequencing for the pregnant mother. Suspecting this might generate much conversation at the IRB, Dr. Pigene responds, "We are just trying to gather as much information on autism as is feasible." Given the massive amount of genomic information generated by sequencing, there is often the temptation to mine as much as possible. However, there are limits to this, especially when including data from pregnant women.

DR. PSYCHLAW: I have great difficulty including pregnant women in this study: we are talking autism, not meningomyelocele. And surely you're not going to give them their results or incidental findings when they're pregnant? Are you?

DR. PIGENE: Of course not...unless it's medically urgent. All other findings about her we can consider disclosing after she gives birth.

DR. PSYCHLAW: Oh, so when the risk of postpartum depression is highest? And what about the impact of all this information on parent-infant bonding?

DR. FARMETH: And what about information on the fetus? What were you all thinking in proposing this? What are you going to do with all that information? Keep in mind, Dr. Pigene, that this is not information for something life-threatening; this is really beyond stretching the limits of acceptable research.

DR. PEDONC: Well, I need to be frank at this point. I don't understand what could possibly be the reason for doing this study on a fetus.

Historically, Subpart B of the human subjects research regulations recognizes the importance of restricting protocols involving fetuses and pregnant women, particularly when there is no, or minimal scientific justification to add risk to vulnerable populations. Specifically, in this context, based on our current knowledge, it is not ethical to include pregnant women in this particular genomic ASD study, exposing fetuses and pregnant women to unreasonable risk in spite of the push to the contrary.[184,185] This technological imperative is illuminated when Dr. Pigene points out to the IRB members, "Look, the genomic sequencing technology is out there and other groups are going to be using it for all types of disorders, so we might as well apply our expertise and do it right ourselves. We can start developing what we hope will eventually be a very good predictive test for autism."[187]

Many questions remain to be addressed, however, and Dr. Pedonc expresses one concern: "What if, even though genetic counseling explains that detection of a particular variant is only a risk factor, the family thinks that definitively means their kid won't turn out to be *normal*?" Dr. Neurow is concerned as well and raises another issue: "But do we not tell them—even though they indicated they want to know everything?—including how this might affect the child's future and their future reproductive planning, as well as the rest of the family's future?"

Questioning how that genomic information can impact bonding and parenting if they find out that something is "outside the range of *normal*— like the newborn will have autism," Dr. Psychlaw adds in exasperation, "And don't give us the line that it's preventing harm because early intervention can be started so much earlier." Dr. Pigene snaps back, "That is exactly why we want to do it!," clarifying that they are not planning to provide results on the fetus during the early phase of the research, and admitting, "We don't even know all the variants and other factors that cause the brain to develop *abnormally*. That's why this whole-genome sequencing research has value." "Actually some folks are proposing we add ASD and fragile X to the newborn screening (NBS) panel right now since we have the technology to do it," [189,190] Dr. Pedonc adds. Along with the imperative to move forward, there is a range of perspectives on the relative value of genomic information to individuals, families, and society to be considered.

While Mr./Ms. Comparent expresses that "the autism community supports this study,"[62] Dr. Farmeth is worried: "What if this protocol gets negative reactions in the press and on the blogs? Don't we want to approve things that can withstand public scrutiny? It's risky business doing WGS research on pregnant women, fetuses, and healthy sibs—particularly for a nonfatal condition like autism!!" Without hesitation, Mr./Ms. Comparent volleys back, "There is no need to overreact. Dr. Pigene, I know I speak for many in the autism community—we appreciate all your research in the field to help families affected by ASD."

Dr. Pedonc asks Dr. Pigene to wait outside while the IRB members finish their deliberations, commenting as the co-PI walks out, "I strongly recommend you consider adding an ELSI consultant to your research team."[194] The co-PI, Dr. Pigene, leaves.

While first acknowledging that the protocol requires "some work," Dr. Neurow remains supportive, asking colleagues, "What's so terrible about trying to collect data to find out if a good predictive measure can be developed for autism? There are many people affected by this disorder." Mr./Ms. Comparent nods in agreement and reminds everyone that the numbers are growing.

DR. PSYCHLAW: But *whole*-genome sequencing? There is no ethical reason WGS should be allowed on fetuses and *unaffected* siblings...for autism research!

DR. NEUROW: But I see these families day in and day out, and there is so much more we need to know. I don't want us to stand in the way if genomic research can give us some answers.

MR./MS. COMPARENT: I couldn't agree more; I think this is a valuable study and should proceed. I have experienced so many years of frustration and heartache watching my son and our family fall apart. Research is the only hope for the autism community.

DR. FARMETH: I understand, but I'm worried you'll be getting unvalidated information. An IRB needs to be objective and concerned with the risk of uncertainty. We need to maintain a critical eye and not be overly swayed by personal interests.

MR./MS. COMPARENT: I'm not just thinking of my son. We have to look out for the next generation of ASD families.

As time runs short, Dr. Pedonc recognizes that these issues will require additional time to sort through institutionally and with this IRB: "We need much more deliberation on this topic, not just this particular protocol. We need more time for this discussion...and we don't have it today." The Chair asks members to vote on whether to approve, reject, or defer the proposal for further revision, first requesting that Dr. Neurow share recommendations. Dr. Neurow comments that this study "has a lot of promise" based on the belief that "we do need to use WGS to answer questions of this nature." Dr. Neurow goes on to recommend that they table this protocol until Dr. Pigene comes back "with details that address our stipulations," concluding that the co-PI has "not provided sufficient scientific justification" to even begin to consider the magnitude of risks associated with the prenatal portion of the study. With respect to the rest of the study, further information is needed, particularly on how Dr. Pigene plans to deal with genomic findings.

As a final thought, Dr. Psychlaw queries whether the IRB has an obligation to monitor an approved genomic protocol when problems arise as investigators start discovering incidental findings, adding, "And I predict they will!" Dr. Farmeth sagely notes, "It depends on the problem," because presently the only mechanism for guidance in West Coastal Children's Hospital is either the IRB or an ethics consult. Recognizing that they can benefit from additional guidance, Dr. Neurow comments, "So maybe our medical center needs to seriously consider establishing a genomic advisory committee, like some of my colleagues are forming at their institutions." Dr. Pedonc motions to table the protocol for further evaluation and calls for a vote: "All in favor? All opposed? Any abstentions?" The motion to table passes, and the Chair invites Dr. Pigene back in.

Dr. Pedonc explains to Dr. Pigene that the members had an opportunity to evaluate the protocol and will be sending the list of stipulations with respect to the main protocol and will not approve the optional prenatal component as part of this protocol. Turning toward fellow IRB colleagues, the Chair ponders aloud: "As I reflect upon this meeting, I'd like to leave us all with a pretty fundamental question: How might whole-genome sequencing reconceptualize the boundaries of *normal*?"

Focus Question: What stipulations would you want to include if you were on this IRB?

SCENE II: THE GENOMIC ADVISORY COMMITTEE

One year later, the drama is set at Pacific University Medical Center, where Dr. Cardio, a cardiologist with a PhD in genetics, is chairing the medical center's inaugural Genomics Advisory Committee meeting. The advisory committee[191,192] was created by the university in response to the growing demand for whole-exome and whole-genome sequencing and the complex issues they anticipate will accelerate now that the medical center has a HiSeq machine and CLIA (Clinical Laboratory Improvement Act) approval. Dr. Cardio explains that advisory committee members are charged with working together to address and advise on both research and clinical genomics sequencing challenges in the context of return of results and, particularly, which incidental findings, if any, should be identified, disclosed, to whom, and under what circumstances. The Chair formally introduces "the other members and guest, as many may not know those from our children's hospital":

Prof. Legaleth, a legal scholar and ethicist

Dr. Biobank, head of the university's joint neurological and psychiatric biobank

Mr./Ms. Geecee, a certified genetic counselor

Dr. Oncohelix, an oncologist specializing in oncogenetics

Dr. Pathoseq, a pathologist and head of the university's personalized medicine lab

Dr. Neurow, a pediatric neurologist who also was the primary reviewer for the IRB

Dr. Cardio welcomes Dr. Pigene, the co-PI who requested the group's guidance and was invited to be the first researcher to present at Pacific U's Genomics Advisory Committee. The Chair notes that they are fortunate to have Dr. Neurow present for this meeting; beyond being a standing member of this new committee, Dr. Neurow had the experience of serving on the IRB that reviewed Dr. Pigene's protocol.

Acknowledging appreciation for being included on this advisory group, Dr. Neurow briefly fills in the other committee members, especially those who may not have read all that was pre-sent online, summarizing that one year ago the IRB gave Dr. Pigene a list of stipulations for the main protocol and rejected the optional prenatal whole-genome sequencing component. Since the PIs wanted to proceed with their research without delay, they did not hesitate to drop "the fetal component," and all the other stipulations were met. "We had many concerns" going into this project, Dr. Neurow reports, "not the least of which were incidental findings."[57] While the informed consent document was reworded to provide that certain incidental findings may be returned if deemed highly significant by the researcher, Dr. Neurow reflects, "We are now discovering" that this language "may be too vague."[59]

Dr. Pigene thanks them in advance for helping, because "this is a bit overwhelming." The co-PI explains that the analysis of whole-genome sequencing results from the pilot group had recently begun, and already several clinically actionable incidental findings of child- and adult-onset diseases were discovered in both kids and parents. Moreover, other findings that might affect reproductive decisions also appeared in the de-identified aggregate data. "I really need this genomics committee to advise me with decisions such as if, what, when, to whom to disclose, and by whom? I was shocked to discover that there were five *affected* and *unaffected* kids and a few adults with *BRCA1, Lynch*, or *PSN1* mutations...and we have hundreds of whole-genome sequences left to analyze. I am beginning to think we actually need to share some of this information with these folks." In fact, there is little consensus and much debate among the genomics community about the extent to which incidental findings should be shared, if at all, and the extent to which participant preferences play a role.[58,100]

Feeling a bit panicky at the prospect of having to return findings to participants, Dr. Biobank pushes, "Are you suggesting that I go to the repository and re-identify some samples that you have annotated some mutations on? Do you all know the havoc that creates?" Whether to require biobanks to accept responsibility for having to return results and incidental findings to professionals, research participants, or their family members remains a controversial issue that has significant implications for resources and role delineation within the research and clinical establishments, generating many practical and ethical dilemmas.

Indeed, Dr. Cardio quickly points out, "First we really need to determine which incidental findings are truly significant." Dr. Pathoseq believes that most of the incidental findings are not going to be relevant: "We can ignore most and not even look at them. We have bioinformatics for that." The reality is that to date we still have to define the parameters of what to include, or "*bin*," as relevant genomic information. Given the enormous amount of data generated by genomic sequencing, everyone is struggling with how best to deal with the "*incidentalome*."[18]

Tensions rise in response to disparate perspectives among the Genomic Advisory Committee members.[193] When Dr. Oncohelix comments, "Unlike you, as a clinician I personally feel obligated to help the patient. Do you expect us to hide a highly penetrant *BRCA* variant?," Dr. Biobank immediately retorts, "Whoa...did you say 'patient'? May I remind everyone that Dr. Pigene and his team are doing human subjects research." "They are participants," Mr./Ms. Geecee emphatically states, while reinforcing the point that these individuals are family members of patients with ASD who volunteered too. "It's their blood and their genes, and they are the relatives living with the *affected* child."

Whether in research or clinical care, geneticists who consider themselves clinicians tend to feel greater obligations toward participant/patients than non-clinical professionals.[31] This difference also plays out in their blurring of distinctions between their duties to research participants and patients, further graying boundaries between research and clinical responsibilities—especially when children are involved.[27,51,97]

DR. ONCOHELIX: Don't we have what's called an "ancillary duty"? I've been reading a lot about that lately.
DR. LEGALETH: There is great debate about that currently. I personally don't think you need to disclose because it is research paradigm.
DR. PIGENE: That's what I thought...until I started seeing so many potentially significant incidentals pop up. I can't sleep at night worrying about whether I am hiding important information.
DR. PATHOSEQ: Oh, you're one of those "duty-to-rescue" dudes?
DR. ONCOHELIX: It is just basic human decency. It's what is ethical.

There is often confusion over what may be an ethical obligation versus a legal duty, especially when no special relationship exists between the geneticist and the individual. And even when there is agreement of some responsibility, there is little consensus over the context. In an increasingly frustrated tone, Dr. Pigene attempts to clarify: "I'm not saying responsible for *everything*—just what is most important." Mr./Ms. Geecee further stresses that information can be both valuable and important to them, to which Dr. Pathoseq ponders, "And who decides what is important?"

The reality is that not all the specifics can be covered in the informed consent document; it is too unwieldy already. In fact, that is one of the reasons genomics advisory committees have been established: to better address the parameters of disclosing genomic findings.

Recognizing that genomic information is changing every day, Dr. Legaleth gives the advisory committee members a real-life example: "One day a particular variant or mutation for colon cancer is a significant finding, and the next day it's not." Dr. Legaleth further points out, "There are so many findings of *unknown* and *uncertain significance* that we will bin differently 5 years, or 5 days from now," to which Dr. Neurow adds: "Not counting all the mitochondrial and epigenetic influences to be uncovered." At the present time, the reality is that we simply don't know the full spectrum of most diseases.[66]

Some practical concerns are raised. Dr. Biobank wonders whether some of the committee members are actually proposing Sanger testing in a CLIA lab to confirm all research findings. After Dr. Pigene quickly asks whether insurance will covers this, Dr. Legaleth voices a troubling concern that still needs to be addressed with better policy: "Even though there is GINA [the Genetic Information Nondiscrimination Act],[196] I still worry that if these research participants are found to have the *BRCA1 mutation* and their employer finds out, the participants risk losing their job when all they were trying to do was advance ASD research. And what about their ability to get life insurance, disability, or long-term care insurance which GINA doesn't even cover? We could ruin somebody's life." Expressing another concern, Dr. Pathoseq remarks, "The last thing I want is to get sued or have the state shut down my lab because I released information that I wasn't specifically testing them for—that goes for clinical and research WGS." The risks are more complicated than just insurance and lawsuits, however. Sharing genomic information can really change interpersonal relationships—and erode trust in the research endeavor.

Many challenging questions continue to be raised by the Genomic Advisory Committee with no simple answers in sight. Dr. Cardio offers his view that if individuals are willing to collaborate by being in research, "Don't we owe it to them to share this information?" Mr./Ms. Geecee responds that all the participants are vulnerable, and highlights that the parents are living with *affected* and *unaffected* kids who need healthy parents to take care of them: "If this can help the mom get surveillance and potentially treatment, then that helps the kids. But we also have to be concerned if they fall apart psychologically with the disclosure. Does that help the family?" And the debate continues over this complex issue among the advisory committee members.

DR. PIGENE: So does that mean we should tell them, or not? And which ones?

DR. ONCOHELIX: Certainly no one here proposes returning nonactionable incidental findings like *APOE*. Right? Who wants to learn about their risk for getting Alzheimer's?

DR. CARDIO: What do you mean by actionable? The initial 2013 ACMG list of incidental findings that they recommended to actively look for and return?

DR. BIOBANK: No, those are for clinical—this is research. We give back far less, if anything at all.

DR. PIGENE: I'm so confused—I thought I knew the distinction between clinical and research, but now I am unsure with these whole-genome sequencing studies.

DR. PATHOSEQ: Aren't they doing the same tests and analysis as my personalized genomics lab downstairs? And mine is a clinical lab, CLIA certified.

In fact, WGS has accelerated the graying of the boundaries between research and clinical practice. Incidentals happen in radiology too, and there will be mounting frequency of secondary findings when using brain imaging and sequencing concurrently on patients in the clinical and research settings. In response to these increasing challenges, oversight boards and genomic advisory committees are being established in major academic institutions to consider both research and clinical applications of genomics, although their membership and missions may vary somewhat and will continue to evolve with more experience.

Along with considering the implications of secondary findings, the genomic advisory committee or oversight board may also serve the functions of identifying the list of incidental findings to be discovered and evaluating preferences among individuals, blood relatives, and other family members. As can be expected, there are varying perspectives among the Genomic Advisory Committee members.

Whereas Dr. Oncohelix thinks the decision is clear-cut, "Well if it's significant, obviously the patient and family would want to know about it and do something," Dr. Cardio recognizes the nuances: "Depends on the individual...and the entire family when you talk about whole-genome sequencing because the information impacts blood relatives." While the medical impact solely affects blood relatives, the psychosocial implications are also borne by members of the family not connected by genetics. Moreover, there are additional challenges to be considered when determining what information is best to share consistent with "the best interests of the child."

MR./MS. GEECEE: And there are parents deciding for the kids. I am concerned what all this may mean for the kids. Not sure which is tougher for the parents—more health problems to deal with in the kids with autism or being told your *unaffected* child is affected with something deleterious that you must now address.

DR. ONCOHELIX: In oncology we must give back difficult news all the time. No one is ready for it, even if we give them the choice to know a little or a lot.

DR. PATHOSEQ: Yeah, but they consult you, knowing beforehand that it's likely cancer or not cancer. I may sequence a girl with ASD, and surely her parents won't expect me to say that the daughter has a *BRCA1* mutation of adult onset—and, by the way, the mom does too!

DR. ONCOHELIX: It's all well and good to worry about incidental findings causing someone distress. But I am worried about keeping them alive!

As the discussion continues among members of the Genomic Advisory Committee, the blurring between research and clinical boundaries becomes more and more evident.[97] "Are you talking about this research project or a clinical diagnostic test?," Dr. Biobank asks. "The study in front of us is research, and repositories are research, so they don't have to return incidental findings," and then reminds the other advisory committee members that the initial 2013 ACMG recommendations are "only clinical." Dr. Neurow quickly responds, "We don't even know if that early attempt to publish recommendations will get followed." Dr. Oncohelix matter-of-factly reminds the committee, "We return all kinds of results in medicine all the time."

In fact, often in clinical practice, patients receive findings that were never anticipated and they were never asked if they wanted to know the results or not. There continues to be a lot of controversy and debate on returning genomic information that is not evidence-based and giving back results that people say they don't want to know, especially the disclosure of incidental findings to children.

Dr. Cardio provides an illustrative example:

> I had a colleague, an infectious disease specialist, who had a middle-aged patient with Lyme Disease and ordered a MRI to check if newly onset memory problems were caused by the bacterium that would alter administration of antibiotic treatment. The radiologist discovered an intracerebral aneurysm but couldn't precisely judge the size. So, for more than a decade now, the patient must get expensive and sometimes invasive surveillance, including repeated MRI angiography. Turned out to be a very small aneurysm that was likely present from birth. This finding was ultimately noted to be unrelated to the memory difficulties. Are patients lucky or not once they are expected to be hypervigilant? And this patient surely was not asked ahead of time if she wanted information concerning secondary or incidental findings.

It is important to point out that, unlike most radiology findings, whole-genome sequencing has implications for the entire family, particularly blood relatives, and raises complex challenges in sorting our relative responsibilities for the geneticist when disclosing information and collaborating in follow-up with various specialties.

The discovery of incidental findings can evoke much confusion and angst for genetic professionals. Dr. Pigene admits, "I'm so torn. I really want to help these families who have kids with ASD. That's why I am doing this research. There is mounting evidence that the infant sibs of kids with ASD are at increased risk for ASD—to the tune of one in five. But we don't know them personally. I mean, I'm not responsible for them like they are my patients." To which Prof. Legaleth declares, "You have an ethical responsibility as a co-PI! To the probands as well as their family members who are also participating in the study." In fact, the ACMG made a first attempt in 2013 for clinical recommendations, outlining an ethical responsibility to return a small group of deleterious mutations that, if adopted and applied by medical professionals, could be considered as strong evidence of standard practice of care. Prof. Legaleth reminds everyone that this is "IRB-approved research and the ACMG recs for returning incidental findings do *not* apply . . . yet."

Dr. Cardio expresses that even though the Genomic Advisory Committee is considering today the reporting of significant IFs in the early analysis of this aggregate ASD research study, "I feel compelled to reflect on my own concern that if this were a clinical case, at least the ACMG would recommend reporting some later onset diseases to *unaffected* child sibs." Mr./Ms. Geecee is concerned that "Those families have so much to deal with already. Our genetic counseling group will really need to spend a ton of time explaining and trying to do psychosocial counseling."[90] Addressing the practicality of that, Dr. Biobank points out, "That is not sustainable" and then declares being "really opposed" to returning genomic research findings.

DR. NEUROW: Maybe it is because I am a pediatric neurologist, but I have concern that children have a right to an *open future* without being straddled by worries about *BRCA1*, for example. There is time for them to find out when they are older.

DR. ONCOHELIX: As for having knowledge that the parent most likely has a *Lynch*, *BRCA1*, or *PSN1* mutation, isn't it in *the best interest of the child* to have a parent alive to care for that child—which might not have happened if the parent was not informed of the incidental finding for a disease that may have been prevented?

DR. PATHOSEQ: That's not the goal of this research study. Anyway, by the time the PIs are done with their ASD study, most people in this country will have the opportunity to be clinically tested for *Lynch*, *BRCA1*, and *PSN1*.

This won't be happening so fast. We are a very long way from knowing what most variants even mean and to whom. Even an incidental finding of a variant for *long QT* is a prediction, a risk factor, not a diagnosis to say definitively, "You will get this condition." At this point in time, the high costs of sequencing preclude most people's access to predictive tests, and this research may be their only opportunity to get this genomic information. Even the ACMG reports that the evidence is not all there yet. So the question remains, how good does the genomic information have to be before it may be returned? And does this decision vary for the researcher versus the clinician? These are questions that the Genomic Advisory Committee must address.

DR. PIGENE: With all due respect, I believe I have a right to share valuable information if they want it.

DR. ONCOHELIX: Personally, I believe we have an obligation—even if they don't want to learn—to share a significant finding that in our medical opinion is in their best interest to know.

MR./MS. GEECEE: This seems very paternalistic. You would override their right not to know?

PROF. LEGALETH: It's not only autonomy—and whose autonomy, child or parent?—that needs to be considered. It is more complex than that.

DR. NEUROW: What about the *unaffected* sibs?

DR. ONCOHELIX: Yes, I'd override their *right not to know* if it is highly penetrant and means that the parent can do something prophylactically or by surveillance.

The costs of absorbing this fiduciary role and not respecting what some believe is *the right not to know* are changing the paradigms established in research ethics and clinical practice, altering traditional relationships. What would be the cost of losing the trust of participants in genomic research if we override their wish not to know incidental findings for themselves or their children, especially after the latest publication of HeLa data without the consent of the family? Many studies have demonstrated over the past few years that we cannot guarantee genomic privacy. The reality is that WGS information can be identified even when we try to keep it de-identified.[108-111]

Furthermore, as we return more and more research results, we need to be mindful about what goes into the electronic medical record, especially as we blur the lines between research and clinical care.[101] Confirming the confusion, Dr. Biobank says, "This is research, so nothing goes in the medical record," while Dr. Cardio cautions, "Well if we start giving research results back, it's just a matter of time before that information will find its way into the medical record." "Isn't that the goal?" asks Dr. Oncohelix. Dr. Pigene reminds them, "There is nothing to place in the record until we determine whether I am supposed to re-identify the data and disclose some of the incidental findings. I thought we had a plan, but this is more difficult than I ever imagined."

Prof. Legaleth then offers this anecdote:

> Let me share with you all an ethics consultation I did elsewhere, in which that medical center initiated a large genomic research project involving many of their clinical patients. The plan was that none of the patients who participated in the research biobank would receive any genomic results, including incidental findings. We determined that the best strategy was to send a monthly newsletter updating everyone on the aggregate results inclusive of incidental findings, and provided that if they had interest in learning more, they could contact the study coordinator for follow-up.

Having run out of time, Dr. Cardio cuts Dr. Pigene off: "We appreciate your struggles with decision making regarding the mounting incidental findings. As you continue your analysis, we anticipate many more genomic findings, some of troubling concern, such as those you expressed today." Recognizing that this is the committee's first official meeting and they need more time for institutional policy deliberation, Dr. Cardio advises Dr. Pigene to hold off from re-identifying and disclosing *any* incidental findings until hearing back from the Genomic Advisory Committee. Dr. Pigene looks a bit stunned that although advice was sought, so litle was actually provided.

The Chair expresses a final thought: "It is my hope that advisory committees like ours, with expertise in genomics and its implications, will provide guidance to benefit the research and clinical community as well as society." Dr. Cardio thanks everyone for coming, and looks forward to the next Genomic

Advisory Committee meeting "as we work together toward anticipating the future with genome sequencing."

Focus Question: If you were Chair, how would you next proceed to improve institutional policy deliberations?

ADDITIONAL QUESTIONS

1. What are the implications of including "*normal*" children in WGS research, and is there a difference if the child is a sibling of an *affected* child?
2. Under what circumstances should an IRB be concerned about having an *unaffected* child participate in genomic research?
3. How would you evaluate whether an IRB should approve a protocol that includes fetal/prenatal WGS?
4. What are the implications of children having "the right"—independent of their parent(s)—to know or not know their genomic information when they are older?
5. What special considerations, if any, should be raised when deciding to disclose genomic research findings?
6. To what extent, and how, should researchers and an IRB accommodate participant preferences for the disclosure of genomic research findings?
7. Should the review process better provide for the inclusion of the range of views from patient communities and families; and if so, how?
8. What obligations, if any, should the researcher have to return findings, and does that vary depending on the relationship with the participant?
9. What factors would help you decide what, when, and to whom to disclose aggregated genomic research?
10. What are your thoughts about the role of genomics advisory committees or genomic oversight boards in contributing to the process of determining whether and what findings to return? Does it matter whether in the research or clinical domain?

CHAPTER 3

Informing the Future

The Process of Consent & Disclosure of Genomic Information

As genomics evolves[1-3] from basic research to clinical research[15] to clinical medicine,[16-17] there are increasingly blurred boundaries[97,106] in the context of expectations and explanations that have implications for both familial and professional relationships.[26-27] Through the lens of a family experiencing a diagnostic odyssey with their longtime clinical genetics team, this dramatic narrative illuminates the challenges they face when trying to make meaningful choices in deciding to attain and share genomic information among family members, each with different values and preferences[28,33,39-42,46,55] as well as differing medical, cognitive, and developmental status.[69,71,74,75,86-88,93,195]

This chapter also brings to life the dialogues and dilemmas for the professional[34,54] trying to determine what genomic information to disclose based on limited or uncertain evidence of predictive value, range of phenotype, penetrance, variability of findings,[92] and the short- and long-term ramifications of these findings[44,62-64,66]—weighing the potential risks and benefits for *affected* pediatric patient-participants and their *unaffected* relatives.[70] We illustrate the difficulties, especially the *therapeutic misconception*,[107] that may arise from the multidimensional roles of the genomics clinician-researcher who has an established clinical relationship with the patient-participant and family.

The dynamics of this fictionalized genomic narrative revolve around the Friedman family as they revisit Dr. Hardy, their clinical geneticist, in the context of the informed consent process and then the return of genomic findings, with dialogue adapted from our plays *It's Not that Simple!* and *It's So Complicated!*, respectively.

SCENE I: THE INFORMED CONSENT PROCESS

The drama opens in a pediatric genetics clinic consultation room at Lakeview, a large academic medical center with:

> Dr. Hardy, MD, PhD, a clinical and molecular pediatric geneticist
> Bobby Friedman, a 19-year-old with an inborn error of metabolism autosomal recessive genetic disorder
> Amy Friedman, 16-year-old sister of Bobby with the same genetic disorder
> Sam Friedman, their *unaffected* 9-year-old sibling
> Ellen Friedman, their mother, who is an elementary school teacher
> Jennifer Smith, CGC, their genetic counselor, working in an adjacent room

Bobby's degenerative symptoms manifested several years ago, and are similar in nature to those beginning to affect Amy. The *affected* brother and sister reside with their mom and younger sibling, neither of whom have the heritable condition. Their dad, Howie, is in good health and lives in another town with his second wife and young son. Although Dr. Hardy requested the entire family be present today if feasible, Mr. Friedman did not attend.

Dr. Hardy has just noted that both Bobby and Amy are clearly experiencing a decline in their health, Bobby more than Amy.

MOM: Isn't there anything new that could be done? I'm always seeing stories in the newspapers about all sorts of tests and treatments being developed for genetic diseases.

AMY: You'll find some way to cure us, won't you Dr. Hardy?

SAM: Why did I have to come? I'm not sick.

DR. HARDY: In fact, the reason I gathered you all here today is that I have some good news. We now have a better chance to understand what's causing your disorder—and you can be part of a new study. That includes you, too, Sam.

SAM: How can I help them if I don't have their bad gene?

The diagnostic odyssey that frequently accompanies rare genetic disorders in children raises special challenges for the pediatric geneticist who often is involved in genomic research. The graying of these roles as both the clinician and researcher heightens the likelihood of the therapeutic misconception and colors the objectivity of risks and benefits when patients and families are recruited by clinical genetic professionals for genomic research studies. This is particularly complex when the participants include children, especially *unaffected* siblings, in part because such studies may alter perceptions of self and other about having "*good*" or "*bad*" genes.[25]

Speaking on behalf of her family, Mom[84-89] expresses their willingness to participate: "We'll do anything you say, Dr. Hardy…as long as it's safe." "There's little danger, just a simple blood draw," responds Dr. Hardy, quickly minimizing any concerns and explaining that the specimens are for a new type of analysis "called genome sequencing used to help understand the causes of genetic disorders by looking at all the human genes we know about."

Excited to proceed, Amy announces, "I know I want this test. I'll sign up for it right now! I don't need to read anything." When her snarky brother snaps back, "Right, another test that probably won't actually help us; don't be so trusting Amy," Mom is clearly annoyed that Bobby is so cynical. Dr. Hardy explains that several institutions are collaborating[163] on a study of adolescent-onset genetic disorders that are known to have increased prevalence in the Ashkenazi population, adding, "Hopefully we'll also be able to learn more about Bobby and Amy's specific heritable defect to help them." "So are you saying that this test is not just about my family but mostly about lots of Jewish teenagers with Jewish diseases?" asks Mom. Targeting genomic testing on certain ethnic and racial groups raises complex ethical and psychosocial questions, such as what it means to have or not have a familial disease associated with ethnic identity.[28,42]

Puzzled to be included, Sam reminds everyone, "But I don't have any disease." Oftentimes in genomic research and clinical medicine, there is variable phenotypic expression, and *unaffected* blood relatives are tested too. This is especially the case in the context of investigating rare disorders[199] with single gene defects in which there tends to be higher prevalence by ethnic origin,[175,198] in contrast to complex disorders (such as autism, which we explored in Chapter 2). Sometimes these family members learn for the very first time based on sequencing whether they may or may not have increased risk for the same disorder with an onset in the future. Although the specific time frame and severity of presentation is unknown,[128,200] the implications are particularly problematic when involving siblings who are children.[67-68,129,136,161,178]

Clarification is obviously needed about the inclusion criteria, including ethnicity and other aspects of the study design.[70] However, trying not to fall too far behind in an overbooked clinic schedule, Dr. Hardy just quickly states that the protocol looks at several groups, including healthy siblings, and then hands Mom five consent forms "to take home and read before signing," adding, "It's highly preferable for dad to participate and have his specimen taken too." Stumbling over her words in hesitation, Mom responds, "It may be…difficult" to include their father, her ex-husband. Bobby bluntly explains, "Dad hates doctor stuff, and anything to do with sick people. That's why he left us." However, Amy expresses that she believes her father will "do it when he hears it can cure us."

The reality is that families have complex dynamics and are not always intact, creating challenges for the genetic professional and family members when seeking consent to attain DNA specimens. There is also the risk that families of pediatric patients with rare or unknown diseases, who typically have long-term relationships with genetics professionals, may too readily consent, especially when they want to show their trust and gratitude, often perpetuating the therapeutic misconception.

Ideally, informed consent for genomic sequencing is part of an ongoing process rather than mere paperwork.[47-50] There is a lot of debate regarding how to best enhance and encourage the informed consent dialogue in light of competing resources, particularly when the nature of genomic medicine, in contrast to other specializations, involves so many family members at once. One impediment is the reality that there are not enough trained professionals to provide adequate genomic counseling.[90-91]

The dramatic narrative continues with Bobby, Amy, Sam, and Mom returning home from Dr. Hardy's office with an array of medical documents and consent forms. Mom expresses hope: "After all these years with so few answers—finally, there's some really powerful genetic technology." While Amy is in a rush to start reading the consent forms, Bobby is not so quick to sign up, and cautions his sister:

BOBBY: I wouldn't be so rushed if I were you or too optimistic. I've been going through all sorts of genetic tests longer than you, Amy. Why do you think this is going to be so different and solve our problem?

AMY: Because Dr. Hardy's consent form says so right here: *"We will use new techniques to read all of the genetic information in your cells that might cause a health problem if it contained a mistake."* See, Dr. Hardy's new test will find our genetic mistakes.

The language used in the informed consent process—describing how genetic technology will find "mistakes," "mutations," and "errors" within your DNA—can intensify the level of psychological distress and the diminished self-integrity that already affects individuals with genetic conditions and their families. *Unaffected* siblings who are sequenced as part of an *affected* sibling's genomic analysis are also at risk when genetic *mistakes* are discovered from their genomic information and labeled as such. Regardless of the label used, current genomic technology does not have capacity to identify all *mistakes*, and not all *mutations* cause disease; most *errors* are *uncertain* or of *unknown* functionality. It is important that these limitations are conveyed and appreciated during the informed consent process to temper the influence of therapeutic misconception, particularly in light of our belief in the power and promise of new technology.

Having read on the internet that a doctor back East used whole-exome sequencing (WES)[197] "to save a baby," Mom wonders aloud whether Dr. Hardy will be doing "all the DNA" or "just the *exome*." Bobby comments that he suspects the exomes will be sequenced first, due to the cost, adding that the consent form says, "*DNA tests can take years....*" Amy responds in a panic, "But we need to get our results sooner than that!" in recognition of their ongoing degenerative process. In spite of Amy's wish to move forward quickly, the fact remains that the informed consent process must raise many challenging issues in order to "inform" sufficiently, though this is often difficult to accomplish without creating further confusion, especially because genomic sequencing involves complex technologies that impact many family members.

"Why are there so many warnings in this consent form?" Mom asks Bobby and Amy. Interrupting her mother, who is preoccupied with completing the informed consent document, Sam, as the *unaffected* sibling, feels no need to be part of the process and asks to walk over and play at a friend's house. Mom lets her, adding, "I'll take care of your consent." The reality is that, according to the framework set in the federal regulations involving human subject protections, *assent* must be provided by Sam and Mom technically cannot grant *consent* for Sam to participate in research. Rather, the parent is asked to provide *permission*, while the child is asked to *assent* depending on age and capacity.[16,117] This "*consent process*" is specifically required under Subpart D for research involving children, and is also often adopted in clinical practice when using diagnostic genomic sequencing.[83] In spite of the *assent* requirement, psychosocial dynamics surrounding guilt and loyalty may make it very difficult for *unaffected* siblings within these families to freely reject the request to share their DNA in either a clinical or research context.[43]

Given the complexity of the issues, the decision-making process, and the number of interested parties involved, Bobby soon recognizes why seven pages are used to explain things and snidely remarks, "They think we should be happy the whole world doesn't see our medical information" and reads aloud portions of the consent document: "*Researchers who have access to genetic information will take measures to maintain the confidentiality of your genetic information.*" "But how much of a measure, a ton or a drop in the bucket?" asks Bobby, reflecting the uncertainty of the degree to which confidentiality[118] and privacy[108,109] can be ensured, especially when involving genomic information.

Afterward, Mom points out, "There's going to be lots of people reading about us when the consent form bluntly says, '*Even investigators at other participating institutions may see your information if they consult with other researchers.*'" "So, other than the janitor, everyone will know about us?" Bobby responds sarcastically, recognizing that increasing numbers of collaborators are interested in sharing genomic data, which increases the risk of misuse of the information.

As Bobby continues to read, he is struck by the wording of another paragraph, which he rapidly calls out to his mother and sister: "*Breaches in confidentiality involving genetic information could impact future insurability, employability, or reproduction plans, or have a negative impact on family relationships.*" This strikes a chord in Amy, who asks, "What does that mean? Reproduction plans? Does that mean it hurts my chances of having a baby?" Mom quickly pushes that issue aside, claiming that reproduction is not something to be worried about now, and then shares her deep concern about the statement of potentially hurting family relationships: "What happens if my sisters discover that our family's genetic information is known to so many people? They'll hate me for that!"

Unlike other medical tests, genomic technology by definition generates information that has many implications that extend beyond the individual to other family members.[26,231] While brushing off her Mom's anxiety, suggesting that there is no reason to care what they think because, "Remember, it's been years since you even spoke to one of your sisters," Amy reveals her immediate fear of how she will be perceived by her peers if she divulges her genomic information, "But do I have to worry that every boyfriend is going to know I have bad genes?"

It is a real challenge for the informed consent process[47–49] to adequately address and articulate risks and conceptualize psychosocial issues that are not quantifiable.[134,153] For example, how should the consent document or genomic counseling convey to participants the speculative risk of rejection by others and potential changes in identity when genomic information is shared? Also, how do you quantify the risk of discrimination and the reach of protection when more and more genomic information may be finding its way into the medical record? In addition, how can the informed consent process effectively convey the protections and limitations of the Genetic Information Nondiscrimination Act (GINA)?[196]

BOBBY: What about me? Is it going to hurt me from getting a job if I get better because of our screwed up DNA? Look at this: *"There may be a risk that genetic information obtained as a result of participation in research could be misused for discriminatory purposes."*

AMY: Don't worry Bobby. See, it says: *"However, state and federal laws provide some protections against genetic discrimination."*

BOBBY: Here it even warns us: *"The Federal Privacy Act allows release of some information from your medical record without your permission..."* And they include *"law enforcement"* ... That's the cops, Amy!

AMY: Well, if you don't get in trouble with the police, then there's no problem.

MOM: I'm not worried about the police; I'm worried about what you and Amy have. We don't want to sound ungrateful and risk losing our chance to get these tests. I don't earn enough to pay for them, and I wouldn't even know where else to go. Anyway, this may be our last hope.

Many engaged in a diagnostic odyssey are desperate to participate in genomic research in order to access new technologies. Even when the informed consent process attempts to explicitly outline risks such as psychosocial harm, can it ever be really a voluntary choice for *unaffected* family members, particularly for children?[43] Moreover, the degree of nonquantifiable risks vary in significance among each individual family member, as does how the perceived harm is handled.

When Bobby shouts out in alarm that since the consent form says their samples are "*stored indefinitely*," that means "everything about us goes into a federal databank. But why?...And forever?"[96,102-105,113-115] Amy is quick to reassure her brother that there is "No need to worry" because she read that everything was being "*coded and locked up*" and all their information is "*password protected.*" Laughing at what he considers his sister's naiveté, Bobby reminds Amy that people hack into computer files all the time and crack codes. Not wanting to give up her trust in the clinician-researchers, Amy lets Bobby know in no uncertain terms that "they make sure to tell us how careful they are: *When results are reported in medical journals or at scientific meetings, study participants are not named and identified.*"

The next page of the consent form is more cautionary, as Mom suggests reading on: "*However,...it may include your family history and other medical information. It is possible but unlikely that you and/or a family member could be recognized.*" Very concerned that "Grandma would be so upset if our family story was out there for others to know," Bobby responds to his mother by voicing concern for himself and his young *unaffected* sibling, "I wouldn't want the world to see that either. And what about Sam?" Indeed, there is mounting concern about the identifiability[111] of genomic information and whether people understand and appreciate the extent to which their data will be shared.[112] Current research confirms that next-gen sequencing information can be identifiable, a reality to be considered in the consent process, IRB deliberations, and the future development of data sharing policy.[100,101,158,181]

As the family continues to review the informed consent document, they note several more passages that add to the complexity of the issues faced when returning results:[23,31,32,45,76-77]

MOM: You know...I have another worry. This says we might get told what's wrong even if we don't want to know. Listen: "*You will be given a choice to learn or not to learn the results of your genome sequencing....The only exception to opting out is if we find a result that has urgent importance to your health. We plan to share this type of result with you.*"

BOBBY: The doctors don't say anywhere in all these pages just how urgent or bad it has to be before they tell us bad news! Does "*urgent importance*" mean you're going to die in a week?

AMY: The form goes on to say, "*In the future, we may contact you to find out if you are interested in learning about your results or gene variants that are important to your health and/or the health of your relatives.*"

BOBBY: They say "*important*," but how will they decide what's really important enough to tell us?

Once again, the informed consent document uses language, "*importance*," to reflect multiple dimensions—in this case, of magnitude, temporal, and relative values. What is the importance of preferences, and what might be the best way to capture them in the informed consent process? Different values within families, as well as between different ethnic groups and other demographic variations, present many challenges when attempts are made to try to craft consent language that adequately captures a variety of values and contexts. Adding to this challenge is that preferences can be overridden in certain circumstances by the genetic professional and family members. Furthermore, who determines what is important enough to not honor the *right not to know* and what values drive that decision?[38,174] Currently, there is no consensus on these questions; nor are these issues answered by lists of check boxes in the consent form:

> AMY: So Mom, how are you going to check this off? "___ *I would like to be contacted about the diagnosis, possible treatment, or genetic causes of my (my child's) disorder . . . or . . . ___ Please do not contact me regarding the progress of this study or any specific gene change you found.*"

Not answering Amy's query, Mom wants to know, "Why isn't there a checklist for us to say exactly which diseases we want to be told or which we really don't want to be told about?" Soon Bobby raises another critical question: "But what if Amy wants to know everything and you don't, and it turns out both you guys have something like the *BRCA* gene you hear about so much? And what about Sam?" Having returned home a few minutes earlier, Sam fires back, "Don't worry about me. I'm the healthy kid in the family." Not wanting to miss any opportunity to gain genomic information she deems valuable, Amy declares, "Of course I want to know everything— we'd all want to know." Uncomfortable with her daughter's response, Mom quickly snaps, "Don't jump to any conclusions Amy. You can't speak for the whole family."

Whether or not connected by blood, or whether or not *affected*, it is difficult to anticipate what individuals want to know in the future and what you believe others would want to know. People often change their minds, which may impact other family members involved, whether tested or not. Since *values* differ among family members, views of being recontacted may vary considerably.[95] Also, because there is discordance among clinician-researchers[100] about *the duty to recontact* and the sharing of genomic information, a specific plan to clarify expectations for return of results should be outlined in the protocol by the research team and incorporated into the informed consent process, with review by the IRB or another advisory committee.[94,98,157] These deliberations can include the evaluation of numerous approaches such as sharing aggregate data[101] and information related to genomic condition in a newsletter and/or online for all family members, whether *affected* or not:

MOM: Your dad and I are healthy. We obviously gave you something bad in our genes, but there's no need for us to know anything. And who knows if your dad will even show up to do his part of the test?

AMY: How could you not want to know what's in your genes? That's so old-fashioned. Well, I checked off that I want to know all the results!

BOBBY: So did I, because I wouldn't want the doctors to know all about me and my genes if I didn't know too.

MOM: I would not want any of us to know if something bad is going to happen way into the future, like *Alzheimer's*, or *breast cancer*. Why would we want to know ahead of time and worry?

Preferences often differ, and decision-making shifts depending on time and context regarding whether an individual truly wants to know genomic information that will affect them in the present or the future. The duty one feels they owe others to disclose individual genomic data within familial relationships is fraught with psychosocial complexity. This challenge is illuminated after Amy reminds her mother that the consent form also said something about relatives learning results. There was no hesitation in her Mom's response this time as she declared, "I certainly wouldn't want my mother hearing about any results, and I wouldn't even know how to begin to tell my sister Rachel. As for my sister Sarah, it's none of her business. If the doctors find something, I'll just keep it a secret." Bobby snickers while reminding his mom that she is terrible at keeping secrets.

Although Amy diplomatically tries to allay her mom's concerns by suggesting that their genetic counselor, Jennifer Smith, can always tell Aunt Rachel and Aunt Sarah, Mom was not about to budge: "They don't need to know anything. If my sisters are curious, they can get tested themselves." What it means to be a blood relative, whether directly participating in genomic testing or not, has implications that raise issues of family responsibilities—to share or not share genomic information. When Amy begs her Mom, "Just sign the paper and keep it simple please," her Mom voices a truism—"It's Not That Simple!"[4]

Focus Question: How might Dr. Hardy improve the informed consent process?

As the application of next-gen sequencing into clinical medicine increases, the pressure to disclose genomic information intensifies, and it will also become increasingly apparent not only that "It's Not That Simple!" but indeed "It's So Complicated!"[4] With this reality in mind, the drama continues, moving from the informed consent process to the return of results and incidental findings.

SCENE II: THE RETURN OF GENOMIC FINDINGS

We now find Bobby, Amy, Sam, and Ellen Friedman again waiting in the pediatric genetics clinic to see their clinical geneticist, Dr. Hardy. Several months have passed since signing the consent forms and having blood drawn for DNA analysis. The family anticipates learning today more about Bobby and Amy's autosomal recessive genetic disorder based upon whole-exome sequencing attained through Dr. Hardy's research protocol.

This scene opens with Dr. Hardy in a pediatric genetics consultation office speaking on the phone with Ms. Jennifer Smith, the genetic counselor, moments before the Friedman family arrives. Dr. Hardy whispers to her, "So we agree with the IRB about what I should tell them. This is not going to be easy...for any of us. I'll send them to your office next," realizing just how critical the genetic counseling team is to everyone involved.[73,200] Dr. Hardy quickly hangs up when a knock is heard at the door. The Friedman family enters Dr. Hardy's office—Mom first, then Bobby and Amy together, with Sam trailing.

Before fully seated, Mom immediately expresses pent-up anticipation: "We're so anxious to hear what you have to say that may help Bobby and Amy." Amy quickly follows up by asking, "What do Bobby and I have?" Dr. Hardy slowly reports, "Well, Amy, as for Bobby and your disorder, unfortunately nothing conclusive was uncovered," explaining that more waiting is necessary "until we gain further knowledge about how some of these genes relate to neurological functioning. Right now there is more we don't know than do—but the field is rapidly evolving." Bobby's cynicism rang true this time, as he reminded everyone: "I told you this high-tech test would be a waste of time," impatiently inquiring, "Now how much longer?" Sam's frustration over missing swim practice at school was palpable when suggesting to Dr. Hardy that the lack of results should have been shared with her on the phone instead. Dr. Hardy responds, "Not exactly, Sam," and then expresses the reality that although we are often not yet able to provide a well-defined genomic explanation for individuals on a diagnostic odyssey, they still all needed to be present.

DR. HARDY: While we didn't get the answers we were hoping for regarding Bobby and Amy's disease, we learned several things that I must discuss with some of you...some potentially significant findings unrelated to what we were looking for.
AMY: Huh? How can you find something if you weren't looking for it?
DR. HARDY: Remember, the consent document explained that we were sequencing all of the protein coding genes that can cause disease. Next-generation sequencing uncovers a lot of information, not like the earlier genetic tests you've had that just targeted very specific genes.

Clearly thrown by Dr. Hardy's statements,[18-24,35-37,57-58] Mom, in a shaky voice, asks, "What do you mean learn my results—I'm not sick!...Am I?," then wants confirmation that she doesn't have breast cancer. Panicked, Sam pleads to Dr. Hardy, "Nothing can happen to Mom—we all need her. I can't take care of Bobby and Amy." Dr. Hardy encourages everyone to stay calm. "Calm?!!" rebounds Amy. "You're telling us we should be worried about Mom, not just me and Bobby." Dr. Hardy expresses understanding of their fears and explains that there will be ample time for each person to meet with Jennifer, the genetic counselor, should any of them wish. The kids go to the waiting room while Dr. Hardy speaks privately with their mom.

MOM: Just remember that I don't want to know if I'm getting *breast cancer* or if other bad things like *Alzheimer's* are going to happen when I get old...or my kids get old.

DR. HARDY: We don't typically report those kinds of findings from a research protocol investigating another disorder.

Currently there is controversy and debate over whether or not preferences should be sought, and in what way, in the informed consent process.[59] This determination may vary depending on a number of factors, whether in a clinical or research context, including type of relationship between participant and professional; what evidentiary standards need to be met before disclosure; and developmental, cognitive, or health issues. The anticipation of getting results can be very disconcerting psychologically, whether in the research or clinical domain. Mom describes having been so nervous in anticipation of coming to find out how Dr. Hardy "can help Bobby and Amy" that the previous day she couldn't remember where she parked her car. Apparently Mom spent so much time searching for the vehicle and "was so frazzled," that she forgot to pick up Sam from her swim practice. After Dr. Hardy recalls Mom mentioning during the last visit that she thought the stress of dealing with Bobby's and Amy's illness was making her forgetful at work and at home, Mom nods in agreement. The disclosure of incidental findings is complex, often involving a multitude of unanticipated specialists, lab tests, and imagings as well as anxiety for patients, families, genetic professionals, and primary care providers.

DR. HARDY: I'd like to recommend that you see a neurologist...and have some neuroimaging done, and have a bit of the genomic test redone by a CLIA lab.[203]

MOM: What does my nervousness have to do with my gene test? Everyone knows it's because of Bobby and Amy's condition. Why does this Dr. Clia neurologist have to redo my test?

DR. HARDY: Sorry for the confusion; this is complicated, and Jennifer can explain more later. There were certain findings from your genomic analysis that hint at the possibility, a susceptibility, to something that we want to check out more clearly. CLIA is not a doctor, but rather a specially certified lab that helps determine if our research results were accurate.

MOM: You don't trust your lab to know if your research is bogus? And what does that have to do with my forgetting to pick up Sam from swim practice? You're not implying that I'm going to go senile when I am 80 years old? I told you I don't want to know that stuff.

DR. HARDY: There are several possibilities that the neurologist will explore, and retesting at a CLIA lab may help shed light as well.

MOM: Well Alzheimer's is for old people. I'll worry about that when I get old; now I need to think about my kids.

Mom leaves, and alone, Dr. Hardy voices relief: "It will be the neurologist having to tell the Mom she very likely has early-onset AD (Alzheimer's disease), assuming that the CLIA test result confirms the incidental finding."[201] Dr. Hardy soon recognizes the need to "brace myself for more" and calls out to speak with Bobby. Upon hearing this in the waiting room, Mom becomes even more worried, asking, "What are you going to tell us now?"

Given the choice as to whether to include Mom in this initial discussion, Bobby requests being informed privately first and expresses his concern: "This sounds serious. I thought you said Amy and me had 'inconclusive' genes?" Dr. Hardy apologizes for any confusion, and attempts to clarify: "I was referring to the disease we were investigating. We found some... extra... concerns... and had the results repeated by a lab to confirm their validity." This repeat of the research test in a CLIA-certified lab further blurs the lines between genomic research and clinical medicine, perpetuating and deepening the therapeutic misconception. When Bobby declares, "Give it to me straight, doc," he has little clue about the distinction between the two spheres and the dual role his geneticist plays.

DR. HARDY: The genome analysis shows that you carry the *BRCA1* mutation. That doesn't necessarily mean you'll get breast cancer; it only indicates a *susceptibility*, the *possibility* for getting a disease. Indeed, your *risk* is quite low, only about 6% lifetime risk for breast cancer. But since it's much higher than the average male, we felt we should share it with you so you can be monitored, now that we know to look.

BOBBY: I think you confused my results with Amy's or Mom's—that's a girl's disease.

DR. HARDY: While prevalent in females, it also occurs in males.

BOBBY: Do Amy and Sam have breast cancer too? And Mom?

DR. HARDY: First off, please let me be clear that I am *not* saying you have breast cancer. Only that you carry the genetic *mutation* associated with the *possibility* for developing the disease. We call that higher *risk*; not definitely getting the disease.

The genetic professionals' decision of what to disclose, how to disclose, and when to disclose is contextually nuanced. For example, in this case, is Dr. Hardy considering the fact that Bobby has an increasingly degenerative terminal disease when weighing the benefits and risks of sharing the *BRCA* findings?

Furthermore, like his mom, Bobby can't hear or process the distinction between *susceptibility* and *disease*.[61] Feeling that this information is "so embarrassing," Bobby inquires if he needs to tell his friends.[202] Aware that this new genomic-based *predictive diagnosis* is layered on top of Bobby having a more immediate medical condition, Dr. Hardy first offers some reassurance that this is private information that doesn't need to be shared with anyone, then asks Bobby to see Jennifer, "while I speak with your mom about something else."

Bobby stumbles out dazed, then blurts out when passing Mom in the hallway, "I have *breast cancer!*"[204] Dr. Hardy quickly tries to alleviate the distress, reminding Bobby, "You don't have breast cancer now and might never even get it. It's only a *potential future possibility*, a slight future possibility." Mom enters the office distraught, telling Dr. Hardy, "Oh my, this is some nightmare! We came here for you to tell us results that can help my kids' disease, and now you're telling Bobby he'll die from breast cancer instead?" Dr. Hardy, feeling somewhat overwhelmed, tries to explain the situation, to little avail as just occurred with Bobby: "I did not say that Bobby had breast cancer, or would die from it. Just that the sequencing showed a small increased risk," reminding her that Jennifer can explain further. "But first," Dr. Hardy continues, "I need to discuss something else with you... about Sam."

Mom never anticipated other findings outside the scope under research.[78] The limits get pushed even further when an incidental finding is discovered in an *unaffected* child.

MOM: Please don't tell me you discovered that she has Amy and Bobby's bad gene.
DR. HARDY: No, absolutely not, please rest assured...
MOM: [*cutting Dr. Hardy off*] Thank heavens she's OK. She's my healthy one.
DR. HARDY: Sam definitely does not carry that genetic defect... However, ...
MOM: Oh my, you're going to tell me she has the breast cancer gene too.
DR. HARDY: I'm not referring to those disorders... and given Sam's age, most geneticists would not report most research results that may possibly have health implications much later in life.

Relieved, Mom exclaims, "So she is OK then." To which Dr. Hardy responds with great hesitation: "We are concerned... about something else that we found in the genomic testing...related to her heart." "You must be mistaken," cries out Mom, justifying that Sam doesn't have a murmur and she's a really good athlete. "She runs and swims like a fish, has since she was little," adding that Sam has been on their Y's swim team and hopes to be on the high school team one day. Dr. Hardy then explains long QT syndrome, associated with rhythm disturbances in the heart, that potentially can lead to sudden death. Kids who have the genetic mutation associated with long QT syndrome are advised to avoid competitive swimming because passing out in the water can result in drowning. Mom is silent as Dr. Hardy further informs her, "Currently we can't perfectly predict when or which patients" with the genetic *predisposition* to long QT syndrome will have an arrhythmia associated with sudden cardiac arrest.[205]

DR. HARDY: So I need to share the seriousness of this with Sam and tell her we very strongly recommend that competitive athletics be forsaken.

MOM: Oh no, you can't tell her anything is wrong.[24] Remember you just said doctors don't tell kids Sam's age. And anyway, remember you told me these tests aren't certain!

DR. HARDY: You are correct that for kids we typically do not report most disease susceptibility that may affect them later in life. This, however, has immediate implications. There is the potential for sudden death without treatment and an excellent outcome with treatment—including taking a medication to protect the heart. We've already confirmed this result in a CLIA lab. Because of the severe ramifications for some kids—and we don't know who—I must inform her so she'll give up competitive swimming.

MOM: No...that would devastate her...let's wait till high school. Then I can just say I have to go to work earlier so can't take her to 6 AM swim practice.[207]

DR. HARDY: She should be closely followed by a cardiologist, who may also consider beta blockers or an implantable defibrillator. We really need to bring Sam into this discussion now.[208]

Dr. Hardy gives Mom tissues and gets Sam. In fact, whether or not it is ethical to share secondary findings with children is controversial and context specific, particularly when there is *uncertainty* of penetrance and phenotype and the medical and psychological implications of proactive interventions.

When Sam enters the office and asks, "Why does my Mom look so sad?," Dr. Hardy replies, "Your mom is concerned because we found something in your test, called long QT syndrome, which has been linked to very serious heart problems in *some* young people. Problem is, *we aren't fully sure* who will be the kid whose heart suddenly stops when doing competitive sports, so I must advise you to immediately stop competitive swimming. There are so many wonderful activities you can do...art, music." Sobbing, Sam responds, "But you're telling me I can't do what I do best."

With tears, Mom looks at Dr. Hardy and says in a quivering voice, "I can't believe this is happening...Sam was my healthy kid this morning..." The drama ends with Dr. Hardy being rather reflective, expressing to them, "I am so sorry...It's So Complicated!"

Focus Question: If you were Dr. Hardy, how would you have handled the disclosure of genomic findings?

ADDITIONAL QUESTIONS

1. What complex ethical and psychosocial issues are raised by next-gen sequencing focused on certain ethnic and racial groups?
2. What is the rationale for so many warnings in the informed consent form, and how, if at all, do you think this impacts the informed consent process? Should the process for genomic research and clinical medicine differ?
3. How does the informed consent process attempt to explicitly outline benefits and risks that are difficult to quantify, such as psychosocial impact?
4. How can we enhance the principle of voluntary choice for *unaffected* family members, particularly children?
5. What is the importance of preferences, and what might be the best way to capture them in the informed consent process?
6. Who determines what is important enough to override the *right not to know*, and what values drive that decision?
7. How would you evaluate the use of a checklist for informing the participant and researcher on preferences and limitations for the disclosure of incidental findings?
8. Would you want to know if you were at increased risk for a serious medical condition discovered through genomic sequencing and likely to occur in the future, such as Alzheimer's or breast cancer? What factors would influence your decision making in varying contexts?
9. How might the process of informed consent and disclosure of findings vary depending on whether we believe a phenotype—like Mom's memory problems—is explained by genetics, other factors, or both?
10. What impact is there when secondary findings require the clinical genetics team or researcher to make referrals to primary care professionals and specialists?
11. What might be the unintended consequences of sharing inconclusive genomic findings or those with an uncertain outcome?
12. How would you evaluate the benefits and risks of sharing genomic information with Sam? with Bobby? with Mom?

CHAPTER 4

Reframing an "Open Future"

The Shifting Landscape from NBS to NBSeq

We recently celebrated the anniversaries of three scientific innovations that have each engendered much ethical debate and now intersect—the 60th anniversary of the elucidation of the double helix structure of DNA, half a century of population-based newborn screening (NBS) [217,225] guided by the tradition of protecting the best interests of young children,[80] and a decade since mapping the human genome.[2,119] As the medical, public health, and bioethical communities currently contemplate the application of whole-genome sequencing in the context of newborn screening (NBSeq), narrative genomics can illuminate this emerging controversial issue to enhance understanding and exploration of the complex challenges ahead—the ethical, legal, psychosocial, and policy implications on children, parents, and our multicultural society.[123,125]

For the last dramatization in Part I, adapted from our shorter vignette-play *The Paradoxes in Pandora's Box*, yet another group of interdisciplinary professionals is situated in an advisory role, this time for the making of public health policy. This chapter brings to life a very contemporary debate: the future of a shifting landscape[120] from NBS to NBSeq and the impact that the implementation of genomic technology—as a primary screening tool on all infants or secondary testing of *affected* infants—may have, particularly on the tradition of a *child's right to an open future*[72,136] and parent-infant attachment.[71,146]

Historically, NBS has been fraught with controversy,[118,121,122,131–133] such as the rationale for screening criteria,[124–127] informed consent,[137–140,142] and social justice,[143–145] and concerns raised will surely accelerate in parallel with the mounting information generated by genomic sequencing. Deliberation among diverse voices seems essential given that the potential benefits associated with the discovery of genomic findings on a newborn coexist with a multitude of potential risks—a Pandora's box replete with many paradoxes.

SCENE I: THE PARADOXES OF NBSEQ

The dramatic narrative is set in a government conference room where the NBSeq Expert Committee has been convened to advise a state agency on whether to consider being the first state program to potentially pilot NBSeq as a screening measure. This is the Expert Committee's initial time together, and the members are seated at the conference table:

> Prof. Chair, MD, JD: a health law policy scholar and chair of this committee
>
> Dr. Pedethic, MD, MS: a pediatrician-ethicist and co-chair
>
> Dr. Clingene, MD, PhD: a clinical geneticist
>
> Mr./Ms. Gencounselor, MS, CGC: a genetic counselor
>
> Dr. Pho, MD, MPH: a public health genetics official from this pilot state
>
> Dr. Labgen, PhD: a lab geneticist
>
> Mr./Ms. Advocate, MBA: a genetic disorder advocacy group representative

To enrich the discourse and policy process, Prof. Chair thought it might be helpful to use their first meeting together—"our only one without a public forum to gain input from the perspective of many parents and advocacy groups"—to list some of the dilemmas they will confront should this expert committee ultimately decide to recommend that this state pilot whole-genome sequencing "for all newborns born here." Hoping to reveal the complexity of this shifting landscape, Prof. Chair tasks fellow committee members: "Let us generate a list of potential challenges—some paradoxical—posed by whole-genome sequencing on newborns in the context of a public health initiative." Encouraging everyone to engage in a "robust discussion, listing paradoxes first," the co-Chair is asked to begin.

After Dr. Pedethic acknowledges appreciation for the opportunity to co-chair "this thought-provoking committee given the group's collective expertise and diversity," recognition is given to this state's long tradition of being "a national leader in expanding the conditions for newborn screening panels and at the forefront of implementing new technologies for evidence-based research."[127,213,219,222-223]

Then, getting to the task at hand, Dr. Pedethic moves forward with the Chair's mental exercise to explore some paradoxes raised when discovering a newborn's genomic information in the context of a potential statewide screening program. One paradox comes quickly to Dr. Pedethic: "When folks speak of whole-genome sequencing as giving us the 'full picture,' it is important to bear in mind that genotypic expression signaling disease for a newborn may ultimately be influenced by many other factors, such as environment and epigenetic influences." Dr. Labgen adds, "And many conditions do not have known phenotypes at birth."[128,166]

DR. CLINGENE: You know, some conditions identified in current NBS secondary panels[211] already resemble what would, in some contexts, be considered incidental findings[154] or false positives.[18-21,22,24,35-37,57-59,78,152]

MR./MS. GENCOUNSELOR: Well, I can guarantee you that both incidental findings and false positives will dramatically increase with NBSeq if we aren't very careful. Not only that, the fact is that we are currently clueless as to the significance of so much of this genomic sequencing data.[62-64]

More basic science and interventional strategies to reduce the harm of psychological distress to the parent, and hence the child, are clearly needed. Not only are we a long way from understanding the function of a multitude of genes, even if we understood what they do, we are a long way from identifying all the genetic variants that may impact the diagnosis, treatment, and prognosis. To be used as a primary screening tool for all newborns in a public health context, the benefit needs to outweigh the challenges and risks,[21,83-86,133,215,220,226] especially in recognition of the potential anxiety for parents when we still poorly communicate current panel results and have so many false positives.[61,147,152,228]

MR./MS. ADVOCATE: Think of the benefits to families—whole-genome sequencing can prevent diagnostic odysseys.

DR. PHO: True, but it can also send families off on painful new odysseys that are ultimately found to be nothing but wild goose chases. Even when successful, we need to keep in mind that by reducing diagnostic odysseys, on the one hand, we will almost certainly be increasing medical surveillance for these individuals, on the other.

MR./MS. GENCOUNSELOR: Yes, and remember that the increased identification of conditions can diminish or heighten distress.[148,151,214,221]

We know from the empirical data and literature that for some families parental anxiety continues well after learning that an initial positive NBS was actually false,[133] often exacerbated by poor communication of results and inadequate counseling.[149-150,200] This will be an even greater challenge as the volume of genomic information stresses the healthcare system as well as the family, and calls into question whether population-based comprehensive NBSeq can ever show clear evidence of greater benefit than risk in a public health context.

As the meeting continues, many paradoxes evolve. Dr. Pedethic shares, "The psychological framework for an infant's *open future* may be at odds when juxtaposed with the imperative to use genomic information now to potentially enhance an infant's future."[136,153] Dr. Clingene offers another point: "Given the enormous quantity of data yielding many anomalies on every individual, we may recognize even more than we currently do that huge variability exists and reframe our conceptualization of *normal*." Concerned with the potential implications of Dr. Clingene's comment, Mr./Ms. Advocate asks, "Are you implying that instead of NBS being there to help kids get 'diagnosed' and given treatment if available,[209] there may be more stigmatizing labeling of children?" The reality is that stigmatization and discrimination[30,68] are always a concern to be aware of, and must be outweighed by clear evidence of benefit—particularly with children. Dr. Clingene and Mr./Ms. Advocate's comments are reminiscent of Chapter 2's narrative on changing perceptions of how we delineate *normalcy*.

Shifting to a different perspective, Dr. Pho raises another paradox: "I am also concerned that NBS as a social justice leveler may be jeopardized by NBSeq if many conditions are identified and neither individuals nor states have economic resources to provide necessary follow-up." In fact, NBS programs are overseen by the states, and while designed to ensure equal access, there is huge variation in the number of tests offered by each state and economic limitations to expansion even without genomic technology. A bit later, Dr. Labgen reminds Mr./Ms. Advocate that NBS is a screening tool and "does not suffice as a diagnostic measure," adding that in fact, "One of the paradoxes of NBSeq is that it may actually be thought of as conferring a diagnosis rather than a prediction."[135]

It is critical that adequate communication be provided to inform families and professionals that NBSeq would be more akin to a research paradigm[15] rather than a diagnostic test in the clinical sphere.[74,75,135] And, as we have seen in the previous narrative with the Friedman family, there are many challenges in clarifying what connotes risk and susceptibility even with a confirmed diagnosis.[60,61]

"We must also be mindful," cautions Dr. Pho, "that any large expansion of conditions outside the scope of the current screening paradigms would raise concerns that even with true positives, there is limited infrastructure to adequately provide counseling to address the confusion with disclosure of NBSeq findings that will require confirmation and follow-up tests." Prof. Chair reflects: "Reason suggests that as such, if NBSeq were to be piloted, it should be limited initially to targeted screening of conditions on the current panel and should still recognize that there needs to be a rigorous, evidence-based process for any additional conditions added later, paralleling the criteria for NBS."[123,189,190,224]

Another paradox, raised by Dr. Pho, is that the Wilson-Jungner 10-point criteria for public health screening developed by WHO in the 1960s—and traditionally used for NBS[124]—"was not even designed to be used for infants and, as noted by the authors, was supposed to be flexible to modification over the years." So changes that many thought were needed with NBS following tandem mass spectroscopy are likely to be even more hotly debated with NBSeq, including reporting adult-onset disorders, carrier status, uncertain benefits for the child, or those that extend beyond the child.[75,125,126,131,132,134] "Clearly more research is needed," states Mr./Ms. Advocate, "to better address these challenges before dramatically increasing the amount of ambiguous genomic information to families."[92,129]

Pondering the issues, Dr. Clingene then reflects: "Speaking of paradoxes, I am afraid that the ability to protect the interests[80] of vulnerable newborns by traditionally mandating NBS may be eroded with NBSeq due to issues of informed consent[47–50,142] and return of results,[7,31,45,76,77] blurring boundaries among a public health screening measure, research, and clinical test."[15,21,81,82] "In fact," Dr. Pedethic comments, "NBS is in a rather privileged place because it can confer such dramatic benefit for both individuals and society. If we start to dilute the benefit, our mandate and our legitimacy are both undermined. And this would do great harm."

Prof. Chair calls for a brief break as the NBSeq Expert Committee is ready to move from the philosophical sphere of generating paradoxes to brainstorming a list of salient concerns and challenges of a more practical nature.

Focus Question: Which paradoxes resonate with you, and what other paradoxes would you raise?

SCENE II: THE PRACTICAL CONCERNS IN PANDORA'S BOX

Returning from the short break after considering some of the more philo-sophical issues raised by this new technology, Prof. Chair thought it worth-while to begin by asking the co-chair to share an insight they discussed during the break. While reflecting upon fellow committee members' earlier thought-ful comments, Dr. Pedethic recalls realizing that the term "criteria"—so often used when discussing NBS—has multiple meanings that have all engendered considerable debate over the years.

"Criteria" of what constitutes a condition to be added to a panel can both reference the public health screening criteria—whether the classical Wilson-Jungner framework or another, more flexible set of criteria such as that proposed more recently by Andermann and colleagues for the World Health Organization (WHO)[124]—as well as reference empirical, biochemical standards that determine criteria for inclusion or exclusion.[210,229] Dr. Pedethic points out, "We should be mindful that all criteria are subject to our values and perspectives perhaps more than we may suspect. What really are our cri-teria for screening, and what, when, and how are those criteria developed and supported?"

Prof. Chair then opines that the opening exercise of highlighting paradoxes stimulated thinking about the complexities of NBSeq and, confident that all committee members are "aware of the potential benefits," tries to move the policy deliberations forward by spending the remaining time sorting out "some major concerns and challenges" that may face the state if piloting NBSeq as a population screen is adopted.

DR. CLINGENE: There are many multisystemic congenital syndromes that are associated with cardiac problems. WES can identify the comorbidities in such syndromes more readily and in a more timely fashion than can cur-rent screening modalities.

DR. LABGEN: More cost effective too, since we won't have to do several tar-geted tests. Greater efficiency, reduced diagnostic odyssey, all for less money—a no-lose situation!

DR. PEDETHIC: Come on...What ever happened to using old-fashioned clinical judgment to diagnose an infant with Williams syndrome? We need whole-genome sequencing to tell us that?

DR. LABGEN: Well, not everyone likely has your clinical acumen, Dr. Pedethic. The more readily we can diagnose conditions the better, in my view.

In fact, it will be a long time, if at all, that comprehensive sequencing can be done quickly enough (including delays in processing and shipping specimens) as a population-based screen to help those babies; many need surgery before any state public health office would have WGS results. Dr. Pedethic reminds the group that most parents of babies who have significant heart problems—like hypoplastic left heart syndrome, which may coincide with extracardiac syndromes—are "worried sick" about going through multiple complex surgeries, and then adds, "You're going to tell these parents all the other things that may be wrong with their baby that are less clinically significant, like short stature?"

Equally concerned with the psychosocial implications, Mr./Ms. Gencounselor asks rhetorically, "You tell them all this when the risk of postpartum depression is highest? And what does the timing of all this genomic information mean for the attachment process, for infant-parent bonding?"[146]

"Why not just use target testing and wait till they are older?" asks Prof. Chair. "We can just tell the parents whatever they would have gotten back from the tandem mass NBS and not report the full sequencing results; certainly we shouldn't return adult-onset conditions," Dr. Labgen opines. Firmly, Dr. Pho raises an important policy consideration: "Why on earth would we do a shotgun test on every newborn instead of targeting our testing and our technology where it can be most beneficial? We'd never dream of getting whole-body MRIs on neonates as a routine measure. It would be equally inane to sequence their whole genome at birth. If there is one thing medicine has taught us, it's that we need to apply complex tests in a thoughtful manner."

From Dr. Pedethic's perspective, "We ought to determine what conditions necessitate early intervention and consider using this genome sequencing technology as a panel first on those, and perhaps a limited number of other disorders, rather than analyzing and reporting every bit of data we can generate on a newborn." This NBSeq Expert Committee's discussion and deliberations are focused on figuring out where to draw the line, recognizing that historically, since the early days of PKU, preferences for reporting will vary.

MR./MS. ADVOCATE: Parents have a right to know...and whatever they want to know. Why are you all being so negative and paternalistic? And it makes no sense to wait a few weeks or months until they get older. It's tough to face bad news about your kid at any time.

DR. CLINGENE: Older? Don't worry about older. I predict whole-genome sequencing will all be done prenatally. [212]

DR. PHO: Maybe so, but that will never happen as a public health measure. It is likely that only the moms-to-be with money will get access to the prenatal technology.

Lessons learned from the past half-century suggest that regardless of whether everyone had access to screening, they did not all have access to treatment. Even after the very first NBS bloodspot, PKU, we still identify conditions but are unable to provide adequate resources for all those *affected* to receive the necessary dietary treatment, particularly after transitioning into adulthood.[143-145]

Moving on in the discussion of practical concerns, Mr./Ms. Gencounselor raises the question: "Will the shift in technology change our perspectives of whether to get informed consent?" We have not had a tradition in NBS of affirmatively obtaining informed consent, and that has been controversial from the early PKU years.[138,139] NBSeq may likely change the model so that parents must opt in.[142] As technology evolves, we need to determine whether informed consent must be given always, never, or sometimes and what "criteria" will be used when deciding what conditions—all, none, some—will be returned.

MR./MS. GENCOUNSELOR: What are we going to do if we find a Lynch mutation in a baby? It has no direct impact on her for decades; however, it probably means that her mom or dad is at a very high risk for a serious, yet preventable disease. Do we look at those genes? Do we return those results?

DR. LABGEN: Well, we'd better figure out these kinds of things ahead of time with NBSeq so we don't risk being ordered to destroy millions of specimens as we had to in Texas and Minnesota where we had lawsuits because a few folks complained about not being asked to give consent.[137,141]

This is really tough terrain. There is much to learn from reflecting back historically, including the need to consider the stress from false positives in NBS that have been reported over the past 50 years.[152, 217] While angst could certainly be reduced with better information and counseling pre- and post-birth,[147,150] the number of false positives and findings of unknown significance are bound to increase exponentially.

When Mr./Ms. Advocate reminds fellow NBSeq Committee members of the value of current NBS using tandem mass spectroscopy, "Think of all the children the screens have helped; let's not throw out the baby with the bathwater," Dr. Labgen offers with enthusiasm, "Newborn whole-genome sequencing will help save more kids." Having a differing opinion, Dr. Pedethic counters, "You've got to be kidding me. From what? There is no way whole-genome sequencing of newborns won't create a massive degree of *patients in waiting*."[65,67,68]

Tension already exists given the prevalence of phenotypic variations with the majority of metabolic conditions on the current core and secondary NBS panels.[229] Further complicating this is the reality that because rare diseases affect very small numbers in the population, it is difficult to generate the power necessary for robust empirical studies, relying instead on natural prospective case histories with inconsistent measures.[13,216] If we don't know when—or if—a condition or symptoms will manifest, or if we cannot predict the severity, we need to be particularly mindful of how we disclose the genomic information to parents.

DR. PHO: And do you know how we plan to give back the whole-genome sequencing results? Do we just analyze and return what is on the current core RUSP [Recommended Uniform Screening Panel] panel and store the bloodspots till newborns reach age of majority?[103–105,116,117]

DR. CLINGENE: By the time kids are old enough to decide for themselves if they want to know, won't the technology and results be out of date? And is there a duty, and whose duty, to recontact the family if the interpretation of genomic information changes?

Many of the practical challenges regarding recontact were explored in the research context in Chapter 2. In fact, there is currently some interest in revisiting and updating the ACMG policy guidelines regarding the *duty to recontact*, written prior to the completion of mapping the human genome.[14]

MR./MS. ADVOCATE: Won't the parent get the whole-genome sequence on a chip to keep at home?

DR. LABGEN: We are not even close to being there yet.

DR. CLINGENE: Most patients don't even remember to prepare an up-to-date list of all the medications they are taking to bring to their doctor's appointment. You think they are going to keep track of where they placed a flash drive with their whole-genome sequence on it, much less remember to bring it to appointments years in the future?

Indeed, there exists a significant practical concern about the process that is currently being investigated as a research priority: how to convey genomic information to the kids upon age of majority and outline their responsibilities to attain research results if desired—such as providing an updated forwarding address for the proband. These are complex challenges calling for creative strategies to generate new ways to share findings from the past well into the future, similar to what would be needed for NBSeq, only on a far greater scale for an entire newborn population. Expressing a more immediate concern, Mr./Ms. Gencounselor asks, "And what if the parent does not want to be recontacted or learn about an adult-onset disease to protect their child's *open future*?" To which Dr. Clingene quickly reacts, "What kind of *open future* is it if the parent closes the box? That screening information could impact the parent's health as well as the child's." Returning to a very practical issue, Dr. Labgen reminds the committee, "Look, regardless of whether we return or not, we need this information to improve our laboratory analysis—for quality improvement."[141,230]

All the focus of discussion on the potential problems and challenges is important. However, it runs the risk of blurring over the fact that we know there are potential benefits in some kind of genome-scale sequencing for screening purposes—if it is applied carefully. What is needed is good empirical data across the board to see how best to apply this new technology—where, when, and for whom it will help, and under what conditions it would cause more harm than good. Dr. Pedethic reminds the committee, "The State is obligated to protect the *'best interest of the child.'*" What gain, if any, does the WGS information provide to benefit the child, parent, and society? As Dr. Pedethic notes, "Maybe it should not be *whole* genome, but rather should be "*part* genome." Even on that somewhat limited scale, we all need to be mindful of the drive of the technological imperative and evaluate the policy implications.

Mr./Ms Advocate reflects: "At the end of the day, after all this debate, actual parents will have to make very real choices given the information they do or do not receive." "So true," responds Mr./Ms Gencounselor, adding, "and since there is no one 'typical' parent or one particular 'condition group' to represent all parents, even within their own group, there will be a wide range of preferences—especially taking into account preferences that may reflect different values, cultures, religious beliefs, and so on. How do we set up effective public engagement to begin to understand these preferences?" Nodding in agreement about the complexity facing the expert committee, Dr. Pedethic states, "Clearly the reality of multiple perspectives—parents as well as professionals—presents a challenge for all of us."[218,227]

After Dr. Pedethic offers the final commentary, Prof. Chair thanks the NBSeq Committee members for sharing their expertise during their first session together, noting that it was indeed productive to discuss the paradoxes and practical concerns and to discover perspectives shared and those debated.

Prof. Chair concludes:

> I look forward to having robust discussions with many parents during the public forum for our next meeting. In addition, more research is needed to explore the scientific validity and ethical implications of engaging in WGS on our newborns. We hope to foster further conversations surrounding the shifting landscape as we better understand many of the ethical and policy paradoxes and the practical challenges that will confront professionals and society when Pandora's box is opened as NBS evolves into NBSeq.

> *Focus Question: By opening Pandora's box, how might newborn sequencing reframe an "open future"?*

ADDITIONAL QUESTIONS

1. How would you analyze the benefits and risks of applying genomic technology for targeted screening on all newborns, as opposed to fully interrogating the whole genome?
2. How would your analysis differ when applying WGS on a newborn who has manifestations of a condition (dysmorphology or disease) of suspected genetic origin?

3. Would your criteria for newborn screening change if NBSeq were integrated in the public health domain? If so, how would the criteria be developed and supported to reach all newborns?
4. How would you determine what findings are clinically significant enough to return to parents?
5. What are some of the psychosocial implications of returning findings beyond the scope of NBS discovered through WGS to parents of newborns?
6. What are the conditions for determining the best timing for returning results generated from NBSeq?
7. How might the shift in genomic technology change our perspective on whether to get informed consent? Would your position differ depending on whether targeted screening or WGS was involved?
8. What is your opinion of WGS being integrated into prenatal care for the population?
9. Relatively speaking, do you think it is better to perform WGS prenatally or during the newborn period? What factors would influence your decision making?
10. How would you evaluate a plan to analyze and return NBSeq results compared to current practice?
11. What is your opinion regarding offering the return of comprehensive WGS findings, which would not have been previously disclosed through the state's newborn screen, to the child upon reaching age of majority?
12. In the context of NBSeq, what is your opinion on a policy of waiting to disclose findings until age of majority for an adult-onset disease? Would your opinion differ if for a non-life-threatening childhood condition?
13. What gain, if any, does newborn WGS information provide to benefit the child; the family; and/or society?

PART TWO

Integrating Narrative Genomics

A Case Study Drama

CHAPTER 5

Reconceptualizing the Past, Present, & Future

Next-Gen Sequencing—"What's Next?!"

Part II integrates most of the issues and themes explored in Part I into a fictionalized genomic case narrative to bring to life the importance of context when considering the potential for genomic research and medicine to reconceptualize our past, present, and future identities and relationships. The drama of DNA in this chapter highlights the implications of next-generation sequencing (next-gen; NGS) for professionals and a family from an IRB deliberation through the informed consent process, to a clinical ethics consultation, and ultimately to the return of genomic findings. This dramatic narrative, an adaptation of our original four-act play, *What's Next?!*, provides an opportunity to imagine and contemplate some of the ethical and psychosocial dilemmas that may be encountered with protocols that apply next-gen sequencing genomic technologies in ways that challenge the boundaries of ethical norms.

On occasion, we also stretch the boundaries of conventional professional interactions to encourage *teachable moments*. The characters, protocol, and disorder to be studied—*Sienna disease*—are all fictitious. However, the consent form excerpts quoted are based on composites of actual documents.

SCENE I: THE IRB DELIBERATION

The setting for this chapter is Midway Health, a mid-size medical center. We enter the IRB meeting, where the drama for Scene I unfolds. The IRB members in attendance include:

Dr. Cardy, a cardiologist and the IRB chair
Dr. Obbie, an obstetrician/ethicist and the primary reviewer
Mr./Ms. Lawcomm, an attorney and IRB community member
Mr./Ms. Pednur, a pediatric nurse practitioner and IRB member

The site co-Investigator (Co-I), Dr. Gene, a pediatric geneticist, is also present.

The Chair, Dr. Cardy, introduces the first protocol on the IRB's agenda,[93,94,98-100,157] titled "Next-Generation Sequencing and 'Sienna' Disease in Children," and explains that because this genomic technology is new to their medical center, they will diverge from their standard practice and instead include the investigator from the onset. Dr. Gene is introduced as the site co-investigator, having "*just* completed" a molecular genetics fellowship at Coastal Medical and now Midway's new pediatric geneticist who will work on this project using next-gen sequencing. Dr. Cardy exclaims "NGS!! Pretty exciting that we're finally getting a chance to play in the big league!" and then the primary reviewer begins to summarize the protocol.

The stated aim of this study, Dr. Obbie informs, is to better understand the natural history and genotype-phenotype variations[44] of Sienna disease, a (fictional) rare[199] neurological disorder characterized by cardiac malformation, muscle degeneration, and severe cognitive decline with onset ranging from birth through adolescence. Dr. Gene interrupts with further details, highlighting that the infantile type results in death by age 2 if no treatment is provided, and the treatment isn't always effective at any age, with significant adverse effects in many patients. Dr. Obbie continues the review, noting the ultimate goal of the research: "knowledge generated by the genomic information that will lead to therapeutic and, hopefully, curative benefit."

The proposed research[21,45,48,94] employs next-gen sequencing[15,49] with pediatric patients[71,72,74-78] already diagnosed with Sienna disease through traditional methods; their immediate family members—siblings and parents—will also be recruited for NGS. The IRB Chair clarifies that this is "one of those multisite studies[163] with part federal funding where we have limited control since Ivy U has the PI, our former Dr. Verde." When Dr. Gene adds that the *Sienna* Foundation is supplying money too, and opines "I'm sure they'll have the patients' interest at heart," Mr./Ms. Lawcomm responds, "Hmmm...," airing some suspicion of potential conflict of interest.[165]

After Dr. Obbie returns to the review, this time quoting directly from the written protocol: "*Along with requiring parental permission for minors,* probands under the age of 18 will be asked to give verbal assent unless lacking cognitive capacity,"[84,116,117] Dr. Cardy reminds the IRB members that Subpart D requires "a risk/benefit analysis if we are involving kids in research—both *affected* and *unaffected*."[83] Mr./Ms. Lawcomm seeks clarification of "who exactly is the *proband* in this study." And when Dr. Gene simply answers, "The kids," more questions ensue. Dr. Cardy inquires, "Which ones, and what about the parents?," followed by Mr./Ms. Pednur asking about the ages of the children and how they will be recruited. Dr. Obbie provides the specifics that the kids—both Sienna patients and their siblings—are between 8 and 18 years old, and adds, "If my understanding of Sienna disease is correct, some patients may lack capacity to assent due to significant decline in neurocognitive functioning."[195]

Raising another potential problem, this time regarding NGS on the *unaffected* siblings, Mr./Ms. Pednur worries: "Does this go beyond our usual concern about what kind of pressure a parent may put on the healthy kids to participate for the sake of their sibs?...And is that truly assent?"[45] Mr./Ms. Lawcomm reminds the IRB that, as always, the investigators need to be sensitive to the suggestion of coercion.[84–87] Looking at Dr. Gene, Dr. Cardy cautions, "Remember, there's a lot of powerful genetic information that can be revealed! Have you really thought through what you will do with any incidental findings?[36,54,59] I mean, on the healthy kids too."[70]

MR./MS. PEDNUR: We have an obligation[35] to help the investigators think about the potential benefits and risks for these siblings. I certainly haven't seen it in this protocol.

DR. GENE: These kinds of things are done all the time; I don't think this looks any different than other genomic studies I've read about.

DR. OBBIE: Well, wait a minute. The massive volume of data from next-gen sequencing is what makes it different. There's going to be a lot of information, and you need to tell us what incidental findings you are considering returning and to whom.

MR./MS. LAWCOMM: Return information? You're confusing the situation...this is *research* not clinical![97,106]

MR./MS. PEDNUR: The investigators have an obligation to return results—certainly if it has *clinical benefit*.

MR./MS. LAWCOMM: Says who? OK, maybe if it is a *"ticking time-bomb."*

DR. GENE: You've got to be kidding me. Don't you read the literature—including from the *Sienna* Foundation—that participants want to know everything whether or not it's *clinically relevant* or *actionable*?[33,39]

Furthering the discussion, Dr. Cardy comments, "That is, until we are ready to tell them bad news.[56,73] Look at Huntington's." Dr. Obbie states the reality that experts can't seem to agree on what is *clinically relevant* or *actionable*.[62–64]

When Dr. Obbie raises "And what about for reproductive decision making? Surely that matters to many of the parents,"[24,232,233,235,250] Mr./Ms. Lawcomm volleys back, "Where does it end—will you give the subjects a CD of their entire genome?"

Acknowledging that "This is neither the time nor place to resolve this debate," Dr. Cardy moves on to another concern. "Given the complexity of this new technology, we need to look carefully at the informed consent forms to see if patients can understand this language" and quotes a passage: "*Heterozygous unclassified variants associated with recessive disorders will not be reported unless a deleterious mutation or a second unclassified variant in the same gene is also detected.*" Shocked at the complexity of the wording, Mr./Ms. Pednur responds, "Seems as if they merged the proband's consent form with a test req explanation for an ordering physician who has a PhD in molecular genetics. There is no way anyone can give an *informed* consent if they can't understand the document." A bit naive, Dr. Gene notes that it won't be problematic because "we require genetic counseling" in advance of the testing to provide explanations and answer questions.[236] However, Dr. Obbie suggests that while a nice concept, "the reality is that we don't have staffs like Ivy, only a couple of certified genetic counselors." Furthermore, as Mr./Ms. Pednur notes, even if there were adequate numbers, "it takes *a lot* of time to explain properly...without much reimbursement."[90,91,200]

Mr./Ms. Pednur goes on to ask, "Do you think the parents are going to be able to understand this part of the consent form?" and quotes the document: "*For probands under the age of 18 the following categories are automatically blinded: late-onset disorders*[74,75] *and autosomal recessive carrier status.*"[250] Dr. Obbie follows with an "even more confusing" passage, "*Probands over the age of 18 must choose whether to blind certain results if they don't want to receive specific secondary incidental findings.*" Looking directly at Dr. Gene, a bewildered Dr. Obbie asks, "You are keeping this open-ended for the parents?" The reality is that no one can ever know all the possible conditions beforehand.

DR. OBBIE: Could we at least provide them with a checklist of diseases so they can decide which boxes to check off?
DR. GENE: If you want us to. But what if it is our medical opinion that it is in their best interest to know, regardless of which box they checked?
MR./MS. LAWCOMM: They have the right not to know.
Mr./Ms. PEDNUR: What if everyone in the family doesn't agree with the doctor's position? And what if the parents don't agree with each other's choices? Even a checklist can't fix that![26,27]

"We also must be sensitive," stresses Mr./Ms. Lawcomm, "that different cultures may have different values about what they want to know and how the genomic information might impact their lives."[28,42] And to further complicate matters, "What if there is little concordance with what should be returned among site co-investigators across the multiple institutions?" asks Dr. Cardy.[34]

MR./MS. LAWCOMM: Dr. Gene, it doesn't seem as if you have thought through a *plan* for reporting incidental findings to the kids later on when they reach the age of majority. You know…the *"ifs* and *hows"* need to be spelled out.

MR./MS. PEDNUR: Are they going to leave it up to the parents to tell their kids when they turn 18, or is the research team supposed to recontact and find the kids?

MR./MS. LAWCOMM: Is that sustainable? Is this our responsibility?

DR. GENE: If it's not ours, whose is it? What about some kid with a *BRCA1* mutation that she never finds out about, and then she gets what may have been a *preventable* breast cancer—or at least one that could have been picked up earlier had she known?

DR. CARDY: We can always leave it up to the sibs and patients to recontact us when they turn 18.

MR./MS. PEDNUR: Wait a second. Even if these patients have not lost significant neurocognitive functioning, how on earth are we going to be sure that the parents told the kids enough for them to know to recontact us?[206,207]

Raising yet another issue, Dr. Obbie expresses concern whether the consent form language is "the best way to set forth our misattributed paternity policy."[8] After quoting the document, *"You will not be informed if family relationship confirmation does not align with the relationship information provided to us, unless it is medically necessary,"* Dr. Obbie turns to the other IRB members and asks, "Who stays up all night coming up with phrases like *does not align?"*[246]

Mr./Ms. Pednur has a more general concern that may impact both the kids and parents. "Is the technology today accurate enough for us to tell someone years later what they do and don't have?" Moreover, Dr. Cardy queries, "Do we have to rerun tests with whatever is the latest and greatest next-gen sequencing program based on our new knowledge at that time? Can we absorb that cost?" In turn, Mr./Ms. Lawcomm asks, "And what if you find out something that demands follow-up and the patient loses their health insurance?"

Cognizant that there is much more to cover, Dr. Cardy asks, "Do we have any control about *retaining* this DNA material that sort of just seems to have been quietly slipped in here?," reading another passage of the informed consent document: *"I understand that my blood specimen may be retained indefinitely for research, test validation, and/or education by Ivy University, as long as my privacy is maintained."*[108,109,113] "Stored *indefinitely*? What *research* are you planning to do with it?," Mr./Ms. LAWCOMM asks the co-investigator. Dr. Gene replies,

"I am not sure—but I do know that my colleagues and I are enthusiastic about the potential to use all these data being generated to help these kids."

With increasing frustration, Dr. Cardy states, "There's mounting concern with all these multisite studies. Does anyone really know who is controlling *privacy*? There's an awful lot of traceable information this study will generate." When Mr./Ms. Pednur reminds colleagues, "This is on healthy kids too," Mr./Ms. Lawcomm inquires, "What's their plan to protect these kids and parents?" Dr. Obbie is quick to note, "There is no guarantee. The data are identifiable even when the consent form says it's de-identified."[111] Looking directly at Dr. Gene, Mr./Ms. Lawcomm wants clarification of whether the families know that, adding, "And it should be spelled out that there is biobanking involved. It's too vague and camouflaged in this document," yet Dr. Gene hedges, "I'm not sure it's clearly stated in any consent form I've seen for next-gen sequencing, but I welcome your suggestions."[58,96,102–105,114]

Dr. Cardy concludes the IRB meeting by stating that they still have another protocol to review that day. Looking at Dr. Gene, the Chair declares, "There is no way we can approve this as it stands. Dr. Gene, you need to be responsive to our concerns and have a more *workable plan*. The IRB will be back in touch with their stipulations."

Focus Question: What stipulations would you outline that must be met before this protocol can be approved by an IRB?

SCENE II: THE INFORMED CONSENT PROCESS

A *month* later, the IRB approves the protocol plan—remember, this is fiction!! We now find Dr. Gene and Mr./Ms. Consuelo, a genetic counselor, beginning their appointment with:

> Monica and Donald Davis, the parents of:
>> Pamela, an 8-year-old patient in the pediatric genetics clinic
>> James, Pamela's 14-year-old brother

Mr./Ms. Consuelo introduces the family to their new geneticist, Dr. Gene, and, after reminding them that their longtime clinical geneticist Dr. Verde went to Ivy Medical Center, acknowledges their travails: "I know it's been a long road for you folks, on this diagnostic odyssey going to so many specialists over the years." After exchanging brief greetings and acknowledging that Mr./Ms. Consuelo was joining in "as you folks all know each other well and I am new here," Dr. Gene explains that based on the muscle biopsy and subsequent tests Dr. Verde ordered before leaving: "I am glad to say that we now have a *definitive diagnosis* for Pamela—Sienna disease."

Dad's attention is piqued: "Isn't that what the kid in that Harrison Ford movie had?" Mom exclaims, "Oh my! You mean *Extraordinary Measures*? But that kid was so young. You must be mistaken because Pamela was okay as a baby." Explaining that symptoms for Sienna can begin anytime from infancy through the teens, Dr. Gene emphasizes that the movie was about Pompe disease, "a fictionalized version actually."[234] Mr./Ms. Consuelo further clarifies that although some similarities exist, there are differences too; so while Sienna is also a rare neurological disease that affects the muscles and sometimes the heart, unlike Pompe, "Sienna always impacts the brain—like you see with Pamela."

MOM: Is there a cure? We prayed that once you found the disease, a cure would come with it.
DR. GENE: Unfortunately, no. Not yet—but we are working really hard to get there.

Sensitive that "this is a lot to absorb,"[73,214] Mr./Ms. Consuelo offers to provide the Davises reading material to take home "after we talk about it some more." Without a pause, Dad emphatically states, "Tell us what we need to do to make this happen." Wanting more information, Mom asks, "What about a treatment like the IV in the movie? How do you make it better?" When Mr./Ms. Consuelo begins to respond, "There's a weekly enzyme replacement infusion," Dr. Gene interrupts, quick to point out: "However, that has had only limited success so far."

DR. GENE: There is an option I would like you to consider ... something that Dr. Verde was working on before she went to Ivy.

DAD: An experimental medicine? We are willing to try it at this point since Pamela is declining so much these days. What about gene therapy?[208]

MR./MS. CONSUELO: It's complex. We're not there yet.

DR. GENE: However, with the diagnosis, the timing is perfect since Dr. Verde's study was just approved. And rest assured that our research team is striving to help find a cure for Sienna.

MOM: There's nothing more we want than that.

DR. GENE: To get to a cure, we need to learn more about the natural history of the disease and variations in genotypes and phenotypes, so that's where you all can help out.[161,220]

DAD: I don't know what "*genos* and *phenos*" are, but we want in.[107,128]

Trying to adequately inform the parents before they decide whether to consent,[38,39,47-49,61,90-92,106,231,237] Mr./Ms. Consuelo goes on to explain that the researchers are looking to see whether differences in the number and arrangement of someone's genes are associated with different features observed in kids with Sienna disease, like age of onset, behaviors, bodily structures, and functioning. "This groundbreaking study," Dr. Gene highlights, "involves the latest in genomic sequencing technology and bioinformatics" at multiple institutions "spearheaded" by Dr. Verde, which would employ "next-generation sequencing of Pamela, both of you, and James." Pausing to think a moment, Mom says "OK, so *all* of us," unlike Dad, who immediately asks, without fully listening or taking time to process the information, "How do we sign up? Will you help us with this?"

Equally eager to have them participate, Dr. Gene informs them, "Since this medical center will be participating in the study, and as I am one of the co-investigators, you can be certain that I will recommend Pamela for this research project." Confused and concerned, Mom questions, "*Research?*[21] Does that mean she might be given sugar water in the infusion instead of the real medicine?" Mr./Ms. Consuelo quickly assures them that it doesn't alter the current treatment with the infusion, while Dr. Gene reports, "Sorry for any confusion. Initially, this is largely just gathering information from blood tests and your medical records. This study is our hope for the future."

Looking at the parents, Mr./Ms. Consuelo explains that before going over the research consent form,[48] more information about Sienna needs to be relayed. Then, glancing at Dr. Gene, the genetic counselor remarks, "I think you are late for your next clinic appointment." Dr. Gene stands and turns to the parents, offering: "Feel free to contact either Mr./Ms. Consuelo or me with any concerns you may have after your meeting today," and then exits.

Having previously counseled Monica and Donald, Mr./Ms. Consuelo briefly reviews genetics with them and then proceeds to discuss Sienna disease. After

Mom asks a series of questions, Dad interrupts and expresses his priority in no uncertain terms: "I don't mean to cut the conversation short, but can we get to the research part so we can sign on before they run out of spots?!" Mr./Ms. Consuelo tries to reassure him, "Sure, but please don't worry about *that*." Handing them each the consent document, Mr./Ms. Consuelo emphasizes that although they both are familiar with the consent forms for targeted clinical genetic sequencing,[50] there are "significant differences in the consent form for whole-genome sequencing, including having you make choices about your preferences for future information."[49]

Mr./Ms. Consuelo systematically reviews the major elements of the genomic research consent process. Intermittently, Dad remarks that he would just like to review the forms and sign them without listening to any more "information"—to which Mom quickly responds, "Let her finish, please." Mr./Ms. Consuelo continues reviewing the major aspects of consent for the genomic sequencing study, before suggesting to the parents: "Take a few minutes alone to discuss the consent amongst yourselves before I obtain your signatures. Should any questions arise, I'll just be next door in my office and can clarify the research further," and then exits.

Mom[99] peruses the informed consent forms while the Dad impatiently turns each page quickly. They remark on several passages. (As a reminder, the consent form excerpts quoted in this dialogue are based on composites of *actual* documents.)

DAD: From what I've read so far, sounds like this research is going to discover *all* the causes of Sienna. This study is bound to put us on the quick path to a cure for Pamela since it says: *"Performing next-gen sequencing for multiple members of an affected family increases the likelihood of finding underlying disease-causing mutations and variants...and allows for allele co-segregation analysis and de novo mutation confirmation."*

MOM: What's an *allele*?

DAD: Don't know. But I think *de novo* is really, really bad.

MOM: Isn't *de novo* that awful kind of breast and colon cancer? I'll double check with Mr./Ms. Consuelo.[60]

Turning a few pages of the consent document, Dad says "Hmm" and then quotes from another paragraph: *"Given the complexity of next-gen sequencing..."* "What do they mean by *complexity*? It's just a blood test and takes like two minutes!" "Unlike the muscle biopsy Pamela had," Mom recalls, when Pamela needed anesthesia for the procedure and it took weeks to recover; "I think they must mean that it's done on hi-tech equipment."

Reading aloud a different passage from the consent forms, Mom worries: *"Next-gen sequencing may also generate information regarding other genetic conditions about which you may or may not want to be informed."*[18–20,22–24]

"'*Other*' conditions. What more can they dump on us?!" Seemingly unfazed, Dad responds, "I guess a lot given this huge checklist of diseases" and then quotes: "*Adults have some options for receiving secondary results not associated with Sienna disease, including carrier status of recessive disorders.*" Looking up at her husband, Mom predicts, "True to your character, I'm sure you want to know everything." Pausing for a moment, she declares, "As for me, all I want to know is that we can help Pamela and other kids with Sienna."

Concerned about the checklist options, Mom asks for Mr./Ms. Consuelo to come back in "to help us figure out what we should check off. I don't want to get it wrong." Dad makes his intention perfectly clear, "Let's just run through this quickly and sign to close the deal." However, when the genetic counselor returns, Dad is first to request clarification of a clause restricting disclosure: "*Many of these categories are automatically omitted for probands under the age of 18.*" Mr./Ms. Consuelo informs them that unless medically necessary, this provision recognizes that children traditionally have the opportunity to make decisions for themselves when they reach adulthood.[16,80]

Considering another passage in the informed consent documents, Mom wonders why it needs to include: "*I understand that the next-gen sequencing may not generate accurate results because of reasons such as sample mix-up or technical problems, but not limited to these.*" Shaking his head at this rationale, Dad declares, "I don't think I realized how little faith these scientists have in this technology, or are these just 'cover your ass' lines from the hospital's attorney?" Acknowledging that while it may sound like that, Mr./Ms. Consuelo suggests that it is rather "an honest recognition that we are in the early stages of the technology and don't always know how to interpret" most of the genomic information generated.

MOM: Oh, are you referring to this statement? "*Finding a specific genetic variant does not predict the onset, severity, or spectrum of human disease with any degree of certainty. Similarly, the absence of a sequence variant may reduce the likelihood of being affected with a specific condition, but in NO way guarantees this.*" But do they really need to hedge their bets this much? If so, maybe they really don't know enough to help Pamela?[62–64,66,236]

MR./MS. CONSUELO: We are all in the process of learning what we know and don't know. That is why good research is so important. In fact, the consent form states, "*New scientific information becomes available every day. At any time, this could significantly alter the interpretation or significance of any sequence variant. It is strongly recommended that you contact Ivy for regular updates on your address.*"

DAD: So by the time the study results are completed, they'll have it all figured out for sure.

MR./MS. CONSUELO: I'm not so sure you can count on that.

Later, when Mr./Ms. Consuelo informs them, "If we find medically important information, we will share it with you," Mom asks whether this was in reference to another proviso that caught her attention: "*Ivy reserves the right to report additional testing results (other than requested) if they are believed to be clinically relevant to the patients and their families, although they may later be found to be less relevant or of unknown certainty.*" Acknowledging confusion, Mom looks at the genetic counselor when voicing concern regarding perceived mixed messages: "Glad they'll keep us posted, but does this mean they can keep changing their minds on what to tell us?"[239]

Perhaps to reassure himself as well as his wife, Dad states his belief that "They'll do what they need to do because they all have our best interests in mind."[248] To further highlight that he thinks "Dr. Verde and Dr. Gene are very thorough," Dad refers directly to the consent form language: "*I understand that my blood specimens may be retained indefinitely for research, test validation, clinical sequencing and/or education by Ivy University, as long as my privacy is maintained.*" Dad, however, seems to misinterpret the process that will in fact be undertaken as he states, "They'll need to have it because, remember, we just read that they keep on reanalyzing all of our DNA, for *free* and *forever.*"

Soon after, when Mr./Ms. Consuelo asks them if they have any additional questions about the consent form or Sienna disease, Dad remains determined to proceed full steam ahead: "Let's just sign the papers so our spots are reserved." However, Mr./Ms. Consuelo feels it necessary to provide more information, and adds, "Since we know Pamela lacks capacity to assent due to cognitive deterioration, you'll need to sign on her behalf. James, though, will need to assent," and gives them the assent form too.[71,93,116,117,195] Pausing, Mr./Ms. Consuelo asks, "How are you managing with everything?"

MOM: As you may remember from the IVF clinic call to you a few months ago— and as you can see—I am now *pregnant*. After having carrier testing on us and testing on the *baby*, it is such a relief that they said everything is fine,[2,40]

MR./MS. CONSUELO: I'm so happy for you. After those two miscarriages, I am glad to know the conditions they tested for were all OK...But I feel obligated to tell you that they wouldn't have included Sienna in their universal carrier screening panel or prenatal testing. Because Sienna disease is so rare, and we were not aware of the Sienna diagnosis until a few days ago, Sienna was not included in any prior testing.[232,238]

MOM: Oh my!!—what does that mean?

DAD: So let's get the test today. We can do that *next.*[200]

Focus Question: How could the informed consent form and process realistically be improved?

SCENE III: THE CLINICAL ETHICS CONSULTATION

After Dr. Gene and Mr./Ms. Consuelo receive research results on the Davis family, they have disparate, and seemingly irreconcilable, perspectives on how disclosure of findings should proceed. Seeking institutional advice and mediation, they request a clinical ethics consultation.[174,242-244] We now find Dr. Gene and Mr./Ms. Consuelo with members of the ethics team on call:

> Dr. Nino, a neonatologist, and the pediatric clinical ethics chair
> Mr./Ms. Critnur, a pediatric critical care nurse
> Dr. Rez, a first-year pediatric resident "shadowing" the ethics service

Following brief introductions, Dr. Nino describes the presenting problem to Mr./Ms. Critnur and Dr. Rez rather succinctly: "Dr. Gene and Mr./Ms. Consuelo need guidance with mediating differing views about returning results from genetic testing, and want our advice prior to seeing the parents of one of their patients." Dr. Gene adds, "There's a lot of information to share with the family and it is difficult trying to balance everyone's needs and wants, particularly given our difference of opinions."

Mr./Ms. Consuelo presents the initial background, describing the Davis family's "strong relationship with Midway's genetics clinical care providers." The genetic counselor emphatically states that 8-year-old Pamela is "a long-time patient of mine. Dr. Verde and I have known the family for years. And I believe Dr. Verde would agree with me that it is not necessary to give back all the results at this time."[36,52] Dr. Gene volleys back, "However, I am the pediatric geneticist at this medical center now and my recent fellowship has kept me abreast of the current consensus on returning results," to which Mr./Ms. Consuelo quickly interjects, "I'm not sure there is much consensus—and there continues to be mounting controversy." Looking at Dr. Nino, Dr. Gene declares, "We tried working this out, but we are at an impasse. I believe there is a medical necessity[35,51] to disclose the findings to family members. I have an obligation to help the adolescent."[207,248] Mr./Ms. Critnur quickly corrects the new attending: "An 8-year-old isn't an adolescent." Clarifying, Mr./Ms. Consuelo explains that Dr. Gene meant James, the 14-year-old sibling, then adds, "But the timing for the mom...," only to get interrupted before being able to provide details.

DR. GENE: We just received their results from next-gen sequencing and...
DR. NINO: [interrupts] Doesn't our medical center still consider NGS to be research?
DR. GENE: Well yes, but it's partly a clinical case.
DR. NINO: Sounds like research to me...on a clinical patient and the family. I would have thought this was for the IRB, and I know you tried to get them

involved, to little avail. I appreciate that you both requested this clinical ethics consultation.[15-17]

Attempting to get back to the specifics of this case, Mr./Ms. Consuelo explains that just before Dr. Verde went to Ivy U, a muscle biopsy was done on 8-year-old Pamela, along with some new targeted tests that revealed Sienna disease. Unfamiliar with this disorder, Dr. Rez requests more information. While Dr. Nino is in the midst of describing Sienna as a very rare neurological disorder with variable genotypic and phenotypic manifestations, including cardiac, muscle, and cognitive involvement, Dr. Gene interjects: "There is a very expensive weekly enzyme infusion that helps reduce some of the progression a bit, though not the neurological decline." Nodding in agreement with these facts, Mr./Ms. Consuelo is nevertheless anxious to return to the reason this ethics consult was called.

DR. GENE: The parents will be so relieved to know the 14-year-old doesn't have Sienna and isn't a carrier...But there are incidental findings...

MR./MS. CONSUELO: The results for this family are a mess...and the mom is pregnant...

DR. GENE: There's misattributed paternity...

MR./MS. CRITNUR: With our patient, the 8-year-old? Or the fetus?

MR./MS. CONSUELO: No, the sib...James.

DR. GENE: ...who, according to the next-gen sequencing, has mutations in the *VHL* gene. Von-Hippel-Lindau syndrome... [*looks at Dr. Rez*] autosomal dominant—not from the mom in this case—and characterized by multisystem tumors and cysts, including renal cell carcinoma—it was a surprise for us.[241]

MR./MS. CONSUELO: And surely will be for them.

After some discussion, Dr. Gene then raises another issue: "Isn't there a responsibility to locate and tell James's biological father that he might also have this disease?"—clearly an ethically complex question mired in controversy.[247] "Yes, and I'd also be concerned about rushing to tell a healthy kid about a condition like that when we don't have 100% certainty—especially when we have these additional psychosocial issues to contend with," adds Mr./Ms. Critnur. Dr. Rez further chimes in, "And maybe it would also matter if it was somatic or germline?"

Reframing the conversation to better understand what prompted this case referral, Dr. Nino asks about going back to the IRB for their advice, stressing, "I think it is important that we continue to evaluate the best processes for ethics reviews—especially when distinctions between research and clinical genomic medicine are graying."[21,106] "I did this morning," a frustrated Dr. Gene responds, and further reports what the IRB chair said: "Since the consent form states we don't disclose misattributed paternity *unless* there is a medical reason, it is up to my judgment—according to Dr. Cardy—to decide what findings raised by misattributed paternity I think are medically necessary to return."[73,249] Mr./Ms. Consuelo emphasizes, "Problem is that Dr. Gene really does not know this family... I do. And based on my years of experience, I have some concerns that this dad might leave the mom if he learns that James inherited Von-Hippel-Lindau syndrome—and *how*. I'm not sure she can deal with any more stress—it is hard enough to have a child with Sienna disease... and now another with Von Hippel."[221,236]

Dr. Gene stresses that Dr. Cardy recommended seeking the clinical ethics consult "since this has clinical implications for the family" and, glancing at Mr./Ms. Consuelo, adds, "We *really disagree* on how this should be handled and seek your guidance."[46] Mr./Ms. Consuelo concurs that they need the ethicists' help, "especially with the Mom being pregnant and now two kids who will need help with serious medical issues."[245] Reflecting a moment on the complexity facing these genetic professionals, Dr. Nino states, "While I think this *ought* to be the IRB's responsibility—to decide what to do with incidental findings before the protocol is approved—I'm glad you approached us to help sort this out."

DR. GENE: The IRB had us plan for many scenarios, even made us revise the consent form with checkboxes and lists... We just weren't anticipating all of these problems in one family, and certainly not in one of our patients.

MR./MS. CRITNUR: With these high tech tests there ought to be a much better plan devised by the med center or it's going to create a huge headache for us when the boundaries with research are blurred like this.

MR./MS. CONSUELO: I know what you mean, but we have a problem to solve. And if we don't decide, who will? This is about an 8-year-old girl under our care, and the family is our responsibility. I really don't think we should tell them about the 14-year-old boy's diagnosis until at least after the baby is born. I'm concerned that the stress will be too great for this mom if the dad can't handle it...

DR. GENE: That's where we disagree! It is my position that there is medical necessity, and therefore I think it's unethical to delay return of findings.

MR./MS. CRITNUR: I think because it's research, you can hold off telling the family about the paternity...

When the young Dr. Rez eagerly suggests, "Can always say it's a *de novo* mutation," Dr. Nino sternly replies, "So you're going to lie to the patient's family? I don't lie to my patients." Stumbling, Dr. Rez tries to recant: "I didn't mean *that*...what I meant was..." Dr. Gene interrupts to clarify for Dr. Rez, "The probability is overwhelming, about 80%, that VHL was inherited from

James's biological father. And Dad could be walking around without a clue that he might have an *early stage renal cancer*. At the very least, he'd have the possibility of being detected if he knew about his *VHL* mutation." Dr. Nino adds, "And Mom may well know who this guy is," while nodding in agreement with Dr. Gene's assessment of the situation.

DR. REZ: But if this research wasn't done, he wouldn't know anyway.
DR. GENE: But we know—even if he doesn't. I believe we have a moral obligation to tell them now.
MR./MS. CONSUELO: [*looking directly at Dr. Gene*] Please...at least wait a few months.

Feeling overwhelmed by the complexity of the implications the clinical ethics team is facing, Dr. Nino declares, "There has to be a *better way* to deal with all this." Trying to impress the team after the earlier gaffe, Dr. Rez shares: "I was recently reading the journal *Genomics and Society* where someone at Ivy U proposed a special oversight board for these kinds of problems that we may want to consider for our hospital." "Yes," Dr. Gene states, "I'm aware that some of my colleagues at larger research institutions are forming such boards or genomics advisory committees." Mr./Ms. Critnur quickly pushes the idea aside, noting, "They have the funds for that sort of stuff; we're already short on staff with no extra money," and urges the ethics team to "get back to this case." When Dr. Nino attempts to recap the scenario, Mr./Ms. Consuelo immediately interrupts to tell the ethicists, "There's more to the story that you all need to know." With a sigh, Mr./Ms. Critnur asks, "What could possibly be *next*?"

More conversation ensues as the saga of this case continues. Speaking rapidly, Mr./Ms. Consuelo reports that the Mom has had two miscarriages and is pregnant again through IVF: "She had universal carrier screening and prenatal testing and thought all was OK, but that was before Pamela was actually diagnosed with Sienna disease—but that wasn't included, so Dad wanted more testing."[99] Interrupting, Dr. Gene adds that Dad was "insisting '*everything like the U Washington test*'—referring to the study mapping the fetus's genetic code via a maternal blood sample and paternal saliva. I convinced him fetal whole-genome sequencing was *not* ready for prime time." Mr./Ms. Consuelo interrupts back, stressing that "Mom was ambivalent" about amnio given her history of miscarriages and IVF. "She really was not sure what she would do if Sienna disease showed up. Dad would have this child only if he knew everything was '*normal*.' Dad persisted, and after some time she contacted our fetal medicine doctor to do the procedure." When Mr./Ms. Critnur inquires, "How far along is she?" Mr./Ms. Consuelo reports "Eighteen weeks," adding that the OB downstairs just called to say that "results on the fetus are due back any day now." Several in the room cross their fingers and sigh.

MR./MS. CRITNUR: Look, the reality is that *if* their research sequencing were still in the pipeline waiting to be analyzed, or reanalyzed in a *CLIA* lab, we would not be having this conversation while the Mom was still pregnant.

MR./MS. CONSUELO: Right. Truth is, they weren't expecting to hear NGS results so soon anyway. Delaying for some months isn't going to matter and at least this extra time will let the family regroup after all they are going through.

DR. GENE: With that strategy, how are you going to feel if they don't return to clinic for awhile because they are too busy with a new baby, and then the teen isn't diagnosed with an early onset of an adrenal tumor that could have been treated...*if* we would have told them!!!

As the meeting concludes, Dr. Nino shares: "Let's hope that the fetal testing is negative for Sienna. We've never had a consult like this; there's a lot to take in." Speaking on behalf of his colleagues, the chair further explains that they will get back to the genetic team shortly—"We need time to reflect and confer with additional colleagues on our Clinical Ethics Committee"—and thanks them for coming.

Focus Question: What would you advise if you were on this clinical ethics committee?

SCENE IV: THE RETURN OF GENOMIC FINDINGS

Dr. Gene and Mr./Ms. Consuelo meet together with Monica and Donald Davis to discuss some results from the next-gen sequencing. Mr./Ms. Consuelo opens the conversation with, "So happy to have heard from Maternal-Fetal Medicine that the amnio results were negative for Sienna," consciously stopping short of finishing the sentence.

MOM: You can imagine how worried we were until they called to tell us that the baby is OK.

DAD: Boy, are we relieved! *Perfectly healthy*, like James.

DR. GENE: Glad you both could make it today. There are some aspects about the study that we'd like to talk to you folks about. The way we typically do this is by first speaking to the parents individually.

MOM: Please tell me you're not going to inform us that James is going to have Sienna too?

MR./MS. CONSUELO: That I will immediately say is not a problem...at least to the best of my knowledge, given our *current understanding* of genomics.

After Dad goes to grab a quick cup of coffee, his wife stays, and Mr./Ms. Consuelo explains to Ms. Davis, "Some information came back that we felt we needed to share with you." Taking over, Dr. Gene stumbles to say, "There seems to be some...confusion...or misunderstanding...about biological relationships in your family."

When Mom reminds them that her father was adopted, Dr. Gene tries to explain: "What I'm thinking about at the moment is your children's father." Clearly confused, Mom responds, "Donald? No, he's not adopted." Mr./Ms. Consuelo offers further clarification: "Findings from the test indicate that your husband is not the father of both children...only Pamela. He is not James's biological father." Stunned, Mom pleads, "Please believe me, I wasn't lying," and describes having a big argument a few days before the wedding and, thinking it was over, spending "just one time" with an old boyfriend. Mom further explains that since she and Donald made up the next day and got married as planned, "I assumed I got pregnant on the honeymoon. I thought James was Donald's all this time." In a nonjudgmental tone, Mr./Ms. Consuelo expresses with empathy, "We understand." Mom panics, then declares, "You can't tell Donald...he'll never understand!"

Feeling the need to push forward, Dr. Gene reports, "There is more we need to discuss related to this...We discovered through the sequencing that James has Von Hippel-Lindau syndrome—it's also called VHL—which is serious." Mom cuts in, "*Von Who* disease?" and Mr./Ms. Consuelo explains, "Von Hippel-Lindau is a genetic disorder that requires careful monitoring—like MRIs—because it can cause someone to have a higher risk of developing tumors and cysts in various parts of the body. Even though many growths may be benign, it is possible that some might need surgical intervention" and offers to provide more detail afterward when she is together with her husband.

MOM: Oh my god... This was my *healthy* child.

DR. GENE: The good thing is that we now know what to keep our eyes open for. We can aggressively go after any lesions. It is almost certainly auto-somal dominant—inherited from one biological parent. And you do not carry that mutation.

MOM: So does that mean James got it from my old boyfriend? You can't tell Donald about this. What if he gets angry at me... and leaves me?

DR. GENE: I feel obliged to tell your son about the VHL gene mutation to protect him from many potential health problems. We can try to figure out a way that does not reveal to your son or husband that James's biological father is not your husband Donald.

MOM: [*without hesitation*] You can't tell them anything—they'll know he's not the real father!

DR. GENE: I cannot ethically hide the information about this disease from your son—James assented to the research protocol.[88]

Recalling the informed consent document, Mom realizes: "Wait, didn't we check off that we didn't want to know *carrier stuff*?" When Mr./Ms. Consuelo tries to clarify, "We are not referring to carrier status," Mom begins to cry and begs, "I need time to let this all sink in. Please let me deal with this my way... and after the baby is born. I can't risk a miscarriage—this may be my only child to survive." As Mr./Ms. Consuelo begins to express in a comforting voice, "I know how much you have been through," Dr. Gene declares, "We *all* understand how upsetting this is—however, I am *obligated* to tell. James must know about the presence of the disease-causing mutation so that MRIs and other evaluations can be initiated." Ms. Davis sobs and tries to catch her breath.

Further clarifying the reality of the situation, Mr./Ms. Consuelo tells Mom, "*Even if* we will tell just James the diagnosis, it would be very difficult to hide from Mr. Davis the kinds of procedures needed to treat James." While expressing understanding of this dilemma, Mom still pleads, "Please promise me you won't tell Donald, or anyone else, that Donald is not James's real dad." Addressing that plea, Dr. Gene states in no uncertain terms, "I also feel strongly that it is immoral not to tell the biological father that he carries the disease-causing mutation, in case he is asymptomatic or on a diagnostic odyssey."

Trying to convince the geneticist that this particular case compels some modification to such a position, Mom points out, "But he has no idea he's the father!" and asks for the geneticist's help, declaring, "You must find a way that no one ever knows Donald is not James's real dad." Rather than taking on that responsibility, Dr. Gene states, "I will leave it up to you to contact James's biological father, but I felt I was ethically obligated to inform you about this, as it could have important medical implications for him." Appreciating the emotional and practical implications facing Mom, Mr./Ms. Consuelo expresses, "I'm sorry; I know you don't need more on your plate right now. I can explain more about the specialists who can help monitor and treat various conditions associated with VHL syndrome at the earliest stages for James."

When Mom and Mr./Ms. Consuelo leave the room to discuss, Dad enters, blurting out, "I'm so relieved that James and the baby are fine and don't have Sienna!" As Dr. Gene awkwardly attempts to disclose other news, "something...about you," Dad unexpectedly responds with, "I know I'm overly pushy at times. Just trying to come up with every possible way to fight Sienna. Sorry if you find me annoying for calling your office so much." Surprised at the remark coming at this point in time, Dr. Gene exclaims, "Oh no, I don't mean *that!*"

DR. GENE: It is about your sequencing. You checked off on your consent form that you wanted us to share with you everything on the list...and...we found variants that have been associated with increased risk of developing adult-onset autosomal dominant leukodystrophy.

DAD: I have *leukemia*?

DR. GENE: No—*leukodystrophy* is a *neurological* condition, and this type is often confused with *multiple sclerosis*. But please understand we are *not* saying you definitely have the disease...only that the sequencing showed some *markers* that are *linked* to the *possibility*...a somewhat greater *risk*...of developing the condition.

DAD: [*after taking a deep breath, he quickly responds*] You need to tell me what to do about this. I want the *best* neurologist...but you can't tell my wife, I don't want to burden her with one more thing...Oh the baby...we need to test the baby for this!...What test can we do next?...*What's Next?!*

Focus Question: How does context matter in considering whether, what, to whom, when, and how to disclose genomic findings?

ADDITIONAL QUESTIONS

1. Does the Sienna protocol pose issues beyond our usual concern for the kind of pressure a parent may put on healthy kids to participate for the sake of their *affected* sibs? If so, is that truly assent?
2. Who has the obligation to think about the potential benefits and risks for these *unaffected* siblings?
3. Do you believe the return of genomic information is dependent on whether it was generated in the research or clinical context?

4. If experts can't seem to agree on what is clinically actionable or relevant, should genomic findings be returned?

5. What is your opinion on whether to return genomic findings that are not clinically actionable or relevant to parents for reproductive decision making?

6. How would you proceed if not all members of the family agree with a clinical researcher's decision to return clinically actionable or relevant genomic information?

7. What if there is little concordance about what should be returned among site co-investigators across the multiple institutions?

8. What would you include in a misattributed paternity policy, and how would you best describe it in the consent form? How might context matter, if at all, regarding disclosure of this misattributed paternity or consanguinity?

9. Should we leave it up to the parents to tell their kids genomic findings when they turn 18, or is the research team supposed to locate and recontact the kids? If the latter, is this sustainable?

10. Is the genomic technology today accurate enough for us to tell a young adult, years later, what they do and don't have?

11. Do we have to rerun tests with the latest genomic technology based on our new knowledge at the time a pediatric patient-participant reaches age of majority? What if you then discover primary or secondary findings that demand follow-up and the young adult has no health insurance?

12. What policy should be in place for retaining DNA material to be stored indefinitely for research? How might that policy differ if the material was initially attained in a clinical context?

13. Is it a reasonable expectation that next-gen sequencing will provide a genomic explanation? And, if so, is there an expectation for an effective medical intervention?

14. How might you design an informed consent process that clarifies reasonable expectations for current genomic technologies?

15. How should our assumptions about genomic literacy be considered when designing the informed consent process and disclosure of findings?

16. When an established clinical patient and family participate in research, does their clinician-researcher have an ancillary obligation to continue to offer emerging genomic technologies? Are these obligations time-dependent, including when a woman is 18 weeks pregnant?

17. Is there a responsibility to tell James's biological father that he might have VHL disease? If so, would multiple psychosocial issues in a family alter your position?

18. In recognition of the real-life complexities of genomic technologies, how might we better anticipate the technical, ethical, psychological, and legal challenges from the outset?

PART THREE

Narrative Genomics on Stage

DNA, Society, and Theatre

CHAPTER 6

Dramatizing the Past, Present, & Future

Theatrical Narratives from Genetics to Genomics

Excerpts from existing theatrical dialogue may also be used to analytically explore ethical and social issues raised by the evolution from genetics to genomics.[i,4] The essence of genetic inheritance and its imagery in theatre have influenced society for many generations. As more than two decades have passed since setting forth to decipher the human genome, we are at an opportune time for reflection—to better understand how we imagine the implications of mapping and manipulating our genomic fate.[1,15-17] Ethical complexities concerning the potentiality to identify and control distinct facets of our humanness through genomic information challenge both professionals and the public, with frequent confusion and misinterpretation of the scientific reality coloring the imagination.

Placed in historical context,[2,3] theatrical narratives[7,10] provide a framework to reflect upon how the implications of emerging genetic technologies evolve over time and how attempts to control fate through genomic science have influenced—and been influenced by—personal and professional relationships. The drama of these human interactions is powerful and has the potential to generate fear, create hope, transform identity, and inspire empathy. These dramatic narratives are a vivid source to observe the complex implications of translating genomic research into clinical practice through the lens of other individuals.

Historically, themes of heritability have attained a place in our imagination that have effectively portrayed in popular culture and theatre.[5] As expressions of social and cultural concerns, plays manipulate the way issues are perceived through characters that evoke sympathy, disdain, or confusion. Dramatic dialogue mirrors the complexity of self-introspection, public opinion, and social policy. Recurrent ethical and societal themes of hereditability are consistently explored by playwrights acting as social commentators—initiating, reflecting, affirming, shaping, and questioning the public perception of genetics and genomics.[11]

By situating theatrical narratives within the evolution of genomic history, we illuminate varying perspectives and reactions—the drama of DNA.

The consistent overtone of concerns expressed decades ago parallel many of today's issues—such as society's search for explanations regarding the nature-nurture dichotomy and the implications of creating "better" living organisms, be they pea plants, livestock, or humans. Such images bring to life the tension and depth of emotions depicted in a broad spectrum of genetic and genomic plays encompassing numerous medical subspecialties, including psychiatry, assisted reproduction, oncology, neuroscience, and regenerative medicine. They also reflect the role that bioethical foundations can play to mediate these tensions in society.

The sensory and visceral impact of experiencing dramatic narrative is powerful, and it is our premise that a longitudinal glimpse into the theatrical arts offers a rich, underutilized vehicle for exploring genomic-related themes. As early as ancient Greek times, theatre provided a stage to promote and engage public discourse on significant societal issues.[5] Plays often highlighted complex relationships, attitudes, and perceived tensions created by attempts to modify hereditability and trump destiny in the nature-nurture dichotomy, and have persisted at least since *Oedipus* and *Electra*.

As the scientific landscape shifts at an ever-increasing pace, it becomes even more essential to search for creative approaches, such as narrative genomics, to better appreciate the issues and to place them in historical and societal context.[ii] With these goals in mind, this chapter explores the evolution of ethical and social issues raised by attempts to understand and manipulate fate by advances in genomic science. Excerpts from a selection of plays are integrated and analyzed chronologically to reflect the context of the era, beginning with the mid-twentieth century, as Rosalind Franklin, James Watson, and Francis Crick were deciphering the mystery of DNA's double helix, as portrayed in *Photograph 51*.[251] This discovery would inspire the genomics revolution and, in turn, playwrights dramatizing the promises and perils of this powerful information, as explored in *Who's Afraid of Virginia Woolf?*,[252] that foreshadows imagining our future with DNA technology and the development of the field of bioethics.

From "chromo*zones*" to codes to clones, through mapping the human genome, theatrical narratives—*The Twilight of the Golds*,[253] *An Experiment with an Air Pump*,[254] *The Sequence*,[255] *Immaculate Misconception*,[256] and *A Number*[257]— bring to life the debate over the use and potential misuse of genetic technology and genomic information. Since the completion of the mapping of the human genome in 2003, contemporary theatre has produced a number of plays, such as *Relativity*,[258] *Lucy*,[259] *Distracted*,[260] *The Good Egg*,[261] and *The Other Place*,[262] illuminating how the genomic revolution may be expanding our understanding of genomic influences on ancestry, on neurological and other disorders, and on the use of reproductive technologies. Even though the power of technology continues to increase dramatically, raising more ethical and societal challenges, the urge to find genetic explanations and medical interventions remains relatively constant and will likely continue to provide dramatic narratives throughout time.

SECTION I: THE THEATRICAL DOUBLE HELIX AND "CHROMOZONES"

The rediscovery in 1900 of Gregor Mendel's seminal work using pea plants to demonstrate inheritance theory led to new research that favored biological inheritance.[263] This growing fascination with hereditability and our potential to intervene to affect future generations has been seized upon by playwrights and has mesmerized audiences.[264] By World War II, the repudiation of eugenics as "pseudoscience" had solidified in the United States, and by the late 1940s, Rosalind Franklin was painstakingly creating the images that would later contribute to the discovery of the double helix, with the Nobel prize awarded after her death to Watson and Crick[265]—so well illuminated in Anna Ziegler's play, *Photograph 51*.[251]

As Franklin reflects, gazing at her early crystallographic visions in her lab: "You know, I think one sees something new each time one looks at truly beautiful things.... But they need to be so much clearer...if we're ever to find the structure.... It's going to get to the heart of everything," Watson is in his lab pondering: "It makes me think—more than ever—that the gene's the thing. I mean, we have to get to the bottom of it—discover how it replicates itself. And so we need its structure.... It's just incredibly exciting.... To be born at the right time. There's an element of fate to it, don't you think? And I don't believe in fate." In a twist of fate, just as the image became clearer to her—"It's a perfect X. It's a helix"—Rosalind runs out of time, both because of her perfectionism and her premature death from ovarian cancer.

The discovery of the double helix in 1953 gave rise to a new scientific framework, creating excitement for genetics and its implications for the future. The "new genetics" field emerged and was followed by prenatal genetic testing, assisted reproduction technologies, and experimentation with gene therapy. And with the promise of new genetic discoveries and technologies came growing concerns about the potential perils for our future.[266]

Although Edward Albee's *Who's Afraid of Virginia Woolf?*[252] is not well known for dramatizing genetic themes, but rather dysfunctional relationships, this 1962 play in fact directly addresses society's concerns about the threat of genetic manipulation and fears of determining the fate of future generations with this new technology, particularly when the field is poorly understood. Set on a college campus, George, the senior history professor, verbally attacks Nick, the young science professor: "You're the one! You're the one's going to make all that trouble...making everyone the same, rearranging the chromozones [*sic*], or whatever that is. Isn't that right?" When Nick corrects him, "Not exactly: chromo*somes*," George fires back, "I'm very mistrustful. Do you believe...that people learn nothing from history?," then adds, "I read somewhere that science fiction is really not fiction at all...that you people are rearranging my genes, so that everyone will be like everyone else. Now, I won't have that!"[252]

Albee dramatizes the disharmony of their disciplines and generations—the historian who reflects on the past as prologue and the biologist who creates and manipulates the future—similar to tensions explored during the same time by C. P. Snow's *The Two Cultures and the Scientific Revolution*.[267] The dichotomy of their professional world views shapes their presumptions about the benefits and risks of applying genetic technology. This inherent tension is frequently witnessed in plays and, in this context, dramatizes potential ethical and societal ramifications of genetic manipulation.

MARTHA (*to Nick*): Georgie-boy here says you're terrifying. Why are you terrifying?

HONEY: It's because of your chromosomes, dear.

MARTHA (*to Nick*): What's all this about chromosomes?

GEORGE: It's very simple, Martha, this young man is working on a system whereby chromosomes can be altered...the genetic makeup of a sperm cell changed, reordered...to order, actually...for hair and eye color, stature, potency...I imagine...hairiness, features, health...and mind. Most important...Mind. All imbalances will be corrected, sifted out...propensity for various diseases will be gone, longevity assured. We will have a race of men...test-tube bred...incubator-born...will tend to look like this young man here.

Albee's narratives bring to life many of the ethical and societal concerns we still face today: the continuum of perspectives on whether and how to modulate the "scientific imperative"; the extent to which scientific innovations will alter relationships; the impact of genetic manipulation on our individual, familial, and cultural identities; and the presumptions we share about the power of emerging technologies and the information generated to decide our future.

This value-laden struggle to modify traits of inheritance and to alter nature in future generations continues as a theme. Over the next 30 years, genetic counseling, newborn screening, and prenatal testing become integrated into practice and generate enthusiasm for better understanding the promise of genetic and genomic science. In response to these, and other medical technologies, the interdisciplinary field of bioethics emerged to examine the complex moral dilemmas raised.

By 1990, the Human Genome Project (HGP) was established with the primary goal of mapping the human genome to generate new information that has the potential to positively contribute to human health.[268] In response to the major societal challenges posed by the HGP, an unprecedented amount of funding was allocated toward research on its ethical, legal, and social implications (ELSI). How do we balance moving the promises of science forward while also being mindful of the perils we have encountered in the past? Notably, contemporary ELSI issues echo debates of an earlier time as society continues to search for biological explanations and solutions. In fact, as technology advances, challenges continue to emerge, including social perceptions of *normalcy* and the potential for discrimination on the basis of race, disability, sexuality, class, and gender.[269]

Although the HGP has provided remarkable technological advances that have put quite a distance between genetics and its maligned predecessor *eugenics*,[270] it continues to raise complex ethical issues ripe for dramatization in theatre. Plays address our hopes for a world free of disease, as well as our fears for life devoid of human individuality.[270] Theatrical dialogue brings to life many questions: What exactly could be inherited? What is determined by the environment? What does it mean to try to change our destiny? What influence might the disclosure of genetic-genomic information have on increasing the risk of discrimination and stigmatization?

Jonathan Tolins' 1992 play *The Twilight of the Golds* introduces characters that raise many questions about who, if anyone, should, or can, determine the fate of future generations through the use of emerging prenatal genetic technology.[253] Tensions rise when Suzanne and her geneticist husband Rob learn she is pregnant, and fear their child will be homosexual like her brother David. They then decide to use (fictionalized) technology to test the fetus for the "gay gene" to see if it was inherited. After learning that the test is positive, Suzanne shares her hopes and disappointments: "This baby was going to change our lives and make everything better. Not that things are bad.... Now the whole thing is tainted. I wish we didn't know, but we do. And it's a problem."

Such applications of genetic-genomic screening or diagnostic testing raise a familiar question as to what limits, if any, should be placed, and in what context, on technologies used to preselect some lives over others? David viscerally reacts to his sister Suzanne's decision to seek prenatal genetic testing: "What if you found out the kid was going to be ugly, or smell bad, or have an annoying laugh, or need really thick glasses?" David continues, "But where do we stop?... So now we have this technology, what are we going to do with it?"

Juxtaposed with David's position is the drive to utilize new scientific tools, as dramatized by his geneticist brother-in-law Rob:

> The power of the creator.... [M]y road to a career in genetic research was paved with Legos. I always had a fascination with components; how things are put together, how to take them apart, how to change them...I sit there in the lab...and I think, why not with people? There's obviously a lot...that needs to be corrected. Or can at least be improved. Just look at the amount of suffering, inward and outward, all around us. Let's use every weapon we have to combat it. Is that such a horrible thing to think?

This moral dilemma is also at the heart of struggles faced by all the characters in *An Experiment with an Air Pump*,[254] Shelagh Stephenson's 1999 play. Ellen, a geneticist, declares that she is having an "ethical crisis" deciding whether to work with her colleague Kate, a cutting-edge fetal researcher. Reminiscent of *Who's Afraid of Virginia Woolf?*, Ellen's husband Tom, a history professor, expresses unease with the implications of this genomic technology, as does Phil, her real estate agent. Kate wants Phil to consider: "If, very very early in your wife's pregnancy, you were able to discover in your child the gene for say, Alzheimer's disease, or asthma, or maybe something more alarming like schizophrenia, would you be grateful for that information?"

A discussion ensues and when Phil raises a critical question, "What's the point of any of it?," Kate quickly responds, "Well, you might want to terminate the pregnancy, for example." Sarcastically, Phil volleys back, "What, because the kid might get asthma?" Kate continues to explain her rationale: "Well, not for something like that, obviously. But eventually we'll be able to apply gene therapy in the womb. We'll be able to eradicate all sorts of things. Schizophrenia, manic-depression—." With caring emotion in his voice, Phil relays his experience, "My uncle Stan was manic-depressive and he was magic. He built us a tree house covered in shells and bits of coloured glass. He used to play the Northumbrian pipes."

Ellen enthusiastically adds, "We're mapping the human gene system at the moment. There's something called the Human Genome Project. Have you heard of it?" "You what?" Phil questions. Kate explains, "It's like a new map of humanity, every element described and understood. It's breathtaking." Kate then describes with utmost enthusiasm that this technology will not only enable scientists "to pinpoint genes" for cancer and other disorders, "but what it really means is we'll understand the shape and complexity of a human being, we'll be able to say this is a man, this is exactly who he is, this is his potential, these are his possible limitations. And manic-depression is genetic. We'll pin it down soon." Unimpressed, Phil wants to know, "And then what? No more Uncle Stans."

The social implications—including the stigmatization that surrounds[30] psychiatric, neurological, and behavioral conditions—become heightened in the context of genomic information.[167,177,183] Phil later points out, "[I]f they can map your genes before you're born, they'll soon be wanting a little plastic card with your DNA details on. And if it says anything dodgy, it'll be like you're credit blacked. And then imagine this, people'll say I can't have this kid because it'll never get a mortgage."

Afterward, Tom accuses Kate of failing to "respect ambiguities." He continues: "You bandy these words about, like manic-depression and schizophrenia, and you don't even know what they mean. Schizophrenia is just a label, it's not a finite quantifiable thing,"[180] adding, "James Joyce probably had a schizophrenia gene, his daughter certainly did. It's a continuum, at one end you get poetry and at the other confusion, you can't just swat it like a fly." In fact, there is no one gene for a complex disorder. And if there were a biological explanation, the psychosocial implications will likely be context-specific, particularly with respect to stigma and identity issues.

Paul Mullin's play *The Sequence*[255] further illuminates issues that may ensue with genomic discovery in the context of the frenetic race between Francis Collins and Craig Venter to be the first to decipher the human genome. In a fictionalized interview, Kellie, a young journalist, captures Collins' strong drive and motivation as he explains: "Because a complete sequence compared to what we have now is like the difference between a high-def satellite image and one of those medieval maps that trails off at the edges with 'Here be monsters.' The better the map, the better we can cure diseases. That's the rational grown-up answer. The other answer is: because it's there...just sitting there waiting to be known." As Kellie ponders the similarity between their two fields, "I mean, what are we after? Truth, right? And why? Well, sometimes because the truth is useful but sometimes just because it's the truth and it's good to know, right?," Collins reflects: "Well, yes, from the scientific perspective—." Kellie offers her perspective: "So we're truth hunters, and how do we do that? Well, we have some golden rules. Objectivity is key, no?"

In reality, the application of knowledge is never that simple in the context of genomics, as Collins points out in the fictional play:

> [W]henever I or colleagues of mine get a little too self-congratulatory about the benefits of genetics, I think of Woody Guthrie....See Woody had Huntington's disease. One of those few diseases that genetics can predict with absolute certainty....Genetic pathology is rarely clear-cut, but when it is, it can be merciless. And it leaves us with a kind of brutal question: once you begin to know a little bit what God knows, do you act on that limited knowledge? Do you abort Woody Guthrie?

Much later in the ficticious interview, Kellie asks Collins to reflect on "What's next?" after the mapping of the human genome is complete. "I've been turning a lot of my attention to the ethical questions," Collins replies,[15-17,26,28] and further clarifies his thoughts: "The sort of scenarios people are most worried about, like designer babies, clones, etc. aren't really very realistic at the moment. The pressing issue right is genetic discrimination." Collins then posits, "If I were to have a genetic test, would that information be used to take away my health insurance or my job? What do you do when you know things that only God knew before?" This fundamental question is, for many, at the heart of the debate surrounding the implications of emerging genomic technologies.[196,269]

Carl Djerassi's 2000 play *Immaculate Misconception*[256] imagines the tangled web of intracytoplasmic sperm injection (ICSI)[256] to bring forth life through modern medical innovations. Its creator Melanie Laidlaw and her collaborator Felix Frankenthaler consider the many ways in which new applications of this technology will be utilized, raising complex ethical challenges for our society over generations. Melanie shares her excitement: "A few more months and I'm ready to try fertilizing a human egg by *direct* injection with a *single* sperm!" She proudly states that thanks to her ICSI innovation: "[W]omen could draw on a bank account of their frozen *young* eggs and have a much better chance of having a *normal* pregnancy later on in life. I'm not talking about *surrogate* eggs." Melanie continues her explanation with enthusiasm:

> Each embryo will be screened genetically *before* the best one is transferred back into the woman's uterus. All we'll be doing is improving the odds over Nature's roll of the dice. Before you know it the 21st century will be called "The Century of Art."...The science of...A ...R...T: assisted reproductive technologies. Young men and women will open reproductive bank accounts full of frozen sperm and eggs. And when they want a baby, they'll go to the bank to check out what they need.

In recognition of the scope of Melanie's innovation, Felix responds, "The Laidlaw Brave New World." Their dialogue stimulates us to question and consider whether this is an ethical practice that we want to promote or regulate.[271] What implications will these new applications have for future generations and our conceptions of *normal* reproduction?

The mammalian cloning of Dolly the sheep, born February 1997,[271] is another example of how genetic reproductive technology can push both the scientific and ethical envelope even further, capturing our public imagination.[271] Reaching beyond Melanie's "Brave New World," Caryl Churchill's 2002 play *A Number*,[257] introduces futuristic characters—the original son of Salter, Bernard 1 (B1), and his many clones, including Bernard 2 (B2)—who explore their origins, their identities, and their destinies. Salter inquires if his sons want to know "how far has this thing gone, how many of these things are there?," to which B2 viscerally reacts, "[Y]ou called them things. I think we'll find they're people"; then Salter adds, "copies of you which some mad scientist...."

A Number vividly provides perspective on what it really means to be a unique human being beyond our genetic blueprint.[257] When B2 queries, "[I]f you're not my father that's fine. If you couldn't have children or my mother, and you did in vitro...," Salter confirms, "I am your father, it was by an artificial [sic] the forefront of science but I am genetically" related to all the Bernards. Later on Salter acknowledges to B1:

> Nobody regrets more than me the completely unforeseen unforeseeable which isn't my fault and does make it more upsetting but what I did...also it's a tribute, I could have had a different one, a new child altogether...but I wanted you again because I thought you were the best.

But as B1 reminds us, "It wasn't me again," even with "the same raw materials," and so the father justifies his actions "because they were perfect." Although A Number is purely fictional, the play brings to life the ethical challenges at stake with technologies that may enable cloning humans—an idea that society has been unwilling to accept.[257]

SECTION III: THE GENOMIC CRYSTAL BALL IN THE POST-MAPPING DECADE

By 2003, the mapping of the human genome was complete and the scientific community was excited to create the technology that has the power to identify and modify our fate, or at least generate the information in an attempt to understand it.[272] A few years later, Cassandra Medley's *Relativity*[258] explored how genomic information can impact impressions of ancestry as well as be manipulated to advance both scientific and political agendas.[258] In this 2006 play, Claire, an African-American psychotherapist and educator, and her colleague-boyfriend, Malik, a sociologist, promote the theory that "people of color, or 'melanated people', possess greater quantities of life-enhancing properties of Melanin" to explain why they "excel athletically, culturally, intellectually, and spiritually." Rejecting this theory, Claire's daughter, Kalima, a Harvard graduate with a PhD in molecular genetics, is more interested in exploring new and exciting genetic technologies.

Presumptions about the power of science and technological innovations to inform and control destiny are influenced by the experiences of different generations with different perspectives. Claire shares her point of view:

> This new technology is potentially a breakthrough for all humanity...but just where will this bold new technology take us? Replicating organs...replicating people....If we do not stay on top of this new cloning technology, our bloodlines will continue to diminish, while the non-melanated will have found a way to preserve theirs.

As Malik reminds Kalima, "Your mom critiques the racist and ethical implications of this new cloning technology....And you'll challenge these latest DNA findings." In turn, Kalima defends her position: "[W]hat am I to challenge, exactly? The human genome is the human genome....Their claim that race has no biological basis in fact. Is so—confirmed." She adds, "[H]ow do 'we' deal with the facts that...the genomic sequencing proves that there's more variation *within* groups, than between the groups we perceive to be different....The sequencing shows humans are all ninety-nine-point-nine percent genetically identical." To which Malik volleys back, "Right. And the same so-called 'data' also 'proves' that humans share ninety-eight percent of their genes with the chimpanzee....Seems like that 'two percent' difference makes *all* the 'difference.'" In fact, as the HGP evolved, so too did the scholarship on race and ethnicity in the context of genomic research—which continues to date.[258]

Over the last decade, particularly in the context of the genomics revolution, expectations have increased to better understand the causes of disease and disorders, as well as the promise of innovative treatments. *Lucy*,[259] the 2009 play by Damien Atkins, examines the frustrations of Vivian, an anthropologist, as she strives to discover the origins of her daughter Lucy's "autistic" behavior telling Morris, Lucy's therapist: "I've been looking at autism triggers...there's a lot of conflicting information." When Morris notes that "it's an evolving study," Vivian adds: "But most scientists agree that there has to be a genetic *component*. They've been able to isolate a couple of potential autism genes...."[73] Morris adds, "But there may be as many as a *hundred* involved, we don't know...there are lots of people trying to figure out where it came from. I'm just trying to figure out how to fix it now that it's here."[164,167-169,171,177,179,180]

The back-and-forth dialogue between Vivian and Morris illustrates the continuing controversy over how to treat a complex disorder when we do not fully understand the interactions between genetic and environmental factors.[259] Moreover, even if we had a clear sense of the scientific basis for the cause of autism spectrum disorder (ASD), challenges would remain, particularly given the variability of expression and permutations in functioning.[259]

Typical of how parents feel with this level of uncertainty, Vivian is puzzled: "You want to fix it, but you don't even know *what it is* yet." When Morris responds defensively: "That's not true, it's just, it's *complicated*.... [T]here are a lot of theories out there and not enough proof," Vivian reacts: "*I'm* confused— you keep telling me that you know what you're doing...that you're on the *cutting edge*...why don't tell me something you *do* know!" Morris later tries to explain further:

> Vivian, look. Lots of people may be carrying the genes that are responsible for autism. It's not your fault. *Many things* have to go wrong to make a person autistic. Even if Lucy was born with the autism gene, or the right combination of autistic genes, even if turned out that she *did* have a, a genetic predisposition, it would have to have been activated or exacerbated by *several* environmental factors, in co-operation, and there was no way you could have stopped that from happening.

Although the scientific landscape changes over time, we are still faced with the reality that there are significant limits to our knowledge.[273] Contentious debate continues on how to categorize the wide spectrum of behavioral and neurological manifestations that have societal and financial implications for medical and education benefits[273] while trying to minimize stigmatizing labels.[273] Theatre vividly captures the dramatic implications of familial struggles as they search for causal explanations and effective treatments[273] to change the fate of individuals with neurodevelopmental and neuropsychiatric disorders.

Our struggle to understand the role of genetics and the nature-nurture dichotomy is also explored in Lisa Loomer's 2009 play *Distracted*.[260] Mama, the main character, questions how heredity and environment factor into determining personality by exploring her son's diagnosis of attention deficit hyperactivity disorder (ADHD/ADD). Mama and Dad blame each other for the genetic roots of the boy's actions at home and at school, as well as their parenting behaviors, placing a further strain on their relationship. Mama yells, "YOU HAVE ADD!...[W]hich is HEREDITARY!...Which is why our son has it!" Dad counters, "Let's talk about ADD. Let's talk about your mother! Can a person get a word in edgewise with that woman? Does she ever finish a thought?" In addition to trying to sort out the cause of their son's behavior, they debate whether he actually needs the treatment alternatives[260] or whether the diagnosis is based on society's need to narrowly define what is considered *normal* and its tendency to label difference as dysfunction.

Through a series of dialogues with each other, and with a revolving door of doctors, they discover the risks and limitations of current approaches for explaining and controlling this disorder—just like autism spectrum disorder in *Lucy*.[259] When Mama goes to Dr. Waller looking for answers, this neuropsychologist opines: "Studies indicate the best course of treatment is a combination of behavior modification and medication." Mama then consults with Dr. Zavala and is glad when this child psychologist confirms, "I think you're right to try everything else first, every conceivable good option." Mama asks, "[L]ike neurofeedback? Orthomolecular therapy? Herbs?...Would Ritalin...get him out of his pajamas?" She continues, "But if it's a real disease—like diabetes—then shouldn't one thing work. Like insulin." This dialogue captures the frustrating reality that there is no simple, one-size-fits-all solution, given the wide variability of etiology with many neuropsychiatric disorders. And so the parents keep searching for a better understanding. They next reach out to another psychiatrist, Dr. Jinks, who explains, "The brain is highly complex....ADD is a neurological condition...a *hereditary* condition."

This quest for genetic explanations and *normalcy* continues to raise complex questions for our society. What role will genetic technology play in shaping and defining our identity, as well as our family relationships? What role will epigenetics have on reframing the nature-nurture dichotomy? What will genetic and environmental information mean for the future? What new promises will genomics bring, and what are the potential perils?

The motivation to use medical innovations to control the fate of future generations has been accelerated by the promise of emerging reproductive, genetic, and genomic technologies.[261] Dorothy Fortenberry's *The Good Egg*[261] examines the complex ethical issues raised by using fictionalized prenatal genetic diagnosis for bipolar disorder, with the goal of preventing heritable transmission of this condition to future generations.[261] The tension set up in this 2010 play revolves around Meg, who wants to become pregnant through assisted reproductive technology, and her brother Matt, who is diagnosed with bipolar disorder, just like their dad who committed suicide.

Distressed upon learning that his sister is considering preimplantation testing, Matt inquires, "What's the risk of you passing it on? Statistically." Catching her breath for a moment, Meg explains, "About fifteen percent, given you. And

Dad." Soon after, Matt declares, "So one of your seven embryos has it." Trying to clarify the uncertainty of the actual risk factor, Meg states, "Statistically, one of the seven embryos is likely to have it. Maybe more. Maybe none. No way to know for sure." After her brother is quick to point out, "Without the testing," Meg nods in agreement, succinctly responding, "Exactly." When Meg tries to justify: "[I]t's done all the time...to make sure the baby's healthy and *normal* and—," Matt quickly interrupts, "Not bipolar." He further adds: "You said they were checking for diseases." Meg confirms, "For Huntington's and Parkinson's and Alzheimer's and MS and—." "Me?" Matt shouts. Meg goes on to explain: "It's a new test. They just located the genes recently, and—." Interrupting again, Matt declares, "You're taking advantage of the technology. Like 'New! Improved! Now with no bipolar!'" Trying to calm Matt down, Meg lets him know: "It is a totally routine, common thing to do, just to be on the safe side."

The dialogue highlights how advances in assisted reproductive technology generate new opportunities for Meg to be able to use innovative genetic tests prior to implantation[261] to select what type of child she would be willing to parent, reminiscent of *Immaculate Misconception*.[261] The dynamic between the utilization of these cutting-edge technologies and the value-laden choices created by these innovations raises complex ethical dilemmas for individuals, families, and society that center on the fundamental question of whether there should be limits on how these genomic technologies are used to change the fate of others.[261]

Wanting his sister to reconsider her pursuit of preimplantation genetic diagnostic testing, Matt tries to make Meg feel guilty: "Mom would never have." Meg snaps back, "You don't know what Mom would have said about it, they hadn't even invented genetic testing." Matt is unrelenting: "Mom just had a kid like normal people have kids," and Meg reminds him, "We don't live in that world anymore." In emotional turmoil, Matt declares, "You are genetically editing me from the code of who we are. You're eliminating me and you're eliminating Dad." As the play concludes, Meg reflects, "I thought about it, calling up to cancel...but I couldn't do it. I couldn't handle the thought, the guilt of saying to a child 'I could have prevented your feeling this way, but I chose not to.'" This technological imperative of "reproductive accountability"[261] and Meg's personal experiences are just too powerful for her to resist.

Because values among individuals are so diverse and fluid, the powerful role of relationships within a family varies across a continuum from gently guiding, to denouncing a woman's choice, to the threat of severing all ties, as we witnessed in *Twilight of the Golds*.[253] Different judgments about "what is *normal*" are shaped by our experiences and cultural expectations, which directly impact how we frame our identities and those of others within the context of families and society—a message that has evolved from the disabilities community.[274] In turn, these perceptions color our presumptions about the power of science and technology to control destiny. Despite Matt's strong feelings, Meg is adamant in her belief that the use of innovative technologies will provide the path to a better place.

As we have witnessed in so many plays, the challenges posed by chronic neuropsychiatric and neurological conditions motivate the quest to identify, prevent, ameliorate, and treat a range of genetic disorders with all modes of medical interventions.[167,183] The last play explored, Sharr White's 2011 *The Other Place*,[262] brings to life many of these themes and images, dramatizing attempts to manipulate genomic fate through medical science. The main character, Julianna, is a brilliant scientist who has devoted her professional life to finding a cure for Alzheimer's disease.[201,262] While presenting at an academic meeting, she suddenly loses her memory and stops talking. Thinking that she has had a stroke or possibly brain cancer, she consults a neurologist.

Juliana explains to Dr. Teller, her neurologist, "Look, my whole family died of cancer, Daddy got it in the brain when he was two years younger than I am now, did all sorts of things, got up one morning made scrambled eggs with half a can of dog food. There's one you never forget." When Dr. Teller inquires, "[H]ow long did it take for him to uh, uh, to pass" and Juliana notes "three or four years," the neurologist voices her medical opinion: "Doesn't sound like brain cancer." Juliana, however, makes certain to have the last word on the subject, "Of course it was, chemo kept him alive." As fate would have it, imaging technology confirms that it was neither stroke nor cancer: Juliana is afflicted with the very genetic disease that was her scientific specialty.[262]

As her neurological condition deteriorates, Juliana experiences a flashback in which she is in the midst of her slide presentation at a professional conference describing the mutation she studies and carries:

Next please. Introducing the synthetic molecule Small Interfering RNA-7 Beta. Look at it, it's a thing of beauty. Next please, first theorized by me almost twenty years ago and developed in my lab with the help of Dr. Richard Sillner, SIRNA SEVEN as I patented it, is designed to infiltrate the transcription process and cleave the mutant APOE4 gene, next, I let myself...leave my body.

In time, with her husband Ian and nurse Bobby, Julianna finds the support to participate in experimental treatment. One can only wonder, when reflecting on the principle of social justice, whether access to experimental treatment for this genetic condition would have been as readily available to patients not connected to the scientific community. Juliana reports, "I've...had my first injection, been given my pill...and suddenly I feel...I don't know. I can't explain it." She rejoices, "It can't be true, I'm just being hopeful.... Well I just feel this morning as if…I'm…as if a…*something*. That was in front of my eyes. Has been lifted…this is why you use a, a, whatever—." Bobby helped her find her words, "Test group? Placebo…?" As a scientist, Juliana clearly recognizes the power of placebo[262] and acknowledges, "Yes; we just want so badly to think we feel better."[262]

As the play ends, Julianna expresses her hopes that the experimental drug will diminish the progression of her disease, while still recognizing its limitations:

> A new version of Identamyl is, we're certain, hard at work. Though neuron death is still occurring, our hope, however, is that it is slowing, or even coming to a halt. Regardless of treatment, the memories I had will never be restored. Neither will my very sense of self.…Not being myself is, oddly, who I am. Very rarely, triggered by who knows what, visions—ghosts really—of my past life *do* appear quite vividly.…I'm also taking a new drug meant to help *clear* these plaques, but because it's made by a competitor, if you ask me what it is…I'll tell you I don't remember.…There are many conversations I do not retain.…I am a woman in-between: The sky and the earth. The past and the future. This place…and the other.

Because of Julianna's firm belief that genomic science can provide the answers and alter the impact of Alzheimer's disease, she holds on to the presumption that these innovations have the power to change her fate by leading her away from "the other place."

From Rosalind's "beautiful" image of the double-helical structure of DNA to Julianna's image of the "beauty" within her synthetic RNA molecule, the complexity of genomic technology and information has evolved over time. However, the dramatic potential evoked by attempts to understand and modify our genomic destiny has remained relatively consistent—as witnessed in these theatrical narratives through the lens of history. This historical perspective provides the broader contextual script as the genomic landscape expands expectations for explanations and medical innovations, and narrative genomics allows us to affectively experience and imagine the characters through a more personal lens.

The drama of DNA in these plays offers a vivid source in which to observe the complex implications of translating genomic research into clinical practice through the lens of other individuals. The use of theatrical excerpts with genetics-genomics themes is another avenue to integrate narrative genomics into teaching and interdisciplinary discourse. Whether the dramatic vignettes are from existing theatre or original plays, narrative genomics can give us both distance and insight into a myriad of difficult issues set within human relationships—where patients, families, researchers, and clinicians routinely confront challenges to ethical and societal norms.

ADDITIONAL QUESTIONS

Consider how the narratives highlighted in these plays have illuminated your thoughts on the following.

1. What role will genomic technology play in shaping and defining our individual, familial, professional, and cultural identities and relationships?
2. What presumptions do we share about the power of emerging technologies and the genetic and genomic information generated to decide our future?
3. How can we balance moving forward with the promises of genomic science while at the same time being sensitive to the perils of what we have learned from the past?
4. What influence might the application of genetic and genomic technologies have in increasing the risk of discrimination and stigmatization?
5. What limits, if any, should be placed on genomic technologies used to preselect some lives over others? How might your thoughts vary depending on the contexts such as serious medical conditions, behavioral traits, gender?
6. What implications will new applications of genomic technologies have for future generations and our conceptions of *normal* reproduction?
7. What role will epigenetics have on reframing the nature-nurture dichotomy? What will genomic and environmental information mean for the future?
8. How have different perspectives on the application of genetic and genomic technologies affected your perspective on the spectrum of *normal*?
9. As we moved historically from genetics to genomics, how have the themes and issues remained constant, and how have they changed over time?

NOTES

i. Parts of this chapter include material from Rothenberg and Bush, "Manipulating Fate"; Rothenberg and Bush, "Genes and Plays"; and Rothenberg, "From Eugenics to the 'New Genetics.'"[4]
ii. See Rothenberg and Bush, "Manipulating Fate,"[4] for our excerpts from Ibsen's *Ghosts*, MacKaye's *To-morrow*, and O'Neill's *Strange Interlude*[275] to illustrate how American theatre portrayed heritable conditions in the early 1880s and at the beginning of the twentieth century, and how dramatization was used to expose the public to inheritance theory. See also Rothenberg, "From Eugenics to the 'New Genetics,'"[4] and Wolff, *Mendel's Theatre*.[11]

REFERENCES

1

Green ED, Guyer MS. Charting a course for genomic medicine from base pairs to bed-side. *Nature.* 2011;470(7333):204–213.

2

Altshuler D, Daly MJ, Lander ES. Genetic mapping in human disease. *Science.* 2008;322(5903):881–888.

Bamshad MJ, Shendure JA, Valle D, et al. The Centers for Mendelian Genomics: a new large-scale initiative to identify the genes underlying rare Mendelian conditions. *Am J Med Genet A.* 2012;158A(7):1523–1525.

Beaudet AL, Belmont JW. Array-based DNA diagnostics: let the revolution begin. *Annu Rev Med.* 2008;59:113–129

Biesecker LG. Exome sequencing makes medical genomics a reality. *Nat Genet.* 2010;42(1):13–14.

Biesecker LG, Mullikin JC, Facio FM, et al. The ClinSeq Project: piloting large-scale genome sequencing for research in genomic medicine. *Genome Res.* 2009;19(9):1665–1674.

Burke W, Psaty BM. Personalized medicine in the era of genomics. *JAMA.* 2007;298(14):1682–1684.

Collins FS, Green ED, Guttmacher AE, Guyer MS. US National Human Genome Research Institute. A vision for the future of genomics research. *Nature.* 2003;422(6934):835–847.

Couzin-Frankel J. Human genome 10th anniversary. What would you do? *Science.* 2011;331(6018):662–665.

Evans JP, Khoury MJ. The arrival of genomic medicine to the clinic is only the begin-ning of the journey. *Genet Med.* 2013;15(4):268–269.

Feero WG, Guttmacher AE, Collins FS. Genomic medicine—an updated primer. *N Engl J Med.* 2010;362(21):2001–2011.

Green ED, Guyer MS. Charting a course for genomic medicine from base pairs to bed-side. *Nature.* 2011;470(7333):204–213.

Guttmacher AE, Collins FS. Genomic medicine—a primer. *N Engl J Med.* 2002;347(19):1512–1520.

Guttmacher AE, McGuire AL, Ponder B, Stefansson K. Personalized genomic information: preparing for the future of genetic medicine. *Nat Rev Genet.* 2010;11(2):161–165.

International HapMap Consortium. Integrating ethics and science in the International HapMap *Project. Nat Rev Genet.* 2004;5(6):467–475.

International HapMap 3 Consortium, Altshuler DM, Gibbs RA, et al. Integrating common and rare genetic variation in diverse human populations. *Nature*. 2010;467(7311):52–58.

Khoury MJ, Gwinn M, Yoon PW, Dowling N, Moore CA, Bradley L. The continuum of translation research in genomic medicine: how can we accelerate the appropriate integration of human genome discoveries into health care and disease prevention? *Genet Med*. 2007;9(10):665–674.

Kitzman JO, Snyder MW, Ventura M, et al. Noninvasive whole-genome sequencing of a human fetus. *Sci Transl Med*. 2012;4(137):137ra176.

Kuehn BM. 1000 Genomes Project finds substantial genetic variation among populations. *JAMA*. 2012;308(22):2322, 2325.

Lander ES. Initial impact of the sequencing of the human genome. *Nature*. 2011;470(7333):187–197.

Lander ES, Linton LM, Birren B, et al. Initial sequencing and analysis of the human genome. *Nature*. 2001;409(6822):860–921.

Manolio TA, Chisholm RL, Ozenberger B, et al. Implementing genomic medicine in the clinic: the future is here. *Genet Med*. 2013;15(4):258–267.

Manolio TA, Collins FS, Cox NJ, et al. Finding the missing heritability of complex diseases. *Nature*. 2009;461(7265):747–753.

Mardis ER. A decade's perspective on DNA sequencing technology. *Nature*. 2011;470(7333):198–203.

Mayer AN, Dimmock DP, Arca MJ, et al. A timely arrival for genomic medicine. *Genet Med*. 2011;13(3):195–196.

Moore CA, Khoury MJ, Bradley LA. From genetics to genomics: using gene-based medicine to prevent disease and promote health in children. *Semin Perinatol*. 2005;29(3):135–143.

National Human Genome Research Institute. All about the Human Genome Project (HGP). http://www.genome.gov/10001772. Updated January 24, 2013. Accessed June 21, 2013.

National Human Genome Research Institute. International consortium completes Human Genome Project [news release]. Bethesda, MD: National Human Genome Research Institute and Department of Energy, April 14, 2003. http://web.ornl.gov/sci/techresources/Human_Genome/project/press4_2003.shtml. Accessed July 26, 2013.

Ng SB, Turner EH, Robertson PD, et al. Targeted capture and massively parallel sequencing of 12 human exomes. *Nature*. 2009;461(7261):272–276.

1000 Genomes Project Consortium, Abecasis GR, Altshuler D, et al. A map of human genome variation from population-scale sequencing. *Nature*. 2010;467(7319):1061–1073.

Pennisi E. Genomics. ENCODE project writes eulogy for junk DNA. *Science*. 2012;337(6099):1159, 1161.

Roach JC, Glusman G, Smit AFA, et al. Analysis of genetic inheritance in a family quartet by whole-genome sequencing. *Science*. 2010;328(5978):636–639.

Saunders CJ, Miller NA, Soden SE, et al. Rapid whole-genome sequencing for genetic disease diagnosis in neonatal intensive care units. *Sci Transl Med*. 2012;4(154):154ra135.

Varmus H. Ten years on—the human genome and medicine. *N Engl J Med*. 2010;362(21):2028–2029.

von Bubnoff A. Next-generation sequencing: the race is on. *Cell*. 2008;132(5):721–723.

Wheeler DA, Srinivasan M, Egholm M, et al. The complete genome of an individual by massively parallel DNA sequencing. *Nature.* 2008;452(7189):872–876.

World Health Organization. *Genomics and World Health: Report of the Advisory Committee on Health Research.* Geneva: World Health Organization; 2002.

3

Bainbridge MN, Wiszniewski W, Murdock DR, et al. Whole-genome sequencing for optimized patient management. *Sci Transl Med.* 2011;3(87):87re3.

Berg JS, Evans JP, Leigh MW, et al. Next generation massively parallel sequencing of targeted exomes to identify genetic mutations in primary ciliary dyskinesia: implications for application to clinical testing. *Genet Med.* 2011;13(3):218–229.

Berg JS, Khoury MJ, Evans JP. Deploying whole genome sequencing in clinical practice and public health: meeting the challenge one bin at a time. *Genet Med.* 2011;13(6):499–504.

Biesecker LG. Opportunities and challenges for the integration of massively parallel genomic sequencing into clinical practice: lessons from the ClinSeq project. *Genet Med.* 2012;14(4):393–398.

Chakravarti A, Kapoor A. Genetics: Mendelian puzzles. *Science.* 2012;335(6071):930–931.

Connolly JJ, Hakonarson H. The impact of genomics on pediatric research and medicine. *Pediatrics.* 2012;129(6):1150–1160.

Drmanac R. Medicine. The ultimate genetic test. *Science.* 2012;336(6085):1110–1112.

Evans JP, Meslin EM, Marteau TM, Caulfield T. Genomics. Deflating the genomic bubble. *Science.* 2011;331(6019):861–862.

Gonzaga-Jauregui C, Lupski JR, Gibbs RA. Human genome sequencing in health and disease. *Annu Rev Med.* 2012;63:35–61.

Hudson KL. Genomics, health care, and society. *N Engl J Med.* 2011;365(11):1033–1041.

Ioannidis JP. Expectations, validity, and reality in omics. *J Clin Epidemiol.* 2010;63(9):945–949.

Jackson L, Pyeritz RE. Molecular technologies open new clinical genetic vistas. *Sci Transl Med.* 2011;3(65):65ps2.

Johnson JO, Mandrioli J, Benatar M, et al. Exome sequencing reveals VCP mutations as a cause of familial ALS. *Neuron.* 2010;68(5):857–864.

Kaiser J. Human genetics. Genetic influences on disease remain hidden. *Science.* 2012;338(6110):1016–1017.

Khoury MJ, Feero WG, Reyes M, et al. The genomic applications in practice and prevention network. *Genet Med.* 2009;11(7):488–494.

Lupski JR, Belmont JW, Boerwinkle E, Gibbs RA. Clan genomics and the complex architecture of human disease. *Cell.* 2011;147(1):32–43.

Lupski JR, de Oca-Luna RM, Slaugenhaupt S, et al. DNA duplication associated with Charcot-Marie-Tooth disease type 1A. *Cell.* 1991;66(2):219–232.

Lupski JR, Reid JG, Gonzaga-Jauregui C, et al. Whole-genome sequencing in a patient with Charcot-Marie-Tooth neuropathy. *N Engl J Med.* 2010;362(13):1181–1191.

Offit K. Personalized medicine: new genomics, old lessons. *Hum Genet.* 2011;130(1):3–14.

Otto EA, Hurd TW, Airik R, et al. Candidate exome capture identifies mutation of SDCCAG8 as the cause of a retinal-renal ciliopathy. *Nat Genet.* 2010;42(10):840–850.

Worthey EA, Mayer AN, Syverson GD, et al. Making a definitive diagnosis: successful clinical application of whole exome sequencing in a child with intractable inflammatory bowel disease. *Genet Med.* 2011;13(3):255–262.

4

Bush LW, Rothenberg KH. Dialogues, dilemmas, and disclosures: genomic research and incidental findings. *Genet Med.* 2012;14(3):293–295.

Bush LW, Rothenberg KH. It's not that simple! Genomic research & the consent process, in Rothenberg KH, Bush LW. *Genet Med.* 2012;14(2):OnlineSuppl.

Bush LW, Rothenberg KH. It's so complicated! Genomic research & incidental findings, in Bush LW, Rothenberg KH. *Genet Med.* 2012;14(3):OnlineSuppl.

Rothenberg KH. From eugenics to the 'new' genetics: "The Play's the Thing." *Fordham Law Rev.* 2010;79(2):407–434.

Rothenberg K, Bush L. Manipulating fate: medical innovations, ethical implications, theatrical illuminations. *Houston J Health Law Policy.* 2012;13(1):1–77.

Rothenberg KH, Bush LW. Genes and plays: bringing ELSI issues to life. *Genet Med.* 2012;14(2):274–277.

5

Caulfield S, Caulfield TA. *Imagining Science: Art, Science, and Social Change.* Edmonton: University of Alberta Press; 2008.

Nelkin D, Lindee MS. *The DNA Mystique: The Gene as a Cultural Icon.* 2nd ed. Ann Arbor, MI: University of Michigan Press; 2004.

van Dijck J. *Imagenation: Popular Images of Genetics.* Basingstoke, UK: Palgrave Macmillan Limited; 1998.

6

Downie RS, Macnaughton J. *Bioethics and the Humanities: Attitudes and Perceptions.* New York: Routledge-Cavendish; 2007.

7

King N, Robeson R. Dramatic arts casuistry in bioethics education and outreach. Paper presented at: ELSI Congress; 2011; Chapel Hill, NC.

Savitt TL. *Medical Readers' Theater: A Guide and Scripts.* Iowa City, IA: University of Iowa Press; 2002.

8

Charon R. *Narrative Medicine: Honoring the Stories of Illness.* Oxford, UK: Oxford University Press; 2006.

9

Anderson CM, Montello M. The reader's response and why it matters in biomedical ethics. In: Charon R, Montello M, eds. *Stories Matter: The Role of Narrative in Medical Ethics.* New York: Routledge; 2002:85–94.

Brody H. Narrative ethics and institutional impact. In: Charon R, Montello M, eds. *Stories Matter: The Role of Narrative in Medical Ethics.* New York: Routledge; 2002:153–157.

Chambers T. *The Fiction of Bioethics: Cases as Literary Texts.* New York: Routledge; 1999. *Reflective Bioethics.*

Chambers T. Literature. In: Sugarman J, Sulmasy DP, eds. *Methods in Medical Ethics.* Washington, DC: Georgetown University Press; 2010:159–174.

Chambers T, Montgomery K. Plot: framing contingency and choice in bioethics. In: Charon R, Montello M, eds. *Stories Matter: The Role of Narrative in Medical Ethics*. New York: Routledge; 2002:79–87.

Charon R, Montello M, eds. *Stories Matter: The Role of Narrative in Medical Ethics*. New York: Routledge; 2002. *Reflective Bioethics*.

Downie RS, Macnaughton J. *Bioethics and the Humanities: Attitudes and Perceptions*. New York: Routledge-Cavendish; 2007.

Frank AW. *The Wounded Storyteller: Body, Illness, and Ethics*. Chicago, IL: University of Chicago Press; 1995.

Hawkins AH. The idea of character. In: Charon R, Montello M, eds. *Stories Matter: The Role of Narrative in Medical Ethics*. New York: Routledge; 2002:70–78.

Lantos J. Reconsidering action: day-to-day ethics in the work of medicine. In: Charon R, Montello M, eds. *Stories Matter: The Role of Narrative in Medical Ethics*. New York: Routledge; 2002:158–163.

Nelson HL. Context: backward, sideways, and forward. In: Charon R, Montello M, eds. *Stories Matter: The Role of Narrative in Medical Ethics*. New York: Routledge; 2002:39–47.

Nelson HL. *Stories and Their Limits: Narrative Approaches to Bioethics*. New York: Routledge; 1997. *Reflective Bioethics*.

Poirier S. Voice in the medical narrative. In: Charon R, Montello M, eds. *Stories Matter: The Role of Narrative in Medical Ethics*. New York: Routledge; 2002:48–59.

Reverby SM. Listening to narratives from the Tuskegee syphilis study. *Lancet*. 2011;377(9778):1646–1647.

Stripling MY. *Bioethics and Medical Issues in Literature*. Westport, CT: Greenwood Press; 2005. *Exploring Social Issues Through Literature*.

Sugarman J, Sulmasy DP, eds. *Methods in Medical Ethics*. 2nd ed. Washington, DC: Georgetown University Press; 2010.

10

Arawi T. Using medical drama to teach biomedical ethics to medical students. *Med Teach*. 2010;32(5):e205–e210.

Bard J, Mayo TW, Tovino SA. Three ways of looking at a health law and literature class. *Drexel Law Rev*. 2009;1(2):512–572.

Case GA, Brauner DJ. Perspective: the doctor as performer: a proposal for change based on a performance studies paradigm. *Acad Med*. 2010;85(1):159–163.

Charon R. Narrative and medicine. *N Engl J Med*. 2004;350(9):862–864.

Charon R. *Narrative Medicine: Honoring the Stories of Illness*. Oxford, UK: Oxford University Press; 2006.

Charon R, Trautmann Banks J, Connelly JE, et al. Literature and medicine: contributions to clinical practice. *Ann Intern Med*. 1995;122(8):599–606.

Colt HG, Quadrelli S, Friedman LD, eds. *The Picture of Health: Medical Ethics and the Movies*. New York: Oxford University Press; 2011.

Czarny MJ, Faden RR, Sugarman J. Bioethics and professionalism in popular television medical dramas. *J Med Ethics*. 2010;36(4):203–206.

Deloney LA, Graham CJ. Wit: using drama to teach first-year medical students about empathy and compassion. *Teach Learn Med*. 2003;15(4):247–251.

Edson M. *Wit*. New York: Dramatists Play Service; 1999.

Fetters MD. The wizard of Osler: a brief educational intervention combining film and medical readers' theater to teach about power in medicine. *Fam Med*. 2006;38(5):323–325.

Gemmette EV. *Law in Literature: Legal Themes in Drama.* Albany, NY: Whitston Publishing; 1995.

Gillis CM. "Seeing the difference": an interdisciplinary approach to death, dying, humanities, and medicine. *J Med Humanit.* 2006;27(2):105–115.

Hawkins AH, Ballard JO, eds. *Time to Go: Three Plays on Death and Dying with Commentary on End-of-Life Issues.* Philadelphia: University of Pennsylvania Press; 1995.

Hunter KM, Charon R, Coulehan JL. The study of literature in medical education. *Acad Med.* 1995;70(9):787–794.

King N, Robeson R. Dramatic arts casuistry in bioethics education and outreach. Paper presented at: ELSI Congress; 2011; Chapel Hill, NC.

Kleinman A. *The Illness Narratives: Suffering, Healing, and the Human Condition.* New York: Basic Books; 1988.

LaCombe MA, Elpern DJ, eds. *Osler's Bedside Library: Great Writers Who Inspired a Great Physician.* Philadelphia, PA: American College of Physicians; 2010.

Lorenz KA, Steckart MJ, Rosenfeld KE. End-of-life education using the dramatic arts: the Wit educational initiative. *Acad Med.* 2004;79(5):481–486.

McCullough M. Bringing drama into medical education. *Lancet.* 2012;379(9815):512–513.

Mitchell GJ, Jonas-Simpson C, Ivonoffski V. Research-based theatre: the making of I'm Still Here! *Nurs Sci Q.* 2006;19(3):198–206.

Nuland SB. *The Soul of Medicine: Tales from the Bedside.* New York: Kaplan Publishing; 2009.

Reynolds RC, Stone J, eds. *On Doctoring: Stories, Poems, Essays.* 3rd ed. New York: Simon & Schuster; 2001.

Robinson WM. The narrative of rescue in pediatric practice. In: Charon R, Montello M, eds. *Stories Matter: The Role of Narrative in Medical Ethics.* New York: Routledge; 2002:100–111.

Savitt TL. *Medical Readers' Theater: A Guide and Scripts.* Iowa City, IA: University of Iowa Press; 2002.

Shapiro J. Walking a mile in their patients' shoes: empathy and othering in medical students' education. *Philos Ethics Humanit Med.* 2008;3:10.

Shapiro J, Hunt L. All the world's a stage: the use of theatrical performance in medical education. *Med Educ.* 2003;37(10):922–927.

Shapiro J, Kasman D, Shafer A. Words and wards: a model of reflective writing and its uses in medical education. *J Med Humanit.* 2006;27(4):231–244.

Shepherd-Barr K. *Science on Stage: From Doctor Faustus to Copenhagen.* Princeton, NJ: Princeton University Press; 2006.

Trillin AS. Of dragons and garden peas: a cancer patient talks to doctors. *N Engl J Med.* 1981;304(12):699–701.

Unalan PC, Uzuner A, Cifcili S, Akman M, Hancioglu S, Thulesius HO. Using theatre in education in a traditional lecture oriented medical curriculum. *BMC Med Educ.* 2009;9:73.

Volandes A. Medical ethics on film: towards a reconstruction of the teaching of healthcare professionals. *J Med Ethics.* 2007;33(11):678–680.

von Heijne G. A Day in the Life of Dr K. or How I Learned to Stop Worrying and Love Lysozyme: a tragedy in six acts. *J Mol Biol.* 1999;293(2):367–379.

Weinstein AL. *A Scream Goes Through the House: What Literature Teaches Us About Life.* New York: Random House; 2003.

11

Bush LW, Rothenberg KH. Dialogues, dilemmas, and disclosures: genomic research and incidental findings. *Genet Med.* 2012;14(3):293–295.

Bush LW, Rothenberg KH. It's not that simple! Genomic research & the consent process, in Rothenberg KH, Bush LW. *Genet Med.* 2012;14(2):OnlineSuppl.

Bush LW, Rothenberg KH. It's so complicated! Genomic research & incidental findings, in Bush LW, Rothenberg KH. *Genet Med.* 2012;14(3):OnlineSuppl.

Capron AM. Human genetic engineering: Gattaca. In: Colt HG, Quadrelli S, Friedman LD, eds. *The Picture of Health : Medical Ethics and the Movies.* New York: Oxford University Press; 2011:351–356.

Churchill LR. Narrative ethics, gene stories, and the hermeneutics of consent forms. In: Charon R, Montello M, eds. *Stories Matter: The Role of Narrative in Medical Ethics.* New York: Routledge; 2002:187–199.

Konrad M. *Narrating the New Predictive Genetics: Ethics, Ethnography, and Science.* Cambridge, UK: Cambridge University Press; 2005.

Latham S. Reproductive cloning: Multiplicity. In: Colt HG, Quadrelli S, Friedman LD, eds. *The Picture of Health: Medical Ethics and the Movies.* New York: Oxford University Press; 2011:357–361.

Marion R. *Genetics Rounds: A Doctor's Encounters in the Field That Revolutionized Medicine.* New York: Kaplan Publishing; 2009.

Nowaczyk, MJM. Narrative medicine in clinical genetics practice. *Am J Med Genet A.* 2012; 158A:1941–1947.

Rothenberg K. Eugenics, genetics and gender: theatre and the role of women. In: Caulfield ST, Gillespie C, Caulfield TA, eds. *Perceptions of Promise: Biotechnology, Society and Art.* Edmonton: University of Alberta; 2011:73–78.

Rothenberg K, Bush L. Manipulating fate: medical innovations, ethical implications, theatrical illuminations. *Houston J Health Law Policy.* 2012;13(1):1–77.

Rothenberg KH. From eugenics to the 'new' genetics: "The Play's the Thing." *Fordham Law Rev.* 2010;79(2):407–434.

Rothenberg KH, Bush LW. Genes and plays: bringing ELSI issues to life. *Genet Med.* 2012;14(2):274–277.

Shepherd-Barr K. *Science on Stage: From Doctor Faustus to Copenhagen.* Princeton, NJ: Princeton University Press; 2006: 122–127.

Wexler A. Mapping Fate: *A Memoir of Family, Risk, and Genetic Research.* New York: Times Books: Random House; 1995.

Wolff T. *Mendel's Theatre: Heredity, Eugenics, and Early Twentieth-Century American Drama.* Palgrave Studies in Theatre and Performance History. New York: Palgrave Macmillan; 2009.

12

Gillis CM. "Seeing the difference": an interdisciplinary approach to death, dying, humanities, and medicine. *J Med Humanit.* 2006;27(2):105–115.

Reeves S, Zwarenstein M, Goldman J, et al. Interprofessional education: effects on professional practice and health care outcomes. *Cochrane Database Syst Rev.* 2008(1):CD002213.

13

Henderson GE, Juengst ET, King NM, Kuczynski K, Michie M. What research ethics should learn from genomics and society research: lessons from the ELSI Congress of 2011. *J Law Med Ethics.* 2012;40(4):1008–1024.

Oliver JM, McGuire AL. Exploring the ELSI universe: critical issues in the evolution of human genomic research. *Genome Med.* 2011;3(6):38.

14

Bush LW, Rothenberg KH. Dialogues, dilemmas, and disclosures: genomic research and incidental findings. *Genet Med.* 2012;14(3):293–295.

Cooke M, Irby DM, O'Brien BC. *A Summary of Educating Physicians: A Call for Reform of Medical School and Residency.* San Francisco: Jossey Bass; 2010. http://www. carnegiefoundation.org/elibrary/summary-educating-physicians#summary. Published January 2011. Accessed July 22, 2013.

Dhar SU, Alford RL, Nelson EA, Potocki L. Enhancing exposure to genetics and genomics through an innovative medical school curriculum. *Genet Med.* 2012;14(1):163–167.

Doukas DJ, McCullough LB, Wear S. Reforming medical education in ethics and humanities by finding common ground with Abraham Flexner. *Acad Med.* 2010;85(2):318–323.

Feero WG, Green ED. Genomics education for health care professionals in the 21st century. *JAMA.* 2011;306(9):989–990.

Guttmacher AE, Porteous ME, McInerney JD. Educating health-care professionals about genetics and genomics. *Nat Rev Genet.* 2007;8(2):151–157.

Korf BR. Genetics and genomics education: the next generation. *Genet Med.* 2011;13(3):201–202.

Miller BM, Moore DE Jr., Stead WW, Balser JR. Beyond Flexner: a new model for continuous learning in the health professions. *Acad Med.* 2010;85(2):266–272.

Reeves S, Zwarenstein M, Goldman J, et al. Interprofessional education: effects on professional practice and health care outcomes. *Cochrane Database Syst Rev.* 2008(1):CD002213.

Rothenberg K, Bush L. Manipulating fate: medical innovations, ethical implications, theatrical illuminations. *Houston J Health Law Policy.* 2012;13(1):1–77.

Rothenberg KH. From eugenics to the 'new' genetics: "The Play's the Thing." *Fordham Law Rev.* 2010;79(2):407–434.

Rothenberg KH, Bush LW. Genes and plays: bringing ELSI issues to life. *Genet Med.* 2012;14(2):274–277.

Siegler M. A legacy of Osler. Teaching clinical ethics at the bedside. *JAMA.* 1978;239(10):951–956.

15

Annas GJ. Rules for research on human genetic variation—lessons from Iceland. *N Engl J Med.* 2000;342(24):1830–1833.

Caulfield T, McGuire AL, Cho M, et al. Research ethics recommendations for whole-genome research: consensus statement. *PLoS Biol.* 2008;6(3):e73.

Juengst ET, Goldenberg A. Genetic diagnostic, pedigree, and screening research. In: Emanuel EJ, Grady C, Crouch RA, et al., eds. *The Oxford Textbook of Clinical Research Ethics.* New York: Oxford University Press; 2008:298–314.

Kaye J, Boddington P, de Vries J, Hawkins N, Melham K. Ethical implications of the use of whole genome methods in medical research. *Eur J Hum Genet.* 2010;18(4):398–403.

Knoppers BM, Chadwick R. Human genetic research: emerging trends in ethics. *Nat Rev Genet.* 2005;6(1):75–79.

McGuire AL, Caulfield T, Cho MK. Research ethics and the challenge of whole-genome sequencing. *Nat Rev Genet.* 2008;9(2):152–156.

Tabor HK, Berkman BE, Hull SC, Bamshad MJ. Genomics really gets personal: how exome and whole genome sequencing challenge the ethical framework of human genetics research. *Am J Med Genet A.* 2011;155A(12):2916–2924.

16

ACMG Board of Directors. Points to consider for informed consent for genome/ exome sequencing. *Genet Med.* 2013;15(9):748–749.

Foster MW, Mulvihill JJ, Sharp RR. Evaluating the utility of personal genomic information. *Genet Med.* 2009;11(8):570–574.

Green MJ, Botkin JR. "Genetic exceptionalism" in medicine: clarifying the differences between genetic and nongenetic tests. *Ann Intern Med.* 2003;138(7):571–575.

Hallowell N, Foster C, Eeles R, Ardern-Jones A, Murday V, Watson M. Balancing autonomy and responsibility: the ethics of generating and disclosing genetic information. *J Med Ethics.* 2003;29(2):74–79; discussion 80–83.

Levy DE, Byfield SD, Comstock CB, et al. Underutilization of BRCA1/2 testing to guide breast cancer treatment: black and Hispanic women particularly at risk. *Genet Med.* 2011;13(4):349–355.

May T. Rethinking clinical risk for DNA sequencing. *Am J Bioeth.* 2012;12(10):24–26.

Ormond KE, Wheeler MT, Hudgins L, et al. Challenges in the clinical application of whole-genome sequencing. *Lancet.* 2010;375(9727):1749–1751.

Parker M. *Ethical Problems and Genetics Practice.* New York: Cambridge University Press; 2012.

Sharp RR. Downsizing genomic medicine: approaching the ethical complexity of whole-genome sequencing by starting small. *Genet Med.* 2011;13(3):191–194.

Veenstra DL, Roth JA, Garrison LP Jr., Ramsey SD, Burke W. A formal risk-benefit framework for genomic tests: facilitating the appropriate translation of genomics into clinical practice. *Genet Med.* 2010;12(11):686–693.

17

ACMG Board of Directors. Points to consider in the clinical application of genomic sequencing. *Genet Med.* 2012;14(8):759–761.

Ali-Khan SE, Daar AS, Shuman C, Ray PN, Scherer SW. Whole genome scanning: resolving clinical diagnosis and management amidst complex data. *Pediatr Res.* 2009;66(4):357–363.

Khoury MJ, Coates RJ, Evans JP. Evidence-based classification of recommendations on use of genomic tests in clinical practice: dealing with insufficient evidence. *Genet Med.* 2010;12(11):680–683.

Schrijver I, Aziz N, Farkas DH, et al. Opportunities and challenges associated with clinical diagnostic genome sequencing: a report of the Association for Molecular Pathology. *J Mol Diagn.* 2012;14(6):525–540.

18

Berg JS, Adams M, Nassar N, et al. An informatics approach to analyzing the incidentalome. *Genet Med.* 2013;15(1):36–44.

Cho MK. Understanding incidental findings in the context of genetics and genomics. *J Law Med Ethics.* 2008;36(2):280–285, 212.

Christenhusz GM, Devriendt K, Dierickx K. To tell or not to tell? A systematic review of ethical reflections on incidental findings arising in genetics contexts. *Eur J Hum Genet.* 2013;21(3):248–255.

Daack-Hirsch S, Driessnack M, Hanish A, et al. 'Information is information': a public perspective on incidental findings in clinical and research genome-based testing. *Clin Genet.* 2013;84(1):11–18.

Johnston JJ, Rubinstein WS, Facio FM, et al. Secondary variants in individuals undergoing exome sequencing: screening of 572 individuals identifies high-penetrance mutations in cancer-susceptibility genes. *Am J Hum Genet.* 2012;91(1):97–108.

Kohane IS, Hsing M, Kong SW. Taxonomizing, sizing, and overcoming the incidentalome. *Genet Med.* 2012;14(4):399–404.

Kohane IS, Masys DR, Altman RB. The incidentalome: a threat to genomic medicine. *JAMA.* 2006;296(2):212–215.

Parens E, Appelbaum P, Chung W. Incidental findings in the era of whole genome sequencing? *Hastings Cent Rep.* 2013;43(4):16–19.

Parker LS. The future of incidental findings: should they be viewed as benefits? *J Law Med Ethics.* 2008;36(2):341–351.

Schwarzbraun T, Obenauf AC, Langmann A, et al. Predictive diagnosis of the cancer prone Li-Fraumeni syndrome by accident: new challenges through whole genome array testing. *J Med Genet.* 2009;46(5):341–344.

Westbrook MJ, Wright MF, Van Driest SL, et al. Mapping the incidentalome: estimating incidental findings generated through clinical pharmacogenomics testing. *Genet Med.* 2013;15(5):325–331.

19

Lyon GJ, Jiang T, Van Wijk R, et al. Exome sequencing and unrelated findings in the context of complex disease research: ethical and clinical implications. Discov Med. 2011;12(62):41–55.

Van Ness B. Genomic research and incidental findings. *J Law Med Ethics.* 2008;36(2):292–297.

Velizara A, Blasimme A, Julia S, Cambon-Thomsen A. Genomic incidental findings: reducing the burden to be fair. *Am J Bioeth.* 2013;13(2):52–54.

20

Evans JP. When is a medical finding "incidental"? *Genet Med.* 2013;15(7):515–516.

Parens E, Appelbaum P, Chung W. Incidental findings in the era of whole genome sequencing? *Hastings Cent Rep.* 2013;43(4):16–19.

21

Beauchamp TL. Methods and principles in biomedical ethics. *J Med Ethics.* 2003;29(5):269–274.

Beauchamp TL, Childress JF. *Principles of Biomedical Ethics.* 6th ed. New York: Oxford University Press; 2009.

Bickenbach JE. *Ethics, Law, and Policy.* Thousand Oaks, CA: Sage Publications; 2012.

Faden RR, Beauchamp TL, King NMP. *A History and Theory of Informed Consent.* New York: Oxford University Press; 1986.

Faden RR, Kass NE, Goodman SN, Pronovost P, Tunis S, Beauchamp TL. An ethics framework for a learning health care system: a departure from traditional research ethics and clinical ethics. *Hastings Cent Rep.* 2013;43(Suppl):S16–27.

Goering S, Holland S, Edwards K. Making good on the promise of genetics: justice in translational science. In: Burke W, Edwards K, Goering S, Holland S, Trinidad SB, eds. *Achieving Justice in Genomic Translation: Rethinking the Pathway to Benefit.* Oxford, UK: Oxford University Press; 2011:3–21.

Grady C, Wendler D. Making the transition to a learning health care system. Commentary. *Hastings Cent Rep.* 2013;43(Suppl):S32–33.

Juengst ET. FACE facts: why human genetics will always provoke bioethics. *J Law Med Ethics.* 2004;32(2):267–275, 191.

Kass NE, Faden RR, Goodman SN, Pronovost P, Tunis S, Beauchamp TL. The research-treatment distinction: a problematic approach for determining which activities should have ethical oversight. *Hastings Cent Rep.* 2013;43(Suppl):S4–S15.

Kaye J, Meslin EM, Knoppers BM, et al. Research priorities. ELSI 2.0 for genomics and society. *Science.* 2012;336(6082):673–674.

Largent EA, Joffe S, Miller FG. Can research and care be ethically integrated? Commentary. *Hastings Cent Rep.* 2011;41(4):37–46.

Largent EA, Miller FG, Joffe S. A prescription for ethical learning. Commentary. *Hastings Cent Rep.* 2013;43(Suppl):S28–S29.

McEwen JE, Boyer JT, Sun KY. Evolving approaches to the ethical management of genomic data. *Trends Genet.* 2013;29(6):375–382.

National Human Genome Research Institute. The Ethical, Legal and Social Implications (ELSI) Research Program. http://www.genome.gov/10001618. Updated April 10, 2013. Accessed June 21, 2013.

Nijsingh N. Blurring boundaries. *Am J Bioeth.* 2012;12(10):26–27.

Wertz DC, Fletcher JC, Berg K, Boulyjenkov V. *Guidelines on Ethical Issues in Medical Genetics and the Provision of Genetics Services.* Geneva: World Health Organization; 1995.

Wilfond B. Predicting our future: lessons from Winnie-the-Pooh. *Hastings Cent Rep.* 2012;42(4):3.

22

Driessnack M, Daack-Hirsch S, Downing N, et al. The disclosure of incidental genomic findings: an "ethically important moment" in pediatric research and practice. *J Community Genet.* 2013. doi: 10.1007/s12687-013-0145-1.

23

Evans JP. Return of results to the families of children in genomic sequencing: tallying risks and benefits. *Genet Med.* 2013;15(6):435–436.

Solomon BD, Hadley DW, Pineda-Alvarez DE, et al. Incidental medical information in whole-exome sequencing. *Pediatrics.* 2012;129(6):e1605–e1611.

24

Clayton EW, Haga S, Kuszler P, Bane E, Shutske K, Burke W. Managing incidental genomic findings: legal obligations of clinicians. *Genet Med.* 2013. doi: 10.1038/gim.2013.7.

Goddard KA, Whitlock EP, Berg JS, et al. Description and pilot results from a novel method for evaluating return of incidental findings from next-generation sequencing technologies. *Genet Med.* 2013. doi: 10.1038/gim.2013.37.

Krier JB, Green RC. Management of incidental findings in clinical genomic sequencing. *Curr Protoc Hum Genet.* 2013;Chapter 9:Unit9.23.

25

Klitzman R. "Am I my genes?" Questions of identity among individuals confronting genetic disease. *Genet Med.* 2009;11(12):880–889.

26

Rhodes R. Genetic links, family ties, and social bonds: rights and responsibilities in the face of genetic knowledge. *J Med Philos.* 1998;23(1):10–30.

27

Kaye J, Curren L, Anderson N, et al. From patients to partners: participant-centric initiatives in biomedical research. *Nat Rev Genet.* 2012;13(5):371–376.

Kohane IS, Mandl KD, Taylor PL, Holm IA, Nigrin DJ, Kunkel LM. Medicine. Reestablishing the researcher-patient compact. *Science.* 2007;316(5826):836–837.

28

Davis DS. Groups, communities, and contested identities in genetic research. *Hastings Cent Rep.* 2000;30(6):38–45.

Dickert N, Sugarman J. Ethical goals of community consultation in research. *Am J Public Health.* 2005;95(7):1123–1127.

Foster MW, Sharp RR. Research with identifiable and targeted communities. In: Emanuel EJ, Grady C, Crouch RA, et al., eds. *The Oxford Textbook of Clinical Research Ethics.* New York: Oxford University Press; 2008:475–480.

Havasupai Tribe v Ariz. Bd. of Regents, 204 P.3d 1063 (Ariz. Ct. App. 2008).

Hensley Alford S, McBride CM, Reid RJ, Larson EB, Baxevanis AD, Brody LC. Participation in genetic testing research varies by social group. *Public Health Genomics.* 2011;14(2):85–93.

Lakes KD, Vaughan E, Jones M, Burke W, Baker D, Swanson JM. Diverse perceptions of the informed consent process: implications for the recruitment and participation of diverse communities in the National Children's Study. *Am J Community Psychol.* 2012;49(1–2):215–232.

Weijer C, Emanuel EJ. Ethics. Protecting communities in biomedical research. *Science.* 2000;289(5482):1142–1144.

29

Duncan RE, Gillam L, Savulescu J, et al. "You're one of us now": young people describe their experiences of predictive genetic testing for Huntington disease (HD) and familial adenomatous polyposis (FAP). *Am J Med Genet C Semin Med Genet.* 2008;148C(1):47–55.

30

Goffman E. *Stigma: Notes on the Management of Spoiled Identity.* Englewood Cliffs, NJ: Prentice-Hall; 1963.

31

Angrist M. You never call, you never write: why return of 'omic' results to research participants is both a good idea and a moral imperative. *Per Med.* 2011;8(6):651–657.

Bredenoord AL, Onland-Moret NC, Van Delden JJ. Feedback of individual genetic results to research participants: in favor of a qualified disclosure policy. *Hum Mutat.* 2011;32(8):861–867.

Cassa CA, Savage SK, Taylor PL, Green RC, McGuire AL, Mandl KD. Disclosing pathogenic genetic variants to research participants: quantifying an emerging ethical responsibility. *Genome Res.* 2012;22(3):421–428.

Knoppers BM, Joly Y, Simard J, Durocher F. The emergence of an ethical duty to disclose genetic research results: international perspectives. *Eur J Hum Genet.* 2006;14(11):1170–1178.

Miller FA, Christensen R, Giacomini M, Robert JS. Duty to disclose what? Querying the putative obligation to return research results to participants. *J Med Ethics.* 2008;34(3):210–213.

Miller FA, Hayeems RZ, Li L, Bytautas JP. One thing leads to another: the cascade of obligations when researchers report genetic research results to study participants. *Eur J Hum Genet.* 2012;20(8):837–843.

Ossorio P. Taking aims seriously: repository research and limits on the duty to return individual research findings. *Genet Med.* 2012;14(4):461–466.

32

Allyse M, Michie M. Not-so-incidental findings: the ACMG recommendations on the reporting of incidental findings in clinical whole genome and whole exome sequencing. *Trends Biotechnol.* 2013. doi: 10.1016/j.tibtech.2013.04.006.

American College of Medical Genetics and Genomics. Incidental findings in clinical genomics: a clarification. *Genet Med.* 2013;15(8):664-666.

Biesecker LG. Incidental variants are critical for genomics. *Am J Hum Genet.* 2013;92(5):648–651.

Burke W, Matheny Antommaria AH, Bennett R, et al. Recommendations for returning genomic incidental findings? We need to talk! *Genet Med.* 2013; doi: 10.1038/gim.2013.113.

Couzin-Frankel J. Genome sequencing. Return of unexpected DNA results urged. *Science.* 2013;339(6127):1507–1508.

Green RC, Berg JS, Grody WW, American College of Medical Genetics and Genomics. ACMG recommendations for reporting of incidental findings in clinical exome and genome sequencing. *Genet Med.* 2013;15(7):565–574.

Lohn Z, Adam S, Birch PH, Friedman JM. Incidental findings from clinical genome-wide sequencing: a review. *J Genet Couns.* 2013. doi: 10.1007/s10897-013-9604-4.

McGuire AL, Joffe S, Koenig BA, et al. Point-counterpoint. Ethics and genomic incidental findings. *Science.* 2013;340(6136):1047–1048.

Wolf SM, Annas GJ, Elias S. Point-counterpoint. Patient autonomy and incidental findings in clinical genomics. *Science.* 2013;340(6136):1049–1050.

33

Beskow LM, Smolek SJ. Prospective biorepository participants' perspectives on access to research results. *J Empir Res Hum Res Ethics.* 2009;4(3):99–111.

Bollinger JM, Scott J, Dvoskin R, Kaufman D. Public preferences regarding the return of individual genetic research results: findings from a qualitative focus group study. *Genet Med.* 2012;14(4):451–457.

Facio FM, Eidem H, Fisher T, et al. Intentions to receive individual results from whole-genome sequencing among participants in the ClinSeq study. *Eur J Hum Genet.* 2013;21(3):261–265.

Lemke AA, Halverson C, Ross LF. Biobank participation and returning research results: perspectives from a deliberative engagement in South Side Chicago. *Am J Med Genet A.* 2012;158A(5):1029–1037.

O'Daniel J, Haga SB. Public perspectives on returning genetics and genomics research results. *Public Health Genomics.* 2011;14(6):346–355.

Parker LS. Returning individual research results: what role should people's preferences play? *Minn JL Sci & Tech*. 2012;13(2):449–484.

Schwartz MD, Rothenberg K, Joseph L, Benkendorf J, Lerman C. Consent to the use of stored DNA for genetics research: a survey of attitudes in the Jewish population. *Am J Med Genet*. 2001;98:336–342.

Yu JH, Jamal SM, Tabor HK, Bamshad MJ. Self-guided management of exome and whole-genome sequencing results: changing the results return model. *Genet Med*. 2013. doi: 10.1038/gim.2013.35.

34

Brandt DS, Shinkunas L, Hillis SL, et al. A closer look at the recommended criteria for disclosing genetic results: perspectives of medical genetic specialists, genomic researchers, and institutional review board chairs. *J Genet Couns*. 2013;22(4):544–553.

Clayton EW, Kelly SE. Let us ask better questions. *Genet Med*. 2013. doi: 10.1038/gim.2013.68.

Hayeems RZ, Miller FA, Li L, Bytautas JP. Not so simple: a quasi-experimental study of how researchers adjudicate genetic research results. *Eur J Hum Genet*. 2011;19(7):740–747.

Ramoni RB, McGuire AL, Robinson JO, Morley DS, Plon SE, Joffe S. Experiences and attitudes of genome investigators regarding return of individual genetic test results. *Genet Med*. 2013. doi: 10.1038/gim.2013.58.

35

Gliwa C, Berkman BE. Do researchers have an obligation to actively look for genetic incidental findings? *Am J Bioeth*. 2013;13(2):32–42.

Miller FG, Mello MM, Joffe S. Incidental findings in human subjects research: what do investigators owe research participants? *J Law Med Ethics*. 2008;36(2):271–279.

Richardson HS. Incidental findings and ancillary-care obligations. *J Law Med Ethics*. 2008;36(2):256–270.

Richardson HS, Cho MK. Secondary researchers' duties to return incidental findings and individual research results: a partial-entrustment account. *Genet Med*. 2012;14(4):467–472.

Wolf SM, Paradise J, Caga-anan C. The law of incidental findings in human subjects research: establishing researchers' duties. *J Law Med Ethics*. 2008;36(2):361–383.

36

Downing NR, Williams JK, Daack-Hirsch S, Driessnack M, Simon CM. Genetics specialists' perspectives on disclosure of genomic incidental findings in the clinical setting. *Patient Educ Couns*. 2013;90(1):133–138.

Green RC, Berg JS, Berry GT, et al. Exploring concordance and discordance for return of incidental findings from clinical sequencing. *Genet Med*. 2012;14(4):405–410.

Lemke A, Bick D, Dimmock D, Simpson P, Veith R. Perspectives of clinical genetics professionals toward genome sequencing and incidental findings: a survey study. *Clin Genet*. 2012. doi: 10.1111/cge.12060.

Lohn Z, Adam S, Birch P, Townsend A, Friedman J. Genetics professionals' perspectives on reporting incidental findings from clinical genome-wide sequencing. *Am J Med Genet A*. 2013;161(3):542–549.

McGuire AL, McCullough LB, Evans JP. The indispensable role of professional judgment in genomic medicine. *JAMA*. 2013;309(14):1465–1466.

37

Bennette CS, Trinidad SB, Fullerton SM, et al. Return of incidental findings in genomic medicine: measuring what patients value—development of an instrument to measure preferences for information from next-generation testing. *Genet Med.* 2013. doi: 10.1038/gim.2013.63.

Townsend A, Adam S, Birch PH, Lohn Z, Rousseau F, Friedman JM. "I want to know what's in Pandora's box": comparing stakeholder perspectives on incidental findings in clinical whole genomic sequencing. *Am J Med Genet A.* 2012;158A(10):2519–2525.

38

Lindor NM, Johnson KJ, McCormick JB, Klee EW, Ferber MJ, Farrugia G. Preserving personal autonomy in a genomic testing era. *Genet Med.* 2013;15(5):408–409.

39

Trinidad SB, Fullerton SM, Ludman EJ, Jarvik GP, Larson EB, Burke W. Research ethics. Research practice and participant preferences: the growing gulf. *Science.* 2011;331(6015):287–288.

Vermeulen E, Schmidt MK, Aaronson NK, et al. Opt-out plus, the patients' choice: preferences of cancer patients concerning information and consent regimen for future research with biological samples archived in the context of treatment. *J Clin Pathol.* 2009;62(3):275–278.

40

Clayton EW. What should the law say about disclosure of genetic information to relatives? *J Health Care Law Policy.* 1998;1(2):373–390.

Coates R, Williams M, Melillo S, Gudgeon J. Genetic testing for Lynch syndrome in individuals newly diagnosed with colorectal cancer to reduce morbidity and mortality from colorectal cancer in their relatives. *PLoS Curr.* 2011;3:RRN1246.

Doukas DJ, Berg JW. The family covenant and genetic testing. *Am J Bioeth.* 2001;1(3):3–10.

Falk MJ, Dugan RB, O'Riordan MA, Matthews AL, Robin NH. Medical geneticists' duty to warn at-risk relatives for genetic disease. *Am J Med Genet A.* 2003;120A(3):374–380.

Lapointe J, Bouchard K, Patenaude AF, Maunsell E, Simard J, Dorval M. Incidence and predictors of positive and negative effects of BRCA1/2 genetic testing on familial relationships: a 3-year follow-up study. *Genet Med.* 2012;14(1):60–68.

41

Anderson RR. Religious traditions and prenatal genetic counseling. *Am J Med Genet C Semin Med Genet.* 2009;151C(1):52–61.

Boudreault P, Baldwin EE, Fox M, et al. Deaf adults' reasons for genetic testing depend on cultural affiliation: results from a prospective, longitudinal genetic counseling and testing study. *J Deaf Stud Deaf Educ.* 2010;15(3):209–227.

Chen LS, Zhao M, Zhou Q, Xu L. Chinese Americans' views of prenatal genetic testing in the genomic era: a qualitative study. *Clin Genet.* 2012;82(1):22–27.

Levy DE, Byfield SD, Comstock CB, et al. Underutilization of BRCA1/2 testing to guide breast cancer treatment: black and Hispanic women particularly at risk. *Genet Med.* 2011;13(4):349–355.

42

Duster T. Lessons from history: why race and ethnicity have played a major role in biomedical research. *J Law Med Ethics*. 2006;34(3):487–496, 479.

Gustafson SL, Gettig EA, Watt-Morse M, Krishnamurti L. Health beliefs among African American women regarding genetic testing and counseling for sickle cell disease. *Genet Med*. 2007;9(5):303–310.

Ossorio P, Duster T. Race and genetics: controversies in biomedical, behavioral, and forensic sciences. *Am Psychol*. 2005;60(1):115–128.

Paasche-Orlow M. The ethics of cultural competence. *Acad Med*. 2004;79(4):347–350.

Reverby SM. Invoking "Tuskegee": problems in health disparities, genetic assumptions, and history. *J Health Care Poor Underserved*. 2010;21(3 Suppl):26–34.

Suther S, Kiros GE. Barriers to the use of genetic testing: a study of racial and ethnic disparities. *Genet Med*. 2009;11(9):655–662.

Wailoo K, Pemberton SG. *The Troubled Dream of Genetic Medicine: Ethnicity and Innovation in Tay-Sachs, Cystic Fibrosis, and Sickle Cell Disease*. Baltimore, MD: Johns Hopkins University Press; 2006.

43

Denny CC, Wilfond BS, Peters JA, Giri N, Alter BP. All in the family: disclosure of "unwanted" information to an adolescent to benefit a relative. *Am J Med Genet A*. 2008;146A(21):2719–2724.

Goodwin M. My sister's keeper? Law, children, and compelled donation. *West New Engl Law Rev*. 2007;29(2):357–404.

Pennings G, Schots R, Liebaers I. Ethical considerations on preimplantation genetic diagnosis for HLA typing to match a future child as a donor of haematopoietic stem cells to a sibling. *Hum Reprod*. 2002;17(3):534–538.

44

Foster MW, Sharp RR. Ethical issues in medical-sequencing research: implications of genotype-phenotype studies for individuals and populations. *Hum Mol Genet*. 2006;15(Spec No 1):R45–R49.

45

Beskow LM, Burke W. Offering individual genetic research results: context matters. *Sci Transl Med*. 2010;2(38):38cm20.

Biesecker LG. The Nirvana fallacy and the return of results. *Am J Bioeth*. 2013;13(2):43–44.

Bookman EB, Langehorne AA, Eckfeldt JH, et al. Comment on "Multidimensional results reporting to participants in genomic studies: getting it right." *Sci Transl Med*. 2011;3(70):70le1.

Bredenoord AL, Kroes HY, Cuppen E, Parker M, van Delden JJ. Disclosure of individual genetic data to research participants: the debate reconsidered. *Trends Genet*. 2011;27(2):41–47.

Clayton EW, McGuire AL. The legal risks of returning results of genomics research. *Genet Med*. 2012;14(4):473–477.

Clayton EW, Ross LF. Implications of disclosing individual results of clinical research. *JAMA*. 2006;295(1):37; author reply 37–38.

Evans JP, Rothschild BB. Return of results: not that complicated? *Genet Med*. 2012;14(4):358–360.

Fabsitz RR, McGuire A, Sharp RR, et al. Ethical and practical guidelines for reporting genetic research results to study participants: updated guidelines from a

National Heart, Lung, and Blood Institute working group. *Circ Cardiovasc Genet.* 2010;3(6):574–580.

Klitzman R. Questions, complexities, and limitations in disclosing individual genetic results. *Am J Bioeth.* 2006;6(6):34–36; author reply W10–W12.

Kohane IS, Taylor PL. Multidimensional results reporting to participants in genomic studies: getting it right. *Sci Transl Med.* 2010;2(37):37cm19.

McGuire AL, Lupski JR. Personal genome research: what should the participant be told? *Trends Genet.* 2010;26(5):199–201.

McGuire AL, Robinson JO, Ramoni RB, Morley DS, Joffe S, Plon SE. Returning genetic research results: study type matters. *Per Med.* 2013;10(1):27–34.

Parker LS. Best laid plans for offering results go awry. *Am J Bioeth.* 2006;6(6):22–23; author reply W10–W12.

Ravitsky V, Wilfond BS. Disclosing individual genetic results to research participants. *Am J Bioeth.* 2006;6(6):8–17.

Shalowitz DI, Miller FG. Communicating the results of clinical research to participants: attitudes, practices, and future directions. *PLoS Med.* 2008;5(5):e91.

Shalowitz DI, Miller FG. Disclosing individual results of clinical research: implications of respect for participants. *JAMA.* 2005;294(6):737–740.

Sharp RR, Foster MW. Clinical utility and full disclosure of genetic results to research participants. *Am J Bioeth.* 2006;6(6):42–44; author reply W10–W12.

46

Black L, McClellan KA. Familial communication of research results: a need to know? *J Law Med Ethics.* 2011;39(4):605–613.

Chan B, Facio FM, Eidem H, et al. Genomic inheritances: disclosing individual research results from whole-exome sequencing to deceased participants' relatives. *Am J Bioeth.* 2012;12(10):1–8.

47

Netzer C, Klein C, Kohlhase J, Kubisch C. New challenges for informed consent through whole genome array testing. *J Med Genet.* 2009;46(7):495–496.

48

Appelbaum PS. Clarifying the ethics of clinical research: a path toward avoiding the therapeutic misconception. *Am J Bioeth.* 2002;2(2):22–23.

Appelbaum PS, Lidz CW, Klitzman R. Voluntariness of consent to research: a conceptual model. *Hastings Cent Rep.* 2009;39(1):30–39.

Rothstein MA. Tiered disclosure options promote the autonomy and well-being of research subjects. *Am J Bioeth.* 2006;6(6):20–21; author reply W10–W12.

Sankar P. Communication and miscommunication in informed consent to research. *Med Anthropol Q.* 2004;18(4):429–446.

49

Beskow LM, Burke W, Merz JF, et al. Informed consent for population-based research involving genetics. *JAMA.* 2001;286(18):2315–2321.

Hull SC, Gooding H, Klein AP, Warshauer-Baker E, Metosky S, Wilfond BS. Genetic research involving human biological materials: a need to tailor current consent forms. *IRB.* 2004;26(3):1–7.

Kronenthal C, Delaney SK, Christman MF. Broadening research consent in the era of genome-informed medicine. *Genet Med.* 2012;14(4):432–436.

McGuire AL, Beskow LM. Informed consent in genomics and genetic research. *Annu Rev Genomics Hum Genet*. 2010;11:361–381.

McGuire AL, Oliver JM, Slashinski MJ, et al. To share or not to share: a randomized trial of consent for data sharing in genome research. *Genet Med*. 2011;13(11):948–955.

Platt J, Bollinger J, Dvoskin R, Kardia SL, Kaufman D. Public preferences regarding informed consent models for participation in population-based genomic research. *Genet Med*. 2013. doi: 10.1038/gim.2013.59.

Tabor HK, Stock J, Brazg T, et al. Informed consent for whole genome sequencing: a qualitative analysis of participant expectations and perceptions of risks, benefits, and harms. *Am J Med Genet A*. 2012;158A(6):1310–1319.

50

Appelbaum PS, Lidz CW, Meisel A. *Informed Consent: Legal Theory and Clinical Practice*. New York: Oxford University Press; 1987.

Ayuso C, Millan JM, Mancheno M, Dal-Re R. Informed consent for whole-genome sequencing studies in the clinical setting. Proposed recommendations on essential content and process. *Eur J Hum Genet*. 2013. doi: 10.1038/ejhg.2012.297.

Potter BK, O'Reilly N, Etchegary H, et al. Exploring informed choice in the context of prenatal testing: findings from a qualitative study. *Health Expect*. 2008;11(4):355–365.

51

Richardson HS, Belsky L. The ancillary-care responsibilities of medical researchers. An ethical framework for thinking about the clinical care that researchers owe their subjects. *Hastings Cent Rep*. 2004;34(1):25–33.

Zusevics K. Ancillary care, genomics, and the need and opportunity for community-based participatory research. *Am J Bioeth*. 2013;13(2):54–56.

52

Borry P, Dierickx K. What are the limits of the duty of care? The case of clinical genetics. *Per Med*. 2008;5(2):101–104.

53

Aronson SJ, Clark EH, Varugheese M, Baxter S, Babb LJ, Rehm HL. Communicating new knowledge on previously reported genetic variants. *Genet Med*. 2012. doi: 10.1038/gim.2012.19.

Bernard LE, McGillivray B, Van Allen MI, Friedman JM, Langlois S. Duty to re-contact: a study of families at risk for fragile X. *J Genet Couns*. 1999;8(1):3–15.

Fitzpatrick JL, Hahn C, Costa T, Huggins MJ. The duty to recontact: attitudes of genetics service providers. *Am J Hum Genet*. 1999;64(3):852–860.

Hirschhorn K, Fleisher LD, Godmilow L, et al. Duty to re-contact. *Genet Med*. 1999;1(4):171–172.

Hunter AG, Sharpe N, Mullen M, Meschino WS. Ethical, legal, and practical concerns about recontacting patients to inform them of new information: the case in medical genetics. *Am J Med Genet*. 2001;103(4):265–276.

Letendre M, Godard B. Expanding the physician's duty of care: a duty to recontact? *Med Law*. 2004;23(3):531–539.

Pyeritz RE. The coming explosion in genetic testing—is there a duty to recontact? *N Engl J Med*. 2011;365(15):1367–1369.

Rothstein M, Siegal G. Health Information Technology and physicians' duty to notify patients of new medical developments. *Houston J Health Law Policy.* 2012;12(1):93–136.

Rothstein MA. Currents in contemporary bioethics: physicians' duty to inform patients of new medical discoveries: the effect of health information technology. *J Law Med Ethics.* 2011;39(4):690–693.

54

Haga SB, Burke W, Agans R. Primary-care physicians' access to genetic specialists: an impediment to the routine use of genomic medicine? *Genet Med.* 2013;15(7):513–514.

Klitzman R, Chung W, Marder K, et al. Attitudes and practices among internists concerning genetic testing. *J Genet Couns.* 2013;22(1):90–100.

Scheuner MT, Edelen MO, Hilborne LH, Lubin IM. Effective communication of molecular genetic test results to primary care providers. *Genet Med.* 2013;15(6):444–449.

55

Gooding HC, Organista K, Burack J, Biesecker BB. Genetic susceptibility testing from a stress and coping perspective. *Soc Sci Med.* 2006;62(8):1880–1890.

Gray SW, Hicks-Courant K, Lathan CS, Garraway L, Park ER, Weeks JC. Attitudes of patients with cancer about personalized medicine and somatic genetic testing. *J Oncol Pract.* 2012;8(6):329–335, 2 p following 335.

Rini C, O'Neill SC, Valdimarsdottir H, et al. Cognitive and emotional factors predicting decisional conflict among high-risk breast cancer survivors who receive uninformative BRCA1/2 results. *Health Psychol.* 2009;28(5):569–578.

Sivell S, Elwyn G, Gaff CL, et al. How risk is perceived, constructed and interpreted by clients in clinical genetics, and the effects on decision making: systematic review. *J Genet Couns.* 2008;17(1):30–63.

Vansenne F, Bossuyt PM, de Borgie CA. Evaluating the psychological effects of genetic testing in symptomatic patients: a systematic review. *Genet Test Mol Biomarkers.* 2009;13(5):555–563.

56

Brehaut JC, O'Connor AM, Wood TJ, et al. Validation of a decision regret scale. *Med Decis Making.* 2003;23(4):281–292.

57

Wolf SM. The past, present, and future of the debate over return of research results and incidental findings. *Genet Med.* 2012;14(4):355–357.

Wolf SM, et al. Symposium: incidental findings in human subjects research: from imaging to genomics. *J Law Med Ethics.* 2008;36(2):211–435.

Wolf SM, Lawrenz FP, Nelson CA, et al. Managing incidental findings in human subjects research: analysis and recommendations. *J Law Med Ethics.* 2008;36(2):219–248.

58

Clayton EW. Incidental findings in genetics research using archived DNA. *J Law Med Ethics.* 2008;36(2):286–291, 212.

Halverson CM, Ross LF. Incidental findings of therapeutic misconception in biobank-based research. *Genet Med.* 2012;14(6):611–615.

Johnson G, Lawrenz F, Thao M. An empirical examination of the management of return of individual research results and incidental findings in genomic biobanks. *Genet Med.* 2012;14(4):444–450.

Terry SF. The tension between policy and practice in returning research results and incidental findings in genomic biobank research. *Minn J Law Sci & Tech.* 2012;13(2):691–736.

59

Klitzman R, Appelbaum PS, Fyer A, et al. Researchers' views on return of incidental genomic research results: qualitative and quantitative findings. *Genet Med.* 2013. doi: 10.1038/gim.2013.87.

Meacham MC, Starks H, Burke W, Edwards K. Researcher perspectives on disclosure of incidental findings in genetic research. *J Empir Res Hum Res Ethics.* 2010;5(3):31–41.

Williams JK, Daack-Hirsch S, Driessnack M, et al. Researcher and institutional review board chair perspectives on incidental findings in genomic research. *Genet Test Mol Biomarkers.* 2012;16(6):508–513.

60

Hurle B, Citrin T, Jenkins JF, et al. What does it mean to be genomically literate?: National Human Genome Research Institute Meeting Report. *Genet Med.* 2013. doi: 10.1038/gim.2013.14.

61

Marteau TM, French DP, Griffin SJ, et al. Effects of communicating DNA-based disease risk estimates on risk-reducing behaviours. *Cochrane Database Syst Rev.* 2010(10):CD007275.

Stack CB, Gharani N, Gordon ES, Schmidlen T, Christman MF, Keller MA. Genetic risk estimation in the Coriell Personalized Medicine Collaborative. *Genet Med.* 2011;13(2):131–139.

62

Cassa CA, Tong MY, Jordan DM. Large numbers of genetic variants considered to be pathogenic are common in asymptomatic individuals. *Human Mutat.* 2013. doi: 10.1002/humu.22375.

63

Greenberg CR, Dilling LA, Thompson GR, et al. The paradox of the carnitine palmitoyltransferase type Ia P479L variant in Canadian Aboriginal populations. *Mol Genet Metab.* 2009;96(4):201–207.

64

Pullman D, Hodgkinson K. Genetic knowledge and moral responsibility: ambiguity at the interface of genetic research and clinical practice. *Clin Genet.* 2006;69(3):199–203.

65

Clark AE, Shim JK, Shostak S, Nelson A. Biomedicalising genetic health, diseases and identities. In: Atkinson P, Glasner P, Lock M, eds. *Handbook of Genetics and Society: Mapping the New Genomic Era.* New York: Routledge; 2009:21–40.

66

Girirajan S, Rosenfeld JA, Coe BP, et al. Phenotypic heterogeneity of genomic disorders and rare copy-number variants. *N Engl J Med.* 2012;367(14):1321–1331.

Gizewska M, Cabalska B, Cyrytowski L, et al. Different presentations of late-detected phenylketonuria in two brothers with the same R408W/R111X genotype in the PAH gene. *J Intellect Disabil Res.* 2003;47(Pt 2):146–152.

Muntoni F, Torelli S, Ferlini A. Dystrophin and mutations: one gene, several proteins, multiple phenotypes. *Lancet Neurol.* 2003;2(12):731–740.

67

Prince AE, Berkman BE. When does an illness begin: genetic discrimination and disease manifestation. *J Law Med Ethics.* 2012;40(3):655–664.

68

Kwon JM, Steiner RD. "I'm fine; I'm just waiting for my disease": the new and growing class of presymptomatic patients. *Neurology.* 2011;77(6):522–523.

Timmermans S, Buchbinder M. Patients-in-waiting: living between sickness and health in the genomics era. *J Health Soc Behav.* 2010;51(4):408–423.

Viera AJ. Predisease: when does it make sense? *Epidemiol Rev.* 2011;33(1):122–134.

69

Macklin R. Bioethics, vulnerability, and protection. *Bioethics.* 2003;17(5–6):472–486.

70

Shah S, Wendler D. Interpretation of the subjects' condition requirement: a legal perspective. *J Law Med Ethics.* 2010;38(2):365–373.

Shah S, Wolitz R, Emanuel E. Refocusing the responsiveness requirement. *Bioethics.* 2013;27(3):151–159.

71

Boyce WT. The vulnerable child: new evidence, new approaches. *Adv Pediatr.* 1992;39:1–33.

Green M. Vulnerable child syndrome and its variants. *Pediatr Rev.* 1986;8(3):75–80.

Green M, Solnit AJ. Reactions to the threatened loss of a child: a vulnerable child syndrome. Pediatric management of the dying child, part III. *Pediatrics.* 1964;34:58–66.

Perrin EC, West PD, Culley BS. Is my child normal yet? Correlates of vulnerability. *Pediatrics.* 1989;83(3):355–363.

72

Bredenoord AL, de Vries MC, van Delden JJ. Next-generation sequencing: does the next generation still have a right to an open future? *Nat Rev Genet.* 2013;14(5):306.

Davis DS. Child's right to an open future. *Hastings Cent Rep.* 2002;32(5):6; author reply 6.

Davis DS. Genetic dilemmas and the child's right to an open future. *Hastings Cent Rep.* 1997;27(2):7–15.

73

Harrison ME, Walling A. What do we know about giving bad news? A review. *Clinical Pediatr.* 2010;49(7):619–626.

74

Ross LF. Predictive genetic testing for conditions that present in childhood. *Kennedy Inst Ethics J.* 2002;12(3):225–244.

75

Harper PS, Clarke A. Should we test children for "adult" genetic diseases? *Lancet.* 1990;335(8699):1205–1206.

Patenaude AF. The genetic testing of children for cancer susceptibility: ethical, legal, and social issues. *Behav Sci Law.* 1996;14(4):393–410.

Robertson S, Savulescu J. Is there a case in favour of predictive genetic testing in young children? *Bioethics.* 2001;15(1):26–49.

Sevick MA, Nativio DG, McConnell T. Genetic testing of children for late onset disease. *Camb Q Healthc Ethics.* 2005;14(1):47–56.

76

Fernandez CV, Gao J, Strahlendorf C, et al. Providing research results to participants: attitudes and needs of adolescents and parents of children with cancer. *J Clin Oncol.* 2009;27(6):878–883.

77

Hens K, Nys H, Cassiman JJ, Dierickx K. The return of individual research findings in paediatric genetic research. *J Med Ethics.* 2011;37(3):179–183.

78

Abdul-Karim R, Berkman BE, Wendler D, et al. Disclosure of incidental findings from next-generation sequencing in pediatric genomic research. *Pediatrics.* 2013;131(3):564–571.

Fernandez CV, Strahlendorf C, Avard D, et al. Attitudes of Canadian researchers toward the return to participants of incidental and targeted genomic findings obtained in a pediatric research setting. *Genet Med.* 2013;15(7):558–564

Knoppers BM. Paediatric research and the communication of not-so incidental findings. *Paediatr Child Health.* 2012;17(4):190–192.

Wilfond BS, Carpenter KJ. Incidental findings in pediatric research. *J Law Med Ethics.* 2008;36(2):332–340, 213.

79

McCullough LB. Contributions of ethical theory to pediatric ethics: pediatricians and parents as co-fiduciaries of pediatric patients. In: Miller G, ed. *Pediatric Bioethics.* Cambridge, UK: Cambridge University Press; 2010:11–21.

Murray TH. Moral obligations to the not-yet born: the fetus as patient. *Clin Perinatol.* 1987;14(2):329–343.

Pelias MZ, Blanton SH. Genetic testing in children and adolescents: parental authority, the rights of children, and duties of geneticists. *Univ Chicago Law School Roundtable.* 1996;3(2):525–544.

80

Downie RS, Randall F. Parenting and the best interests of minors. *J Med Philos.* 1997;22(3):219–231.

Goldstein J, Freud A, Solnit A. *Before the Best Interests of the Child.* New York: Free Press; 1979.

Goldstein J, Freud A, Solnit AJ. *Beyond the Best Interests of the Child.* New York: Free Press; 1973; 1979.

Goldstein J, Freud A, Solnit A, Goldstein S. *In the Best Interests of the Child: Professional Boundaries*. New York: Free Press; 1986.

Kopelman LM. Using the best-interests standard in treatment decisions for young children. In: Miller G, ed. *Pediatric Bioethics*. New York: Cambridge University Press; 2010:22–37.

Kopelman LM. Using the best interests standard to decide whether to test children for untreatable, late-onset genetic diseases. *J Med Philos*. 2007;32(4):375–394.

Macklin R. Return to the best interests of the child. In: Gaylin W, Macklin R, eds. *Who Speaks for the Child: The Problems of Proxy Consent*. New York: Plenum; 1982:265–301.

81

Diekema DS. Conducting ethical research in pediatrics: a brief historical overview and review of pediatric regulations. *J Pediatr*. 2006;149(1 Suppl):S3–S11.

Diekema DS, Mercurio MR, Adam MB, eds. *Clinical Ethics in Pediatrics: A Case-Based Textbook*. Cambridge, UK: Cambridge University Press; 2011.

82

American Academy of Pediatrics, Committee on Bioethics, Committee on Genetics, American College of Medical Genetics. Ethical and policy issues in genetic testing and screening of children. *Pediatrics*. 2013;131(3):620–622.

Quaid KA. Presymptomatic genetic testing in children. In: Miller G, ed. *Pediatric Bioethics*. New York: Cambridge University Press; 2010:125–140.

Ross LF. Ethical and policy issues in pediatric genetics. *Am J Med Genet C Semin Med Genet*. 2008;148C(1):1–7.

Ross LF, Moon MR. Ethical issues in genetic testing of children. *Arch Pediatr Adolesc Med*. 2000;154(9):873–879.

Ross LF, Saal HM, David KL, Anderson RR. Technical report: ethical and policy issues in genetic testing and screening of children. *Genet Med*. 2013;15(3):234–245.

Wade CH, Wilfond BS, McBride CM. Effects of genetic risk information on children's psychosocial wellbeing: a systematic review of the literature. *Genet Med*. 2010;12(6):317–326.

Wertz DC. Testing children and adolescents. In: Burley J, Harris J, eds. *A Companion to Genethics*. Malden, MA: Blackwell Publishers; 2002:92–113.

83

Botkin JR. Preventing exploitation in pediatric research. *Am J Bioeth*. 2003;3(4):31–32.

Field MJ, Behrman RE, eds. Institute of Medicine. *Ethical Conduct of Clinical Research Involving Children*. Washington, DC: National Academies Press; 2004.

Fleischman AR, Collogan LK. Research with children. In: Emanuel EJ, Grady C, Crouch RA, et al., eds. *The Oxford Textbook of Clinical Research Ethics*. New York: Oxford University Press; 2008:446–460.

Kodish E. Ethics and research with children: an introduction. In: Kodish E, ed. *Ethics and Research with Children: A Case-Based Approach*. Oxford; New York: Oxford University Press; 2005:3–25.

Moreno JD, Kravitt A. The ethics of pediatric research. In: Miller G, ed. *Pediatric Bioethics*. Cambridge, UK: Cambridge University Press; 2010:54–72.

National Commission for the Protection of Human Subjects of Biomedical and Behavioral Research. *Research Involving Children: Report and Recommendations*. Bethesda, MD: National Commission for the Protection of Human Subjects of Biomedical and Behavioral Research; 1977.

U.S. Department of Health and Human Services. Protection of human subjects: sub-part d—additional protections for children involved as subjects in research. 45 CFR §46.401–46.409 (2012).

Varma S, Wendler D. Risk-benefit assessment in pediatric research. In: Emanuel EJ, Grady C, Crouch RA, et al., eds. *The Oxford Textbook of Clinical Research Ethics*. New York: Oxford University Press; 2008:527–540.

Wendler D, Varma S. Minimal risk in pediatric research. *J Pediatr*. 2006;149(6):855–861.

84

Dove ES, Avard D, Black L, Knoppers BM. Emerging issues in paediatric health research consent forms in Canada: working towards best practices. *BMC Med Ethics*. 2013;14:5.

Ross LF. Informed consent in pediatric research. *Camb Q Healthc Ethics*. 2004;13(4):346–358.

85

Burke W, Diekema DS. Ethical issues arising from the participation of children in genetic research. *J Pediatr*. 2006;149(1 Suppl):S34–S38.

Kohane IS. No small matter: qualitatively distinct challenges of pediatric genomic studies. *Genome Med*. 2011;3(9):62.

McBride CM, Guttmacher AE. Commentary: trailblazing a research agenda at the interface of pediatrics and genomic discovery—a commentary on the psychological aspects of genomics and child health. *J Pediatr Psychol*. 2009;34(6):662–664.

86

Hester DM. Ethical issues in *Pediatrics*. In: Hester DM, Schonfeld T, eds. *Guidance for Healthcare Ethics Committees*. Cambridge, UK: Cambridge University Press; 2012:114–121.

Miller G, ed. *Pediatric Bioethics*. Cambridge, UK: Cambridge University Press; 2010.

Murray TH. *The Worth of a Child*. Berkeley, CA: University of California Press; 1996.

Ross LF. *Children, Families, and Health Care Decision-Making*. Oxford, UK: Oxford University Press; 1998.

Sayeed SA. The moral and legal status of children and parents. In: Miller G, ed. *Pediatric Bioethics*. Cambridge, UK: Cambridge University Press; 2010:38–53.

Unguru Y. Pediatric decision-making: informed consent, parental permission, and child assent. In: Diekema DS, Mercurio MR, Adam MB, eds. *Clinical Ethics in Pediatrics: A Case-Based Textbook*. Cambridge, UK: Cambridge University Press; 2011:1–6.

United Nations. United Nations Convention on the Rights of the Child, GA Res 44/736. Art. 18.01, 1989.

Wilfond B, Ross LF. From genetics to genomics: ethics, policy, and parental decision-making. *J Pediatr Psychol*. 2009;34(6):639–647.

87

Gaylin W. Who speaks for the child. In: Gaylin W, Macklin R, eds. *Who Speaks for the Child: The Problems of Proxy Consent*. New York: Plenum; 1982:3–26.

Gaylin W, Macklin R, eds. *Who Speaks for the Child: The Problems of Proxy Consent*. New York: Plenum Press; 1982. *The Hastings Center Series in Ethics*.

88

Goodlander EC, Berg JW. Pediatric decision-making: adolescent patients. In: Diekema DS, Mercurio MR, Adam MB, eds. *Clinical Ethics in Pediatrics: A Case-Based Textbook*. Cambridge, UK: Cambridge University Press; 2011:7–13.

89

Ross LF. Genetic testing of children: who should consent? In: Burley J, Harris J, eds. *A Companion to Genethics*. Oxford: Blackwell; 2002:114–126.

Wertz DC, Fanos JH, Reilly PR. Genetic testing for children and adolescents. Who decides? *JAMA*. 1994;272(11):875–881.

90

Anderson RR. Religious traditions and prenatal genetic counseling. *Am J Med Genet C Semin Med Genet*. 2009;151C(1):52–61.

Boudreault P, Baldwin EE, Fox M, et al. Deaf adults' reasons for genetic testing depend on cultural affiliation: results from a prospective, longitudinal genetic counseling and testing study. *J Deaf Stud Deaf Educ*. 2010;15(3):209–227.

Uhlmann W, Schuette J, Yashar B, eds. *A Guide to Genetic Counseling*. 2nd ed. Hoboken, NJ: Wiley-Blackwell; 2011.

91

Roche MI. A case of genetic counselling for Dr Watson. *Nature*. 2008;453(7193):281.

92

Fox RC. The evolution of medical uncertainty. *Milbank Mem Fund Q*. 1980;58(1):1–49.

Pullman D, Hodgkinson K. Genetic knowledge and moral responsibility: ambiguity at the interface of genetic research and clinical practice. *Clin Genet*. 2006;69(3):199–203.

93

Levine C, Faden R, Grady C, Hammerschmidt D, Eckenwiler L, Sugarman J. The limitations of "vulnerability" as a protection for human research participants. *Am J Bioeth*. 2004;4(3):44–49.

U.S. Department of Health and Human Services. *Institutional Review Board Guidebook*, Chapter VI: Special Classes of Subjects. Updated 1993. http://www.hhs.gov/ohrp/archive/irb/irb_chapter6.htm. Accessed August 15, 2013.

94

Danis M, Largent E, Grady C, et al. *Research Ethics Consultation: A Casebook*. Oxford, UK: Oxford University Press; 2012.

Emanuel EJ, Grady C, Crouch RA, et al., eds. *The Oxford Textbook of Clinical Research Ethics*. New York: Oxford University Press; 2008.

Emanuel EJ, Wendler D, Grady C. What makes clinical research ethical? *JAMA*. 2000;283(20):2701–2711.

Henry LM. Introduction: Revising the common rule: prospects and challenges. *J Law Med Ethics*. 2013;41(2):386–389.

Hoffmann DE, Fortenberry JD, Ravel J. Are changes to the common rule necessary to address evolving areas of research? A case study focusing on the human microbiome project. *J Law Med Ethics*. 2013;41(2):454–469.

King NMP, Churchill LR. Assessing and comparing potential benefits and risks of harm. In: Emanuel EJ, Grady C, Crouch RA, et al., eds. *The Oxford Textbook of Clinical Research Ethics*. New York: Oxford University Press; 2008:514–526.

Klitzman R, Appelbaum PS. Research ethics. To protect human subjects, review what was done, not proposed. *Science.* 2012;335(6076):1576–1577.

Kupersmith J. Advances in the research enterprise. Commentary. *Hastings Cent Rep.* 2013;43(Suppl):S43–S44.

Levine RJ. The nature, scope, and justification of clinical research: what is research? Who is a subject? In: Emanuel EJ, Grady C, Crouch RA, et al., eds. *The Oxford Textbook of Clinical Research Ethics.* New York: Oxford University Press; 2008:211–221.

Platt R, Grossmann C, Selker HP. Evaluation as part of operations: reconciling the common rule and continuous improvement. Commentary. *Hastings Cent Rep.* 2013;43(Suppl):S37–S39.

Puglisi T. Reform within the common rule? Commentary. *Hastings Cent Rep.* 2013;43(Suppl):S40–S42.

Shah SK. Outsourcing ethical obligations: should the revised common rule address the responsibilities of investigators and sponsors? *J Law Med Ethics.* 2013;41(2):397–410.

95

Facio FM, Brooks S, Loewenstein J, Green S, Biesecker LG, Biesecker BB. Motivators for participation in a whole-genome sequencing study: implications for translational genomics research. *Eur J Hum Genet.* 2011;19(12):1213–1217.

Fisher R. A closer look revisited: are we subjects or are we donors? *Genet Med.* 2012;14(4):458–460.

Harris J. Scientific research is a moral duty. *J Med Ethics.* 2005;31(4):242–248.

Kaufman D, Murphy J, Scott J, Hudson K. Subjects matter: a survey of public opinions about a large genetic cohort study. *Genet Med.* 2008;10(11):831–839.

96

Kaufman D, Geller G, Leroy L, Murphy J, Scott J, Hudson K. Ethical implications of including children in a large biobank for genetic-epidemiologic research: a qualitative study of public opinion. *Am J Med Genet C Semin Med Genet.* 2008;148C(1):31–39.

97

Flamm AL. Developing effective ethics policy. In: Hester DM, Schonfeld T, eds. *Guidance for Healthcare Ethics Committees.* Cambridge, UK: Cambridge University Press; 2012:130–138.

Hester DM, ed. *Ethics by Committee: A Textbook on Consultation, Organization, and Education for Hospital Ethics Committees.* Lanham, MD: Rowman & Littlefield Publishers; 2008.

Hester DM, Schonfeld T, eds. *Guidance for Healthcare Ethics Committees.* Cambridge, UK: Cambridge University Press; 2012.

Solomon MZ, Bonham AC. Ethical oversight of research on patient care. *Hastings Cent Rep.* 2013;43(Suppl):S2–S3.

98

National Commission for the Protection of Human Subjects of Biomedical and Behavioral Research. *The Belmont Report: Ethical Principles and Guidelines for the Protection of Human Subjects of Research.* Bethesda, MD: National Commission for the Protection of Human Subjects of Biomedical and Behavioral Research; 1978.

Presidential Commission for the Study of Bioethical Issues. *Moral Science: Protecting Participants in Human Subjects Research.* http://bioethics.gov/sites/default/files/

Moral%20Science%20June%202012.pdf. Published December 2011. Accessed July 9, 2013.

U.S. Department of Health and Human Services. Human subjects research protections: enhancing protections for research subjects and reducing burden, delay, and ambiguity for investigators—advance notice of proposed rulemaking. *Fed Regist.* 2011;76(143):44512–44531.

U.S. Department of Health and Human Services. *Institutional Review Board Guidebook,* Chapter VI: Special Classes of Subjects. Updated 1993. http://www.hhs.gov/ohrp/archive/irb/irb_chapter6.htm. Accessed August 15, 2013.

U.S. Department of Health and Human Services. Protection of human subjects. 45 CFR Pt. 46. Updated October 1, 2012.

World Medical Association. WMA Declaration of Helsinki: Ethical Principles for Medical Research Involving Human Subjects, *JAMA.* 2013;310(20):2191–2194.

World Medical Association. *WMA Declaration of Helsinki—Ethical Principles for Medical Research Involving Human Subjects.* WMA. http://www.wma.net/en/30publications/10policies/b3/. Amended October 2008. Accessed July 26, 2013.

99

Grady C, Denny C. Research involving women. In: Emanuel EJ, ed. *The Oxford Textbook of Clinical Research Ethics.* New York: Oxford University Press; 2008:407–422.

Green RM. Research with fetuses, embryos and stem cells. In: Emanuel EJ, Grady C, Crouch RA, eds. *The Oxford Textbook of Clinical Research Ethics.* New York: Oxford University Press; 2008:488–499.

U.S. Department of Health and Human Services. Protection of human subjects: subpart b—additional protections for pregnant women, human fetuses, and human neonates involved in research. 45 CFR § 46.201–46.207 (2012).

Walters L. Ethical and public policy issues in fetal research. *Research on the Fetus: Appendix. National Commission for the Protection of Human Subjects of Biomedical and Behavioral Research,* DHEW Publication No. (OS) 76–128. Bethesda, MD: Department of Health, Education and Welfare; 1975:8-1 to 8-18.

100

Simon C, Shinkunas LA, Brandt D, Williams JK. Individual genetic and genomic research results and the tradition of informed consent: exploring US review board guidance. *J Med Ethics.* 2012;38(7):417–422.

Simon CM, Williams JK, Shinkunas L, Brandt D, Daack-Hirsch S, Driessnack M. Informed consent and genomic incidental findings: IRB chair perspectives. *J Empir Res Hum Res Ethics.* 2011;6(4):53–67.

Wolf LE, Catania JA, Dolcini MM, Pollack LM, Lo B. IRB chairs' perspectives on genomics research involving stored biological materials: ethical concerns and proposed solutions. *J Empir Res Hum Res Ethics.* 2008;3(4):99–111.

101

Fullerton SM, Wolf WA, Brothers KB, et al. Return of individual research results from genome-wide association studies: experience of the Electronic Medical Records and Genomics (eMERGE) Network. *Genet Med.* 2012;14(4):424–431.

102

Brisson AR, Matsui D, Rieder MJ, Fraser DD. Translational research in pediatrics: tissue sampling and biobanking. *Pediatrics.* 2012;129(1):153–162.

Brothers KB. Biobanking in pediatrics: the human nonsubjects approach. *Per Med.* 2011;8(1):79.

Gurwitz D, Fortier I, Lunshof JE, Knoppers BM. Research ethics. Children and population biobanks. *Science.* 2009;325(5942):818–819.

Hens K, Nys H, Cassiman JJ, Dierickx K. Biological sample collections from minors for genetic research: a systematic review of guidelines and position papers. *Eur J Hum Genet.* 2009;17(8):979–990.

Samuel J, Knoppers BM, Avard D. Paediatric biobanks: what makes them so unique? *J Paediatr Child Health.* 2012;48(2):E1–E3.

103

Goldenberg AJ, Hull SC, Botkin JR, Wilfond BS. Pediatric biobanks: approaching informed consent for continuing research after children grow up. *J Pediatr.* 2009;155(4):578–583.

Hens K, Cassiman JJ, Nys H, Dierickx K. Children, biobanks and the scope of parental consent. *Eur J Hum Genet.* 2011;19(7):735–739.

Holm S. Informed consent and the bio-banking of material from children. *Genomics Soc Policy.* 2005;1(1):16–26.

104

Klima J, Fitzgerald-Butt SM, Kelleher KJ, et al. Understanding of informed consent by parents of children enrolled in a genetic biobank. *Genet Med.* 2013. doi: 10.1038/gim.2013.86.

105

Harris ED, Ziniel SI, Amatruda JG, et al. The beliefs, motivations, and expectations of parents who have enrolled their children in a genetic biorepository. *Genet Med.* 2012;14(3):330–337.

Hens K, Nys H, Cassiman JJ, Dierickx K. Genetic research on stored tissue samples from minors: a systematic review of the ethical literature. *Am J Med Genet A.* 2009;149A(10):2346–2358.

Hens K, Nys H, Cassiman JJ, Dierickx K. Risks, benefits, solidarity: a framework for the participation of children in genetic biobank research. *J Pediatr.* 2011;158(5):842–848.

106

Lockhart NC, Yassin R, Weil CJ, Compton CC. Intersection of biobanking and clinical care: should discrepant diagnoses and pathological findings be returned to research participants? *Genet Med.* 2012;14(4):417–423.

Miller FA, Giacomini M, Ahern C, Robert JS, de Laat S. When research seems like clinical care: a qualitative study of the communication of individual cancer genetic research results. *BMC Med Ethics.* 2008;9:4.

107

Appelbaum PS, Lidz CW. The therapeutic misconception. In: Emanuel EJ, Grady C, Crouch RA, et al., eds. *The Oxford Textbook of Clinical Research Ethics.* New York: Oxford University Press; 2008:633–644.

Appelbaum PS, Roth LH, Lidz CW, Benson P, Winslade W. False hopes and best data: consent to research and the therapeutic misconception. *Hastings Cent Rep.* 1987;17(2):20–24.

de Melo-Martin I, Ho A. Beyond informed consent: the therapeutic misconception and trust. *J Med Ethics.* 2008;34(3):202–205.

King NM, Henderson GE, Churchill LR, et al. Consent forms and the therapeutic misconception: the example of gene transfer research. *IRB.* 2005;27(1):1–8.

Lidz CW, Appelbaum PS. The therapeutic misconception: problems and solutions. *Med Care.* 2002;40(9 Suppl):V55–V63.

108

Gutmann A, Wagner JW. Found your DNA on the web: reconciling privacy and progress. *Hastings Cent Rep.* 2013;43(3):15–18.

Heeney C, Hawkins N, de Vries J, Boddington P, Kaye J. Assessing the privacy risks of data sharing in genomics. *Public Health Genomics.* 2010;14(1):17–25.

Kaye J, Wilbanks J. Privacy II—control, access, and human genome sequence data. *Presentation to the Presidential Commission for the Study of Bioethical Issues.* http://bioethics.gov/cms/node/659. Presented February 2, 2013. Accessed July 26, 2013.

Knoppers BM, Dove ES, Litton JE, Nietfeld JJ. Questioning the limits of genomic privacy. *Am J Hum Genet.* 2012;91(3):577–578; author reply 579.

Lewis MH. Laboratory specimens and genetic privacy: evolution of legal theory. *J Law Med Ethics.* 2013;41(Suppl 1):65–68.

Lunshof JE, Chadwick R, Vorhaus DB, Church GM. From genetic privacy to open consent. *Nat Rev Genet.* 2008;9(5):406–411.

Presidential Commission for the Study of Bioethical Issues. *Privacy and Progress in Whole Genome Sequencing.* http://bioethics.gov/sites/default/files/PrivacyProgress508_1.pdf. Published October 2012. Accessed July 23, 2013.

Warren S, Brandeis LD. The right to privacy. *Harvard Law Rev.* 1890;15(4):193–220.

109

Church G, Heeney C, Hawkins N, et al. Public access to genome-wide data: five views on balancing research with privacy and protection. *PLoS Genet.* 2009;5(10):e1000665.

Im HK, Gamazon ER, Nicolae DL, Cox NJ. On sharing quantitative trait GWAS results in an era of multiple-omics data and the limits of genomic privacy. *Am J Hum Genet.* 2012;90(4):591–598.

Lin Z, Owen AB, Altman RB. Genetics. Genomic research and human subject privacy. *Science.* 2004;305(5681):183.

Loukides G, Denny JC, Malin B. The disclosure of diagnosis codes can breach research participants' privacy. *J Am Med Inform Assoc.* 2010;17(3):322–327.

Ramos EM, Din-Lovinescu C, Bookman EB, et al. A mechanism for controlled access to GWAS data: experience of the GAIN Data Access Committee. *Am J Hum Genet.* 2013;92(4):479–488.

Rothstein MA. Disclosing decedents' research results to relatives violates the HIPAA Privacy Rule. *Am J Bioeth.* 2012;12(10):16–17.

110

Hudson KL, Collins FS. Biospecimen policy: family matters. *Nature.* 2013;500(7461):141–142.

Nyholt DR, Yu CE, Visscher PM. On Jim Watson's APOE status: genetic information is hard to hide. *Eur J Hum Genet.* 2009;17(2):147–149.

Williams BA, Wolf LE. Biobanking, consent, and certificates of confidentiality: does the ANPRM muddy the water? *J Law Med Ethics.* 2013;41(2):440–453.

Wjst M. Caught you: threats to confidentiality due to the public release of large-scale genetic data sets. *BMC Med Ethics*. 2010;11:21.

111

Bohannon J. Genetics. Genealogy databases enable naming of anonymous DNA donors. *Science*. 2013;339(6117):262.

Cassa CA, Schmidt B, Kohane IS, Mandl KD. My sister's keeper?: genomic research and the identifiability of siblings. *BMC Med Genomics*. 2008;1:32.

Couzin J. Genetic privacy. Whole-genome data not anonymous, challenging assumptions. *Science*. 2008;321(5894):1278.

Greenbaum D, Du J, Gerstein M. Genomic anonymity: have we already lost it? *Am J Bioeth*. 2008;8(10):71–74.

Gymrek M, McGuire AL, Golan D, Halperin E, Erlich Y. Identifying personal genomes by surname inference. *Science*. 2013;339(6117):321–324.

Hull SC, Sharp RR, Botkin JR, et al. Patients' views on identifiability of samples and informed consent for genetic research. *Am J Bioeth*. 2008;8(10):62–70.

Lowrance WW, Collins FS. Ethics. Identifiability in genomic research. *Science*. 2007;317(5838):600–602.

Rodriguez LL, Brooks LD, Greenberg JH, Green ED. Research ethics. The complexities of genomic identifiability. *Science*. 2013;339(6117):275–276.

Skloot R. *The Immortal Life of Henrietta Lacks*. New York: Crown Publishers; 2010.

Weil CJ, Mechanic LE, Green T, et al. NCI think tank concerning the identifiability of biospecimens and "omic" data. *Genet Med*. 2013. doi: 10.1038/gim.2013.40.

112

McGuire AL, Fisher R, Cusenza P, et al. Confidentiality, privacy, and security of genetic and genomic test information in electronic health records: points to consider. *Genet Med*. 2008;10(7):495–499.

113

Maschke KJ. Wanted: human biospecimens. *Hastings Cent Rep*. 2010;40(5):21–23.

Master Z, Claudio JO, Rachul C, Wang JC, Minden MD, Caulfield T. Cancer patient perceptions on the ethical and legal issues related to biobanking. *BMC Med Genomics*. 2013;6:8.

114

Beskow LM, Dean E. Informed consent for biorepositories: assessing prospective participants' understanding and opinions. *Cancer Epidemiol Biomarkers Prev*. 2008;17(6):1440–1451.

Caulfield T. Biobanks and blanket consent: the proper place of the public good and public perception rationales. *Kings Law J*. 2007;18(2):209–226.

Caulfield T, Kayet J. Broad consent in biobanking: reflections on seemingly insurmountable dilemmas. *Med Law Int*. 2009;10(2):85–100.

115

Murphy J, Scott J, Kaufman D, Geller G, LeRoy L, Hudson K. Public perspectives on informed consent for biobanking. *Am J Public Health*. 2009;99(12):2128–2134.

Nobile H, Vermeulen E, Thys K, Bergmann MM, Borry P. Why do participants enroll in population biobank studies? A systematic literature review. *Expert Rev Mol Diagn*. 2013;13(1):35–47.

Ormond KE, Cirino AL, Helenowski IB, Chisholm RL, Wolf WA. Assessing the understanding of biobank participants. *Am J Med Genet A.* 2009;149A(2):188–198.

116

Ashcroft R, Goodenough T, Williamson E, Kent J. Children's consent to research participation: social context and personal experience invalidate fixed cutoff rules. *Am J Bioeth.* 2003;3(4):16–18.

Diekema DS. Taking children seriously: what's so important about assent? *Am J Bioeth.* 2003;3(4):25–26.

Miller VA, Drotar D, Kodish E. Children's competence for assent and consent: a review of empirical findings. *Ethics Behav.* 2004;14(3):255–295.

Sibley A, Sheehan M, Pollard AJ. Assent is not consent. *J Med Ethics.* 2012;38(1):3.

Ungar D, Joffe S, Kodish E. Children are not small adults: documentation of assent for research involving children. *J Pediatr.* 2006;149(1 Suppl):S31–S33.

Unguru Y, Coppes MJ, Kamani N. Rethinking pediatric assent: from requirement to ideal. *Pediatr Clin North Am.* 2008;55(1):211–222.

Wendler D. The assent requirement in pediatric research. In: Emanuel EJ, Grady C, Crouch RA, et al., eds. *The Oxford Textbook of Clinical Research Ethics.* New York: Oxford University Press; 2008:661–672.

Wendler D, Shah S. Should children decide whether they are enrolled in nonbeneficial research? *Am J Bioeth.* 2003;3(4):1–7.

Wendler DS. Assent in paediatric research: theoretical and practical considerations. *J Med Ethics.* 2006;32(4):229–234.

Wilkinson D. Dissent about assent in paediatric research. *J Med Ethics.* 2012;38(1):2.

117

Wilfond BS, Diekema DS. Engaging children in genomics research: decoding the meaning of assent in research. *Genet Med.* 2012;14(4):437–443.

118

Paul DB. A double-edged sword. *Nature.* 2000;405(6786):515.

Potter BK, Avard D, Entwistle V, et al. Ethical, legal, and social issues in health technology assessment for prenatal/preconceptional and newborn screening: a workshop report. *Public Health Genomics.* 2009;12(1):4–10.

119

Guthrie R, Susi A. A simple phenylalanine method for detecting phenylketonuria in large populations of newborn infants. *Pediatrics.* 1963;32:338–343.

Rosenberg LE. Legacies of Garrod's brilliance: one hundred years—and counting. *J Inherit Metab Dis.* 2008;31(5):574–579.

120

Harris R. Overview of screening: where we are and where we may be headed. *Epidemiol Rev.* 2011;33(1):1–6.

Hasegawa LE, Fergus KA, Ojeda N, Au SM. Parental attitudes toward ethical and social issues surrounding the expansion of newborn screening using new technologies. *Public Health Genomics.* 2011;14(4–5):298–306.

Hiraki S, Green NS. Newborn screening for treatable genetic conditions: past, present and future. *Obstet Gynecol Clin North Am.* 2010;37(1):11–21.

Hoffmann GF, Cornejo V, Pollitt RJ. Newborn screening—progress and challenges. *J Inherit Metab Dis.* 2010;33(Suppl 2):S199–S200.

Hoffmann GF, Fang-Hoffmann J, Lindner M, Burgard P. Clinical advances and challenges of extended newborn screening. [abstract]. *J Inherit Metab Dis.* 2011;34(Suppl 1): S1.

International Congress on Prevention of Congenital Diseases. Screening newborns: current state and future challenges. Abstracts of the International Congress on Prevention of Congenital Diseases. Vienna, Austria. May 13-14, 2011. *J Inherit Metab Dis.* 2011;34(Suppl 1):S1–S16.

Levy HL. Newborn screening conditions: what we know, what we do not know, and how we will know it. *Genet Med.* 2010;12(12 Suppl):S213–S214.

Roe AM, Shur N. From new screens to discovered genes: the successful past and promising present of single gene disorders. *Am J Med Genet C Semin Med Genet.* 2007;145C(1):77–86.

Tarini BA. The current revolution in newborn screening: new technology, old controversies. *Arch Pediatr Adolesc Med.* 2007;161(8):767–772.

Therrell BL. U.S. newborn screening policy dilemmas for the twenty-first century. *Mol Genet Metab.* 2001;74(1–2):64–74.

Therrell BL, Johnson A, Williams D. Status of newborn screening programs in the United States. *Pediatrics.* 2006;117(5 Pt 2):S212–S252.

Vockley J. Newborn screening: after the thrill is gone. *Mol Genet Metab.* 2007;92(1–2):6–12.

Watson MS. Current status of newborn screening: decision-making about the conditions to include in screening programs. *Ment Retard Dev Disabil Res Rev.* 2006;12(4):230–235.

Wilfond BS, Gollust SE. Policy issues for expanding newborn screening programs: the cystic fibrosis newborn screening experience in the United States. *J Pediatr.* 2005;146(5):668–674.

121

Alexander D, van Dyck PC. In reply: neonatal screening: old dogma or sound principle? *Pediatrics.* 2007;119(2):407.

Alexander D, van Dyck PC. A vision of the future of newborn screening. *Pediatrics.* 2006;117(5 Pt 2):S350–S354.

Clayton EW. Lessons to be learned from the move toward expanded newborn screening. In: Baily MA, Murray TH, eds. *Ethics and Newborn Genetic Screening: New Technologies, New Challenges.* Baltimore: Johns Hopkins University Press; 2009:125–135.

Fearing MK, Levy HL. Expanded newborn screening using tandem mass spectrometry. *Adv Pediatr.* 2003;50:81–111.

Fleischman AR, Lin BK, Howse JL. A commentary on the President's Council on Bioethics report: the changing moral focus of newborn screening. *Genet Med.* 2009;11(7):507–509.

Hiraki S, Ormond KE, Kim K, Ross LF. Attitudes of genetic counselors towards expanding newborn screening and offering predictive genetic testing to children. *Am J Med Genet A.* 2006;140(21):2312–2319.

Levy HL. Lessons from the past—looking to the future. Newborn screening. *Pediatric Annals.* 2003;32(8):505–508.

Levy HL. Newborn screening by tandem mass spectrometry: a new era. *Clin Chem.* 1998;44(12):2401–2402.

Millington DS, Kodo N, Norwood DL, Roe CR. Tandem mass spectrometry: a new method for acylcarnitine profiling with potential for neonatal screening for inborn errors of metabolism. *J Inherit Metab Dis.* 1990;13(3):321–324.

Rinaldo P, Matern D. Newborn screening for inherited metabolic disease. In: Hoffman GF, Zschocke J, Nyhan WL, eds. *Inherited Metabolic Diseases: A Clinical Approach.* Berlin: Springer-Verlag; 2010:251–261.

Wald N. Neonatal screening: old dogma or sound principle? *Pediatrics.* 2007;119(2):406–407; author reply 407.

122

American Academy of Pediatrics Committee on Fetus and Newborn. Screening of newborn infants for metabolic disease. *Pediatrics.* 1965;35(3):499–501.

American College of Medical Genetics Newborn Screening Expert Group. Newborn screening: toward a uniform screening panel and system. *Genet Med.* 2006;8(Suppl 1):1S–252S.

American College of Obstetricians and Gynecologists. ACOG Committee Opinion No. 393, December 2007. Newborn screening. *Obstet Gynecol.* 2007;110(6):1497–1500.

Howell RR, Lloyd-Puryear MA. From developing guidelines to implementing legislation: actions of the US Advisory Committee on Heritable Disorders in Newborns and Children toward advancing and improving newborn screening. *Semin Perinatol.* 2010;34(2):121–124.

President's Council on Bioethics. *The Changing Moral Focus of Newborn Screening: An Ethical Analysis by the President's Council on Bioethics.* Washington, DC: President's Council on Bioethics; 2008.

President's Panel on Mental Retardation. *A Proposed Program for National Action to Combat Mental Retardation.* Washington, DC: The President's Panel on Mental Retardation; 1962.

Trotter TL, Fleischman AR, Howell RR, Lloyd-Puryear M. Secretary's Advisory Committee on Heritable Disorders in Newborns and Children response to the President's Council on Bioethics report: the changing moral focus of newborn screening. *Genet Med.* 2011;13(4):301–304.

U.S. Department of Health and Human Services. Secretary's Advisory Committee on Heritable Disorders and Genetic Diseases in Newborns and Children. Briefing paper—considerations and recommendations for a national policy regarding the retention and use of dried blood spot specimens after newborn screening. http://www.hrsa.gov/advisorycommittees/mchbadvisory/heritabledisorders/recommendations/correspondence/briefingdriedblood.pdf. Published September 2010. Accessed July 17, 2013.

World Health Organization Scientific Group on Screening for Inborn Errors of Metabolism. *Screening for Inborn Errors of Metabolism.* World Health Organization Technical Report Series. Geneva: World Health Organization; 1968.

123

Comeau AM, Parad RB, Dorkin HL, et al. Population-based newborn screening for genetic disorders when multiple mutation DNA testing is incorporated: a cystic fibrosis newborn screening model demonstrating increased sensitivity but more carrier detections. *Pediatrics.* 2004;113(6):1573–1581.

Goldenberg AJ, Dodson DS, Davis MM, Tarini BA. Parents' interest in whole-genome sequencing of newborns. *Genet Med.* 2013. doi 10.1038/gim.2013.76.

Goldenberg AJ, Sharp RR. The ethical hazards and programmatic challenges of genomic newborn screening. *JAMA.* 2012;307(5):461–462.

Green NS, Pass KA. Neonatal screening by DNA microarray: spots and chips. *Nature Rev Genet.* 2005;6(2):147–151.

Grosse SD, Rogowski WH, Ross LF, Cornel MC, Dondorp WJ, Khoury MJ. Population screening for genetic disorders in the 21st century: evidence, economics, and ethics. *Public Health Genomics*. 2010;13(2):106–115.

Kemper AR, Trotter TL, Lloyd-Puryear MA, Kyler P, Feero WG, Howell RR. A blueprint for maternal and child health primary care physician education in medical genetics and genomic medicine: recommendations of the United States secretary for health and human services advisory committee on heritable disorders in newborns and children. *Genet Med*. 2010;12(2):77–80.

Khoury MJ. Public health genomics: the end of the beginning. *Genet Med*. 2011;13(3):206–209.

McCandless SE, Chandrasekar R, Linard S, Kikano S, Rice L. Sequencing from dried blood spots in infants with "false positive" newborn screen for MCAD deficiency. *Mol Genet Metab*. 2013;108(1):51–55.

Welch HG, Schwartz L, Woloshin S. *Overdiagnosed: Making People Sick in the Pursuit of Health*. Boston, MA: Beacon Press; 2011.

124

Andermann A, Blancquaert I, Beauchamp S, Dery V. Revisiting Wilson and Jungner in the genomic age: a review of screening criteria over the past 40 years. *Bull World Health Organ*. 2008;86(4):317–319.

Andermann A, Blancquaert I, Dery V. Genetic screening: a conceptual framework for programmes and policy-making. *J Health Serv Res Policy*. 2010;15(2):90–97.

Petros M. Revisiting the Wilson-Jungner criteria: how can supplemental criteria guide public health in the era of genetic screening? *Genet Med*. 2012;14(1):129–134.

Ross LF. Newborn screening for conditions that do not meet the Wilson and Jungner criteria: the case of Duchenne muscular dystrophy. In: Baily MA, Murray TH, eds. *Ethics and Newborn Genetic Screening: New Technologies, New Challenges*. Baltimore: Johns Hopkins University Press; 2009:106–124.

Wilson JMG. Current trends and problems in health screening. *J Clin Pathol*. 1973;26(8):555–563.

Wilson JMG, Jungner G. *Principles and Practice of Screening for Disease*. Public Health Papers No. 34. Geneva: WHO; 1968. http://whqlibdoc.who.int/php/WHO_PHP_34.pdf. Accessed July 26, 2013.

125

Baily MA, Murray TH. Ethics, evidence, and cost in newborn screening. *Hastings Cent Rep*. 2008;38(3):23–31.

Baily MA, Murray TH, eds. *Ethics and Newborn Genetic Screening: New Technologies, New Challenges*. Baltimore: Johns Hopkins University Press; 2009.

Bayer R. Stigma and the ethics of public health: not can we but should we. *Soc Sci Med*. 2008;67(3):463–472.

Botkin JR, Clayton EW, Fost NC, et al. Newborn screening technology: proceed with caution. *Pediatrics*. 2006;117(5):1793–1799.

Childress JF, Faden RR, Gaare RD, et al. Public health ethics: mapping the terrain. *J Law Med Ethics*. 2002;30(2):170–178.

Colgrove J, Bayer R. Manifold restraints: liberty, public health, and the legacy of Jacobson v Massachusetts. *Am J Public Health*. 2005;95(4):571–576.

Gonzales JL. Ethics for the pediatrician: genetic testing and newborn screening. *Pediatr Rev*. 2011;32(11):490–493.

Green N. Every child is priceless: debating effective newborn screening policy. *Hastings Cent Rep.* 2009;39(1):6–7; author reply 7–8.

Green NS, Dolan SM, Murray TH. Newborn screening: complexities in universal genetic testing. *Am J Public Health.* 2006;96(11):1955–1959.

Grosse SD, Boyle CA, Kenneson A, Khoury MJ, Wilfond BS. From public health emergency to public health service: the implications of evolving criteria for newborn screening panels. *Pediatrics.* 2006;117(3):923–929.

Hoffmann DE, Rothenberg KH. Whose duty is it anyway? The Kennedy Krieger opinion and its implications for public health research. *J Health Care Law Policy.* 2002;6(1):109–147.

Howell RR. Every child is priceless: debating effective newborn screening policy. *Hastings Cent Rep.* 2009;39(1):4–6; author reply 7–8.

Jennings B. Frameworks for ethics in public health. *Acta Bioethica.* 2003;9(2):165–176.

Levin BW, Fleischman AR. Public health and bioethics: the benefits of collaboration. *Am J Public Health.* 2002;92(2):165–167.

Mastroianni AC, Kahn JP. Risk and responsibility: ethics, Grimes v Kennedy Krieger, and public health research involving children. *Am J Public Health.* 2002;92(7):1073–1076.

McCabe LL, Therrell BL Jr, McCabe ERB. Newborn screening: rationale for a comprehensive, fully integrated public health system. *Mol Genet Metab.* 2002;77(4):267–273

Moyer VA, Calonge N, Teutsch SM, Botkin JR. Expanding newborn screening: process, policy, and priorities. *Hastings Cent Rep.* 2008;38(3):32–39.

Ross LF. Newborn screening. In: Miller G, ed. *Pediatric Bioethics.* Cambridge, UK: Cambridge University Press; 2010:111–124.

Wilcken B. The consequences of extended newborn screening programmes: do we know who needs treatment? *J Inherit Metab Dis.* 2008;31(2):173–177.

Wilcken B. Expanded newborn screening: reducing harm, assessing benefit. *J Inherit Metab Dis.* 2010;33(Suppl 2):S205–S210.

Wilfond BS, Parad RB, Fost N. Balancing benefits and risks for cystic fibrosis newborn screening: implications for policy decisions. *J Pediatr.* 2005;147(3 Suppl):S109–S113.

Wilfond BS, Thomson EJ. Models of public health genetic policy development. In: Khoury MJ, Burke W, Thomson EJ, eds. *Genetics and Public Health in the 21st Century: Using Genetic Information to Improve Health and Prevent Disease.* New York: Oxford University Press; 2000:61–81.

126

Bailey DB Jr. The blurred distinction between treatable and untreatable conditions in newborn screening. *Health Matrix.* 2009;19(1):141–153.

Plass AMC, van El CG, Pieters T, Cornel MC. Neonatal screening for treatable and untreatable disorders: prospective parents' opinions. *Pediatrics.* 2010;125(1):e99–e106.

127

Botkin JR. Evidence-based reviews of newborn-screening opportunities. *Pediatrics.* 2010;125(5):e1265–e1266.

Calonge N, Green NS, Rinaldo P, et al. Committee report: method for evaluating conditions nominated for population-based screening of newborns and children. *Genet Med.* 2010;12(3):153–159.

Ewart RM. Primum non nocere and the quality of evidence: rethinking the ethics of screening. *J Am Board Fam Pract.* 2000;13(3):188–196.

Fleischman AR, Howse JL. Newborn screening—the unique role of unique evidence. *Genet Med.* 2010;12(3):160–161.

Holtzman NA. Expanding newborn screening: how good is the evidence? *JAMA.* 2003;290(19):2606–2608.

Kemper AR, Knapp AA, Green NS, Comeau AM, Metterville DR, Perrin JM. Weighing the evidence for newborn screening for early-infantile Krabbe disease. *Genet Med.* 2010;12(9):539–543.

Lipstein EA, Vorono S, Browning MF, et al. Systematic evidence review of newborn screening and treatment of severe combined immunodeficiency. *Pediatrics.* 2010;125(5):e1226–e1235.

Marsden D, Levy H. Newborn screening of lysosomal storage disorders. *Clin Chem.* 2010;56(7):1071–1079.

Perrin JM, Knapp AA, Browning MF, et al. An evidence development process for newborn screening. *Genet Med.* 2010;12(3):131–134.

128

Andresen BS, Dobrowolski SF, O'Reilly L, et al. Medium-chain acyl-CoA dehydrogenase (MCAD) mutations identified by MS/MS-based prospective screening of newborns differ from those observed in patients with clinical symptoms: identification and characterization of a new, prevalent mutation that results in mild MCAD deficiency. *Am J Hum Genet.* 2001;68(6):1408–1418.

Arnold GL, Saavedra-Matiz CA, Galvin-Parton PA, et al. Lack of genotype-phenotype correlations and outcome in MCAD deficiency diagnosed by newborn screening in New York State. *Mol Genet Metab.* 2010;99(3):263–268.

Ensenauer R, Vockley J, Willard J-M, et al. A common mutation is associated with a mild, potentially asymptomatic phenotype in patients with isovaleric acidemia diagnosed by newborn screening. *Am J Hum Genet.* 2004;75(6):1136–1142.

Puckett RL, Lorey F, Rinaldo P, et al. Maple syrup urine disease: further evidence that newborn screening may fail to identify variant forms. *Mol Genet Metab.* 2010;100(2):136–142.

Smith EH, Thomas C, McHugh D, et al. Allelic diversity in MCAD deficiency: the biochemical classification of 54 variants identified during 5 years of ACADM sequencing. *Mol Genet Metab.* 2010;100(3):241–250.

Tluczek A, Chevalier McKechnie A, Lynam PA. When the cystic fibrosis label does not fit: a modified uncertainty theory. *Qual Health Res.* 2010;20(2):209–223.

van Calcar SC, Gleason LA, Lindh H, et al. 2-methylbutyryl-CoA dehydrogenase deficiency in Hmong infants identified by expanded newborn screen. *WMJ.* 2007;106(1):12–15.

Waddell L, Wiley V, Carpenter K, et al. Medium-chain acyl-CoA dehydrogenase deficiency: genotype-biochemical phenotype correlations. *Mol Genet Metab.* 2006;87(1):32–39.

129

Whitmarsh I, Davis AM, Skinner D, Bailey DB Jr. A place for genetic uncertainty: parents valuing an unknown in the meaning of disease. *Soc Sci Med.* 2007;65(6):1082–1093.

130

Brosco JP, Sanders LM, Dharia R, Guez G, Feudtner C. The lure of treatment: expanded newborn screening and the curious case of histidinemia. *Pediatrics*. 2010;125(3):417–419.

Lantos JD. Dangerous and expensive screening and treatment for rare childhood diseases: the case of Krabbe disease. *Dev Disabil Res Rev*. 2011;17(1):15–18.

Malm HM. Medical screening and the value of early detection. When unwarranted faith leads to unethical recommendations. *Hastings Cent Rep*. 1999;29(1):26–37.

131

Carmichael M. Newborn screening: a spot of trouble. *Nature*. 2011;475(7355):156–158.

Clayton EW. Currents in contemporary ethics. State run newborn screening in the genomic era, or how to avoid drowning when drinking from a fire hose. *J Law Med Ethics*. 2010;38(3):697–700.

Malpas PJ. Predictive genetic testing of children for adult-onset diseases and psychological harm. *J Med Ethics*. 2008;34(4):275–278.

Pelias MK. Genetic testing of children for adult-onset diseases: is testing in the child's best interests? *Mt Sinai J Med*. 2006;73(3):605–608.

Pollitt RJ. Introducing new screens: why are we all doing different things? *J Inherit Metab Dis*. 2007;30(4):423–429.

132

Clayton EW. Ten fingers, ten toes: newborn screening for untreatable disorders. *Health Matrix*. 2009;19(1):199–203.

133

Dunn CT, Skrypek MM, Powers ALR, Laguna TA. The need for vigilance: the case of a false-negative newborn screen for cystic fibrosis. *Pediatrics*. 2011;128(2):e446–e449.

Ficicioglu C, Coughlin CR 2nd, Bennett MJ, Yudkoff M. Very long-chain acyl-CoA dehydrogenase deficiency in a patient with normal newborn screening by tandem mass spectrometry. *J Pediatr*. 2010;156(3):492–494.

Fritz A, Farrell P. Estimating the annual number of false negative cystic fibrosis newborn screening tests. *Pediatr Pulmonol*. 2012;47(2):207–208.

Gurian E, Waisbren S. The physical, emotional, and financial trauma incurred by infants and their families when an existing condition is not detected by newborn screening: in reply. *Pediatrics*. 2006;118(4):1802.

134

Hayeems RZ, Bytautas JP, Miller FA. A systematic review of the effects of disclosing carrier results generated through newborn screening. *J Genet Couns*. 2008;17(6):538–549.

Lewis C, Skirton H, Jones R. Can we make assumptions about the psychosocial impact of living as a carrier, based on studies assessing the effects of carrier testing? *J Genet Couns*. 2011;20(1):80–97.

McClaren BJ, Aitken M, Massie J, Amor D, Ukoumunne OC, Metcalfe SA. Cascade carrier testing after a child is diagnosed with cystic fibrosis through newborn screening: investigating why most relatives do not have testing. *Genet Med*. 2013;15(7):533–540.

Miller FA, Paynter M, Hayeems RZ, et al. Understanding sickle cell carrier status identified through newborn screening: a qualitative study. *Eur J Hum Genet.* 2010;18(3):303–308.

Miller FA, Robert JS, Hayeems RZ. Questioning the consensus: managing carrier status results generated by newborn screening. *Am J Public Health.* 2009;99(2):210–215.

National Human Genome Research Institute. Summary of population-based carrier screening for single gene disorders: lessons learned and new opportunities. Rockville, MD: NIH, February 6–7, 2008. http://www.genome.gov/27026048. Accessed July 25, 2013.

Wilfond BS. Ethical and policy implications of conducting carrier testing and newborn screening for the same condition. In: Baily MA, Murray TH, eds. *Ethics and Newborn Genetic Screening: New Technologies, New Challenges.* Baltimore, MD: Johns Hopkins University Press; 2009:292–311.

135

Tarini BA, Singer D, Clark SJ, Davis MM. Parents' interest in predictive genetic testing for their children when a disease has no treatment. *Pediatrics.* 2009;124(3):e432–e438.

Tarini BA, Tercyak KP, Wilfond BS. Commentary: Children and predictive genomic testing: disease prevention, research protection, and our future. *J Pediatr Psychol.* 2011;36(10):1113–1121.

136

Bredenoord AL, de Vries MC, van Delden JJ. Next-generation sequencing: does the next generation still have a right to an open future? *Nat Rev Genet.* 2013;14(5):306.

Feinberg J. The child's right to an open future. In: Aiken W, Lafollette H, eds. *Whose Child? Children's Rights, Parental Authority, and State Power.* Totowa, NJ: Littlefield, Adams; 1980:124–153.

137

Botkin JR, Rothwell E, Anderson R, et al. Public attitudes regarding the use of residual newborn screening specimens for research. *Pediatrics.* 2012;129(2):231–238.

Couzin-Frankel J. Newborn blood collections. Science gold mine, ethical minefield. *Science.* 2009;324(5924):166–168.

Hens K, Nys H, Cassiman JJ, Dierickx K. The storage and use of biological tissue samples from minors for research: a focus group study. *Public Health Genomics.* 2011;14(2):68–76.

Lewis MH, Goldenberg A, Anderson R, Rothwell E, Botkin JR. State laws regarding the retention and use of residual newborn screening blood samples. *Pediatrics.* 2011;127(4):703–712.

Maschke KE. Ethical and policy issues involving research with newborn screening blood samples. In: Baily MA, Murray TH, eds. *Ethics and Newborn Genetic Screening: New Technologies, New Challenges.* Baltimore, MD: Johns Hopkins University Press; 2009:237–254.

Olney RS, Moore CA, Ojodu JA, Lindegren ML, Hannon WH. Storage and use of residual dried blood spots from state newborn screening programs. *J Pediatr.* 2006;148(5):618–622.

Rothwell E, Anderson R, Goldenberg A, et al. Assessing public attitudes on the retention and use of residual newborn screening blood samples: a focus group study. *Soc Sci Med.* 2012;74(8):1305–1309.

Rothwell EW, Anderson RA, Burbank MJ, et al. Concerns of newborn blood screening advisory committee members regarding storage and use of residual newborn screening blood spots. *Am J Public Health.* 2011;101(11):2111–2116.

Tarini BA. Storage and use of residual newborn screening blood spots: a public policy emergency. *Genet Med.* 2011;13(7):619–620.

Therrell BL, Hannon WH, Bailey DB, et al. Committee report: considerations and recommendations for national guidance regarding the retention and use of residual dried blood spot specimens after newborn screening. *Genet Med.* 2011;13(7):621–624.

138

Miller FA, Hayeems RZ, Carroll JC, et al. Consent for newborn screening: the attitudes of health care providers. *Public Health Genomics.* 2010;13(3):181–190.

Newson A. Should parental refusals of newborn screening be respected? *Camb Q Healthc Ethics.* 2006;15(2):135–146.

Press N, Clayton EW. Genetics and public health: informed consent beyond the clinical encounter. In: Khoury MJ, Burke W, Thomson EJ, eds. *Genetics and Public Health in the 21st Century: Using Genetic Information to Improve Health and Prevent Disease.* New York: Oxford University Press; 2000:505–526.

Ross LF. Mandatory versus voluntary consent for newborn screening? *Kennedy Inst Ethics J.* 2010;20(4):299–328.

Tarini BA, Burke W, Scott CR, Wilfond BS. Waiving informed consent in newborn screening research: balancing social value and respect. *Am J Med Genet C Semin Med Genet.* 2008;148C(1):23–30.

Tarini BA, Goldenberg A, Singer D, Clark SJ, Butchart A, Davis MM. Not without my permission: parents' willingness to permit use of newborn screening samples for research. *Public Health Genomics.* 2010;13(3):125–130.

Whitehead NS, Brown DS, Layton CM. *Survey of Parental Attitudes Regarding Voluntary Newborn Screening.* [pamphlet]. Research Triangle Park, NC: RTI Press; 2010.

139

Annas GJ. Mandatory PKU screening: the other side of the looking glass. *Am J Public Health.* 1982;72(12):1401–1403.

Faden R, Chwalow AJ, Holtzman NA, Horn SD. A survey to evaluate parental consent as public policy for neonatal screening. *Am J Public Health.* 1982;72(12):1347–1352.

Faden RR, Holtzman NA, Chwalow AJ. Parental rights, child welfare, and public health: the case of PKU screening. *Am J Public Health.* 1982;72(12):1396–1400.

Holtzman NA, Faden R, Chwalow AJ, Horn SD. Effect of informed parental consent on mothers' knowledge of newborn screening. *Pediatrics.* 1983;72(6):807–812.

Kopelman L. Genetic screening in newborns: voluntary or compulsory? *Perspect Biol Med.* 1978;22(1):83–89.

Paul DB. Contesting consent: the challenge to compulsory neonatal screening for PKU. *Perspect Biol Med.* 1999;42(2):207–219.

140

Bearder et al. v State of Minnesota et al., No. A10–101 (Minn. 2011).

Beleno et al. v Texas Department of State Health Services et al., Case No. 5:2009cv00188 (W.D. Tex. 2009).

141

Benkendorf J, Goodspeed T, Watson MS. Newborn screening residual dried blood spot use for newborn screening quality improvement. *Genet Med.* 2010;12(12 Suppl):S269–S272.

142

Botkin JR. Parental permission for research in newborn screening. In: Baily MA, Murray TH, eds. *Ethics and Newborn Genetic Screening: New Technologies, New Challenges.* Baltimore, MD: Johns Hopkins University Press; 2009:255–273.

143

Daniels N, Kennedy BP, Kawachi I. Why justice is good for our health: the social determinants of health inequalities. *Daedalus.* 1999;128(4):215–251.

Lurie N. Health disparities—less talk, more action. *N Engl J Med.* 2005;353(7):727–729.

Powers M, Faden RR. *Social Justice: The Moral Foundations of Public Health and Health Policy.* Oxford, UK: Oxford University Press; 2006. Issues in Biomedical Ethics.

Ross LF. Newborn screening for cystic fibrosis: a lesson in public health disparities. *J Pediatr.* 2008;153(3):308–313.

144

Berry SA, Brown C, Grant M, et al. Newborn screening 50 years later: access issues faced by adults with PKU. *Genet Med.* 2013. doi: 10.1038/gim.2013.10.

145

Berry SA, Lloyd-Puryear MA, Watson MS. Long-term follow-up of newborn screening patients. *Genet Med.* 2010;12(12 Suppl):S267–S268.

Hoff T, Hoyt A, Therrell B, Ayoob M. Exploring barriers to long-term follow-up in newborn screening programs. *Genet Med.* 2006;8(9):563–570.

James PM, Levy HL. The clinical aspects of newborn screening: importance of newborn screening follow-up. *Ment Retard Dev Disabil Res Rev.* 2006;12(4):246–254.

La Pean A, Collins JL, Christopher SA, et al. A qualitative secondary evaluation of statewide follow-up interviews for abnormal newborn screening results for cystic fibrosis and sickle cell hemoglobinopathy. *Genet Med.* 2012;14(2):207–214.

Lloyd-Puryear MA, Brower A. Long-term follow-up in newborn screening: A systems approach for improving health outcomes. *Genet Med.* 2010;12(12 Suppl):S256–S260.

146

Bowlby J. *Attachment.* New York: Basic Books; 1969. *Attachment and Loss*; vol 1.

Brazelton TB, Koslowski B, Main M. The origins of reciprocity: the early mother-infant interaction. In: Lewis M, Rosenblum L, eds. *The Effect of the Infant on Its Caregiver.* New York: Wiley; 1974:49–76.

Zelkowitz P, Papageorgiou A, Bardin C, Wang T. Persistent maternal anxiety affects the interaction between mothers and their very low birthweight children at 24 months. *Early Hum Dev.* 2009;85(1):51–58.

147

Davis TC, Humiston SG, Arnold CL, et al. Recommendations for effective newborn screening communication: results of focus groups with parents, providers, and experts. *Pediatrics.* 2006;117(5 Pt 2):S326–S340.

Farrell MH, Christopher SA, Tluczek A, et al. Improving communication between doctors and parents after newborn screening. *WMJ.* 2011;110(5):221–227.

Farrell MH, Speiser J, Deuster L, Christopher S. Child health providers' precautionary discussion of emotions during communication about results of newborn genetic screening. *Arch Pediatr Adolesc Med.* 2012;166(1):62–67.

La Pean A, Farrell MH. Initially misleading communication of carrier results after newborn genetic screening. *Pediatrics.* 2005;116(6):1499–1505.

Tarini BA. Communicating with parents about newborn screening: the skill of eliciting unspoken emotions. *Arch Pediatr Adolesc Med.* 2012;166(1):95–96.

148

Dillard JP, Shen L, Robinson JD, Farrell PM. Parental information seeking following a positive newborn screening for cystic fibrosis. *J Health Commun.* 2010;15(8):880–894.

Larsson AK, Svalenius E, Lundqvist A, Dykes AK. Parents' experiences of an abnormal ultrasound examination—vacillating between emotional confusion and sense of reality. *Reprod Health.* 2010;7(1):10.

Waisbren SE, Rones M, Read CY, Marsden D, Levy HL. Brief report: predictors of parenting stress among parents of children with biochemical genetic disorders. *J Pediatr Psychol.* 2004;29(7):565–570.

149

Cavanagh L, Compton CJ, Tluczek A, Brown RL, Farrell PM. Long-term evaluation of genetic counseling following false-positive newborn screen for cystic fibrosis. *J Genet Couns.* 2010;19(2):199–210.

Kladny B, Williams A, Gupta A, Gettig EA, Krishnamurti L. Genetic counseling following the detection of hemoglobinopathy trait on the newborn screen is well received, improves knowledge, and relieves anxiety. *Genet Med.* 2011;13(7):658–661.

Lantos JD. Maybe we are getting better at counseling. [eLetter]. *Pediatrics.* http://pediatrics.aappublications.org/content/128/4/715.abstract/reply#pediatrics_el_51684. Published September 26, 2011. Accessed July 18, 2013.

Tluczek A, Zaleski C, Stachiw-Hietpas D, et al. A tailored approach to family-centered genetic counseling for cystic fibrosis newborn screening: the Wisconsin model. *J Genet Couns.* 2011;20(2):115–128.

Wheeler PG, Smith R, Dorkin HL, Parad RB, Comeau AM, Bianchi DW. Genetic counseling after implementation of statewide cystic fibrosis newborn screening: Two years' experience in one medical center. *Genet Med.* 2001;3(6):411–415.

150

Lang CW, McColley SA, Lester LA, Ross LF. Parental understanding of newborn screening for cystic fibrosis after a negative sweat-test. *Pediatrics.* 2011;127(2):276–283.

Lang CW, Stark AP, Acharya K, Ross LF. Maternal knowledge and attitudes about newborn screening for sickle cell disease and cystic fibrosis. *Am J Med Genet A.* 2009;149A(11):2424–2429.

151

Merelle ME, Huisman J, Alderden-van der Vecht A, et al. Early versus late diagnosis: psychological impact on parents of children with cystic fibrosis. *Pediatrics.* 2003;111(2):346–350.

152

Beucher J, Leray E, Deneuville E, et al. Psychological effects of false-positive results in cystic fibrosis newborn screening: a two-year follow-up. *J Pediatr.* 2010;156(5):771–776, 776.e1.

Fyro K. Neonatal screening: life-stress scores in families given a false-positive result. *Acta Paediatr Scand.* 1988;77(2):232–238.

Gurian EA, Kinnamon DD, Henry JJ, Waisbren SE. Expanded newborn screening for biochemical disorders: the effect of a false-positive result. *Pediatrics.* 2006;117(6):1915–1921.

Hewlett J, Waisbren SE. A review of the psychosocial effects of false-positive results on parents and current communication practices in newborn screening. *J Inherit Metab Dis.* 2006;29(5):677–682.

Howell RR. The high price of false positives. *Mol Genet Metab.* 2006;87(3):180–183.

Kwon C, Farrell PM. The magnitude and challenge of false-positive newborn screening test results. *Arch Pediatr Adolesc Med.* 2000;154(7):714–718.

Lipstein EA, Perrin JM, Waisbren SE, Prosser LA. Impact of false-positive newborn metabolic screening results on early health care utilization. *Genet Med.* 2009;11(10):716–721.

Matern D, Tortorelli S, Oglesbee D, Gavrilov D, Rinaldo P. Reduction of the false-positive rate in newborn screening by implementation of MS/MS-based second-tier tests: the Mayo Clinic experience (2004–2007). *J Inherit Metab Dis.* 2007;30(4):585–592.

Morrison DR, Clayton EW. False positive newborn screening results are not always benign. *Public Health Genomics.* 2011;14(3):173–177.

Prosser LA, Ladapo JA, Rusinak D, Waisbren SE. Parental tolerance of false-positive newborn screening results. *Arch Pediatr Adolesc Med.* 2008;162(9):870–876.

Schmidt JL, Castellanos-Brown K, Childress S, et al. The impact of false-positive newborn screening results on families: a qualitative study. *Genet Med.* 2012;14(1):76–80.

Tarini BA, Christakis DA, Welch HG. State newborn screening in the tandem mass spectrometry era: more tests, more false-positive results. *Pediatrics.* 2006;118(2):448–456.

Tarini BA, Clark SJ, Pilli S, et al. False-positive newborn screening result and future health care use in a state Medicaid cohort. *Pediatrics.* 2011;128(4):715–722.

Tluczek A, Orland KM, Cavanagh L. Psychosocial consequences of false-positive newborn screens for cystic fibrosis. *Qual Health Res.* 2011;21(2):174–186.

153

Anthony KK, Gil KM, Schanberg LE. Brief report: Parental perceptions of child vulnerability in children with chronic illness. *J Pediatr Psychol.* 2003;28(3):185–190.

Green M. Vulnerable child syndrome and its variants. *Pediatr Rev.* 1986;8(3):75–80.

Green M, Solnit AJ. Reactions to the threatened loss of a child: a vulnerable child syndrome. Pediatric management of the dying child, part III. *Pediatrics.* 1964;34:58–66.

Rothenberg MB, Sills EM. Iatrogenesis: the PKU anxiety syndrome. *J Am Acad Child Psychiatry.* 1968;7(4):689–692.

Shonkoff CJ. Reactions to the threatened loss of a child: a vulnerable child syndrome, by Morris Green, MD, and Albert A. Solnit, MD, Pediatrics, 1964;34:58–66. *Pediatrics.* 1998;102(1 Pt 2):239–241.

Tluczek A, McKechnie AC, Brown RL. Factors associated with parental perception of child vulnerability 12 months after abnormal newborn screening results. *Res Nurs Health*. 2011;34(5):389–400.

154

Miller FA, Hayeems RZ, Bombard Y, et al. Clinical obligations and public health programmes: healthcare provider reasoning about managing the incidental results of newborn screening. *J Med Ethics*. 2009;35(10):626–634.

155

ACOG Committee on Ethics. ACOG Committee Opinion #321: Maternal decision making, ethics, and the law. *Obstet Gynecol*. 2005;106(5 Pt 1):1127–1137.
Strong C. Abortion decisions as inclusion and exclusion criteria in research involving pregnant women and fetuses. *J Med Ethics*. 2012;38(1):43–47.

156

Chervenak FA, McCullough LB. A comprehensive ethical framework for fetal research and its application to fetal surgery for spina bifida. *Am J Obstet Gynecol*. 2002;187(1):10–14.

157

Candilis PJ, Lidz CW, Appelbaum PS, et al. The silent majority: who speaks at IRB meetings? *IRB*. 2012;34(4):15–20.
Lidz CW, Garverich S. What the ANPRM missed: additional needs for IRB reform. *J Law Med Ethics*. 2013;41(2):390–396.
Saleem T, Khalid U. Institutional review boards—a mixed blessing. *Int Arch Med*. 2011;4:19.
Shah S, Whittle A, Wilfond B, Gensler G, Wendler D. How do institutional review boards apply the federal risk and benefit standards for pediatric research? *JAMA*. 2004;291(4):476–482.

158

Dressler LG, Smolek S, Ponsaran R, et al. IRB perspectives on the return of individual results from genomic research. *Genet Med*. 2012;14(2):215–222.
Edwards KL, Lemke AA, Trinidad SB, et al. Genetics researchers' and IRB professionals' attitudes toward genetic research review: a comparative analysis. *Genet Med*. 2012;14(2):236–242.

159

State MW, Levitt P. The conundrums of understanding genetic risks for autism spectrum disorders. *Nat Neurosci*. 2011;14(12):1499–1506.

160

Mefford HC, Batshaw ML, Hoffman EP. Genomics, intellectual disability, and autism. *N Engl J Med*. 2012;366(8):733–743.

161

Helgesson G. Children, longitudinal studies, and informed consent. *Med Health Care Philos*. 2005;8(3):307–313.
Hirschfeld S, Kramer B, Guttmacher A. Current status of the National Children's Study. *Epidemiology*. 2010;21(5):605–606.

Ries NM, LeGrandeur J, Caulfield T. Handling ethical, legal and social issues in birth cohort studies involving genetic research: responses from studies in six countries. *BMC Med Ethics*. 2010;11(1):4.

162

Bemmels HR, Wolf SM, Van Ness B. Mapping the inputs, analyses, and outputs of biobank research systems to identify sources of incidental findings and individual research results for potential return to participants. *Genet Med*. 2012;14(4):385–392.

Karp DR, Carlin S, Cook-Deegan R, et al. Ethical and practical issues associated with aggregating databases. *PLoS Med*. 2008;5(9):e190.

163

Loo KK. Procedural challenges in international collaborative research. *Acad Psychiatry*. 2009;33(3):229–233.

Lord C, Petkova E, Hus V, et al. A multisite study of the clinical diagnosis of different autism spectrum disorders. *Arch Gen Psychiatry*. 2012;69(3):306–313.

164

Gurrieri F. Working up autism: the practical role of medical genetics. *Am J Med Genet C Semin Med Genet*. 2012;160C(2):104–110.

Schaefer GB, Mendelsohn NJ. Clinical genetics evaluation in identifying the etiology of autism spectrum disorders: 2013 guideline revisions. *Genet Med*. 2013;15(5):399–407.

Shen Y, Dies KA, Holm IA, et al. Clinical genetic testing for patients with autism spectrum disorders. *Pediatrics*. 2010;125(4):e727–e735.

Warren ZE, Stone WL. Clinical best practices: diagnosis and assessment of young children. In: Amaral D, Dawson G, Geschwind DH, eds. *Autism Spectrum Disorders*. New York: Oxford University Press; 2011:1269–1280.

165

Emanuel EJ, Thompson DF. The concept of conflicts of interest. In: Emanuel EJ, Grady C, Crouch RA, et al., eds. *The Oxford Textbook of Clinical Research Ethics*. New York: Oxford University Press; 2008:758–766.

166

Dresser R. The role of patient advocates and public representatives in research. In: Emanuel EJ, Grady C, Crouch RA, et al., eds. *The Oxford Textbook of Clinical Research Ethics*. New York: Oxford University Press; 2008:231–244.

Stockdale A, Terry S. Advocacy groups and the new genetics. In: Alper JS, Ard C, Asch A, eds. *The Double-Edged Helix: Social Implications of Genetics in a Diverse Society*. Baltimore, MD: Johns Hopkins University Press; 2002:80–101.

167

Betancur C. Etiological heterogeneity in autism spectrum disorders: more than 100 genetic and genomic disorders and still counting. *Brain Res*. 2011;1380:42–77.

Campbell DB, Datta D, Jones ST, et al. Association of oxytocin receptor (OXTR) gene variants with multiple phenotype domains of autism spectrum disorder. *J Neurodev Disord*. 2011;3(2):101–112.

Horev G, Ellegood J, Lerch JP, et al. Dosage-dependent phenotypes in models of 16p11.2 lesions found in autism. *Proc Natl Acad Sci USA*. 2011;108(41):17076–17081.

Kim SJ, Silva RM, Flores CG, et al. A quantitative association study of SLC25A12 and restricted repetitive behavior traits in autism spectrum disorders. *Mol Autism.* 2011;2(1):8.

Vieland VJ, Hallmayer J, Huang Y, et al. Novel method for combined linkage and genome-wide association analysis finds evidence of distinct genetic architecture for two subtypes of autism. *J Neurodev Disord.* 2011;3(2):113–123.

168

Shen Y, Chen X, Wang L, et al. Intra-family phenotypic heterogeneity of 16p11.2 deletion carriers in a three-generation Chinese family. *Am J Med Genet B Neuropsychiatr Genet.* 2011;156(2):225–232.

Sousa I, Clark TG, Holt R, et al. Polymorphisms in leucine-rich repeat genes are associated with autism spectrum disorder susceptibility in populations of European ancestry. *Mol Autism.* 2010;1(1):7.

169

O'Roak BJ, Deriziotis P, Lee C, et al. Exome sequencing in sporadic autism spectrum disorders identifies severe de novo mutations. *Nat Genet.* 2011;43(6):585–589.

Sanders SJ, Ercan-Sencicek AG, Hus V, et al. Multiple recurrent de novo CNVs, including duplications of the 7q11.23 Williams syndrome region, are strongly associated with autism. *Neuron.* 2011;70(5):863–885.

170

Affleck P. Is it ethical to deny genetic research participants individualised results? *J Med Ethics.* 2009;35(4):209–213.

171

Anney R, Klei L, Pinto D, et al. Individual common variants exert weak effects on the risk for autism spectrum disorders. *Hum Mol Genet.* 2012;21(21):4781–4792.

Wang K, Zhang H, Ma D, et al. Common genetic variants on 5p14.1 associate with autism spectrum disorders. *Nature.* 2009;459(7246):528–533.

172

Wendler D. One-time general consent for research on biological samples. *BMJ.* 2006;332(7540):544–547.

173

Chen LS, Xu L, Huang TY, Dhar SU. Autism genetic testing: a qualitative study of awareness, attitudes, and experiences among parents of children with autism spectrum disorders. *Genet Med.* 2013;15(4):274–281.

174

Dubler NN, Liebman CB. *Bioethics Mediation: A Guide to Shaping Shared Solutions.* Revised ed. Nashville, TN: Nashville University Press; 2011.

175

Matsunami N, Hadley D, Hensel CH, et al. Identification of rare recurrent copy number variants in high-risk autism families and their prevalence in a large ASD population. *PLoS One.* 2013;8(1):e52239.

Ozonoff S, Young GS, Carter A, et al. Recurrence risk for autism spectrum disorders: a Baby Siblings Research Consortium study. *Pediatrics.* 2011;128(3):e488–e495.

176

Lidz CW, Simon LJ, Seligowski AV, et al. The participation of community members on medical institutional review boards. *J Empir Res Hum Res Ethics.* 2012;7(1):1–6.

177

Fischbach RL, Fischbach GD. Neuroethicists needed now more than ever. *Am J Bioeth.* 2008;8(1):47–48.

Illes J, Sahakian BJ, eds. *The Oxford Handbook of Neuroethics.* Oxford, UK: Oxford University Press; 2011.

Jordan BR, Tsai DF. Whole-genome association studies for multigenic diseases: ethical dilemmas arising from commercialization—the case of genetic testing for autism. *J Med Ethics.* 2010;36(7):440–444.

178

Ozonoff S, Young GS, Carter A, et al. Recurrence risk for autism spectrum disorders: a Baby Siblings Research Consortium study. *Pediatrics.* 2011;128(3):e488–e495.

179

Miller FA, Hayeems RZ, Bytautas JP. What is a meaningful result? Disclosing the results of genomic research in autism to research participants. *Eur J Hum Genet.* 2010;18(8):867–871.

180

American Psychiatric Association. *Diagnostic and Statistical Manual of Mental Disorders: DSM-5.* Washington, DC: American Psychiatric Publishing; 2013.

Frances AJ, Nardo JM. ICD-11 should not repeat the mistakes made by DSM-5. *Br J Psychiatry.* 2013;203:1–2.

Mattila ML, Kielinen M, Linna SL, et al. Autism spectrum disorders according to DSM-IV-TR and comparison with DSM-5 draft criteria: an epidemiological study. *J Am Acad Child Adolesc Psychiatry.* 2011;50(6):583–592 e511.

Sanders JL. Qualitative or quantitative differences between Asperger's disorder and autism? Historical considerations. *J Autism Dev Disord.* 2009;39(11):1560–1567.

Timimi S. Autism is not a scientifically valid or clinically useful diagnosis. *BMJ.* 2011;343:D5105.

Tsai LY, Ghaziuddin M. DSM-5 ASD moves forward into the past. *J Autism Dev Disord.* 2013. doi: 10.1007/s10803-013-1870-3.

Wing L, Gould J, Gillberg C. Autism spectrum disorders in the DSM-V: better or worse than the DSM-IV? *Res Dev Disabil.* 2011;32(2):768–773.

181

Emanuel EJ, Grady C. Four paradigms of clinical research and research oversight. In: Emanuel EJ, Grady C, Crouch RA, et al., eds. *The Oxford Textbook of Clinical Research Ethics.* New York: Oxford University Press; 2008:222–230.

Holm IA, Taylor PL. The Informed Cohort Oversight Board: from values to architecture. *Minn J Law Sci Technol.* 2012;13:669–690.

182

Crepel A, Steyaert J, De la Marche W, et al. Narrowing the critical deletion region for autism spectrum disorders on 16p11.2. *Am J Med Genet B Neuropsychiatr Genet.* 2011;156(2):243–245.

183

Cross-Disorder Group of the Psychiatric Genomics Consortium. Identification of risk loci with shared effects on five major psychiatric disorders: a genome-wide analysis. *Lancet*. 2013;381(9875):1371–1379.

Guilmatre A, Dubourg C, Mosca AL, et al. Recurrent rearrangements in synaptic and neurodevelopmental genes and shared biologic pathways in schizophrenia, autism, and mental retardation. *Arch Gen Psychiatry*. 2009;66(9):947–956.

Lionel AC, Vaags AK, Sato D, et al. Rare exonic deletions implicate the synaptic organizer Gephyrin (GPHN) in risk for autism, schizophrenia and seizures. *Hum Mol Genet*. 2013;22(10):2055–2066.

Rosenberg RN, DiMauro S, Paulson HL, Ptacek L, Nestler E, eds. *The Molecular and Genetic Basis of Neurologic and Psychiatric Disease*. 4th ed. Philadelphia: Wolters Kluwer Health/Lippincott Williams & Wilkins; 2008.

Rosenfeld JA, Ballif BC, Torchia BS, et al. Copy number variations associated with autism spectrum disorders contribute to a spectrum of neurodevelopmental disorders. *Genet Med*. 2010;12(11):694–702.

184

Burke W, Zimmern RL, Kroese M. Defining purpose: a key step in genetic test evaluation. *Genet Med*. 2007;9(10):675–681.

185

Marchant GE, Robert JS. Genetic testing for autism predisposition: ethical, legal and social challenges. *Houston J Health Law Policy*. 2009;9:203–236.

186

Dicker S, Bennett E. Engulfed by the spectrum: the impact of autism spectrum disorders on law and policy. *Valparaiso Univ Law Rev*. 2011;45:415–456.

187

Appelbaum PS, Lidz CW, Grisso T. Therapeutic misconception in clinical research: frequency and risk factors. *IRB*. 2004;26(2):1–8.

Appelbaum PS, Roth LH, Lidz C. The therapeutic misconception: informed consent in psychiatric research. *Int J Law Psychiatry*. 1982;5(3–4):319–329.

188

Murphy J, Scott J, Kaufman D, Geller G, LeRoy L, Hudson K. Public expectations for return of results from large-cohort genetic research. *Am J Bioeth*. 2008;8(11):36–43.

189

Bailey DB Jr, Skinner D, Davis AM, Whitmarsh I, Powell C. Ethical, legal, and social concerns about expanded newborn screening: fragile X syndrome as a prototype for emerging issues. *Pediatrics*. 2008;121(3):e693–704.

Hill MK, Archibald AD, Cohen J, Metcalfe SA. A systematic review of population screening for fragile X syndrome. *Genet Med*. 2010;12(7):396–410.

Levenson D. A majority of parents accept newborn screening for fragile X. *Am J Med Genet A*. 2011;155A(9):viii–ix.

Skinner D, Choudhury S, Sideris J, et al. Parents' decisions to screen newborns for FMR1 gene expansions in a pilot research project. *Pediatrics*. 2011;127(6):e1455–e1463.

Skinner D, Sparkman KL, Bailey DB Jr. Screening for fragile X syndrome: parent attitudes and perspectives. *Genet Med.* 2003;5(5):378–384.

190

Botkin JR. Newborn screening for fragile X syndrome: do we care what parents think? *Pediatrics.* 2011;127(6):e1593–e1594.

191

Hester DM, Schonfeld T. Introduction to healthcare ethics committees. In: Hester DM, Schonfeld T, eds. *Guidance for Healthcare Ethics Committees.* Cambridge, UK: Cambridge University Press; 2012:1–8.

192

Horton R, Brody H. Informed consent, shared decision-making, and the ethics committee. In: Hester DM, Schonfeld T, eds. *Guidance for Healthcare Ethics Committees.* Cambridge, UK: Cambridge University Press; 2012:48–54.

193

Murphy TF. Hospital ethics committees and research with human beings. In: Hester DM, ed. *Ethics by Committee: A Textbook on Consultation, Organization, and Education for Hospital Ethics Committees.* Lanham, MD: Rowman & Littlefield Publishers; 2008:215–230.

194

Shelton W, Bjarnadottir D. Ethics consultation and the committee. In: Hester DM, ed. *Ethics by Committee: A Textbook on Consultation, Organization, and Education for Hospital Ethics Committees.* Lanham, MD: Rowman & Littlefield Publishers; 2008:49–78.

Smith ML. Mission, vision, goals: defining the parameters of ethics consultation. In: Hester DM, Schonfeld T, eds. *Guidance for Healthcare Ethics Committees.* Cambridge, UK: Cambridge University Press; 2012:32–40.

Spike J. Ethics consultation process. In: Hester DM, Schonfeld T, eds. *Guidance for Healthcare Ethics Committees.* Cambridge, UK: Cambridge University Press; 2012:41–47.

195

Angell M. Respecting the autonomy of competent patients. *N Engl J Med.* 1984;310(17):1115–1116.

Buchanan AE, Brock DW. *Deciding for Others: The Ethics of Surrogate Decision Making.* New York: Cambridge University Press; 1989.

Capron AM. The authority of others to decide about biomedical interventions with incompetents. In: Gaylin W, Macklin R, eds. *Who Speaks for the Child: The Problems of Proxy Consent.* New York: Plenum; 1982:115–152.

Knoppers BM, Avard D, Cardinal G, Glass KC. Science and society: children and incompetent adults in genetic research: consent and safeguards. *Nat Rev Genet.* 2002;3(3):221–225.

Kopelman LM. On the evaluative nature of competency and capacity judgments. *Int J Law Psychiatry.* 1990;13(4):309–329.

196

Genetic Information Nondiscrimination Act (GINA), Pub L No. 110-233, 122 Stat 881 (2008).

McGuire AL, Majumder MA. Two cheers for GINA? *Genome Med.* 2009;1(1):6.

197

Bamshad MJ, Ng SB, Bigham AW, et al. Exome sequencing as a tool for Mendelian disease gene discovery. *Nat Rev Genet.* 2011;12(11):745–755.

198

Edvardson S, Shaag A, Zenvirt S, et al. Joubert syndrome 2 (JBTS2) in Ashkenazi Jews is associated with a TMEM216 mutation. *Am J Hum Genet.* 2010;86(1):93–97.

199

Lipinski SE, Lipinski MJ, Biesecker LG, Biesecker BB. Uncertainty and perceived personal control among parents of children with rare chromosome conditions: the role of genetic counseling. *Am J Med Genet C Semin Med Genet.* 2006;142C(4):232–240.

200

Lipinski SE, Lipinski MJ, Biesecker LG, Biesecker BB. Uncertainty and perceived personal control among parents of children with rare chromosome conditions: the role of genetic counseling. *Am J Med Genet C Semin Med Genet.* 2006;142C(4):232–240.

201

Arribas-Ayllon M. The ethics of disclosing genetic diagnosis for Alzheimer's disease: do we need a new paradigm? *Br Med Bull.* 2011;100(1):7–21.
Green RC, Roberts JS, Cupples LA, et al. Disclosure of APOE genotype for risk of Alzheimer's disease. *N Engl J Med.* 2009;361(3):245–254.

202

Benkendorf JL, Reutenauer JE, Hughes CA, et al. Patients' attitudes about autonomy and confidentiality in genetic testing for breast-ovarian cancer susceptibility. *Am J Med Genet.* 1997;73(3):296–303.

203

Johnson AD, Bhimavarapu A, Benjamin EJ, et al. CLIA-tested genetic variants on commercial SNP arrays: potential for incidental findings in genome-wide association studies. *Genet Med.* 2010;12(6):355–363.

204

Ashida S, Koehly LM, Roberts JS, Chen CA, Hiraki S, Green RC. The role of disease perceptions and results sharing in psychological adaptation after genetic susceptibility testing: the REVEAL Study. *Eur J Hum Genet.* 2010;18(12):1296–1301.
Bosch N, Junyent N, Gadea N, et al. What factors may influence psychological well being at three months and one year post BRCA genetic result disclosure? *Breast.* 2012;21(6):755–760.

205

Kaltman JR, Thompson PD, Lantos J, et al. Screening for sudden cardiac death in the young: report from a national heart, lung, and blood institute working group. *Circulation.* 2011;123(17):1911–1918.

Lieve KV, Williams L, Daly A, et al. Results of genetic testing in 855 consecutive unre-
    lated patients referred for long QT syndrome in a clinical laboratory. *Genet Test
    Mol Biomarkers.* 2013;17(7):553–561.
Refsgaard L, Holst AG, Sadjadieh G, Haunsø S, Nielsen JB, Olesen MS. High preva-
    lence of genetic variants previously associated with LQT syndrome in new exome
    data. *Eur J Hum Genet.* 2012;20(8):905–908.

206

Metcalfe A, Coad J, Plumridge GM, Gill P, Farndon P. Family communication between
    children and their parents about inherited genetic conditions: a meta-synthesis
    of the research. *Eur J Hum Genet.* 2008;16(10):1193–1200.

207

Harrison C. Fidelity and truthfulness in the pediatric setting: witholding information
    from children and adolescents. In: Diekema DS, Mercurio MR, Adam MB, eds.
    Clinical Ethics in Pediatrics: A Case-Based Textbook. Cambridge, UK: Cambridge
    University Press; 2011:32–36.
Harrison C. Truth telling in pediatrics: what they don't know might hurt them.
    In: Miller G, ed. *Pediatric Bioethics.* New York: Cambridge University Press;
    2010:73–86.
Lantos JD. Should we always tell children the truth? *Perspect Biol Med.*
    1996;40(1):78–92.
Liberati A, Mosconi P, Meyerowitz B. Truth telling: a cultural or individual choice?
    JAMA. 1993;269(8):989.

208

Lipstein EA, Brinkman WB, Britto MT. What is known about parents' treatment
    decisions? A narrative review of pediatric decision making. *Med Decis Making.*
    2012;32(2):246–258.

209

Sermet-Gaudelus I, Mayell SJ, Southern KW. Guidelines on the early management of
    infants diagnosed with cystic fibrosis following newborn screening. *J Cyst Fibros.*
    2010;9(5):323–329.

210

McHugh DMS, Cameron CA, Abdenur JE, et al. Clinical validation of cutoff target
    ranges in newborn screening of metabolic disorders by tandem mass spectrom-
    etry: a worldwide collaborative project. *Genet Med.* 2011;13(3):230–254.
Rinaldo P, Cowan TM, Matern D. Acylcarnitine profile analysis. *Genet Med.*
    2008;10(2):151–156.
Rinaldo P, Zafari S, Tortorelli S, Matern D. Making the case for objective performance
    metrics in newborn screening by tandem mass spectrometry. *Ment Retard Dev
    Disabil Res Rev.* 2006;12(4):255–261.

211

Shigematsu Y, Hata I, Tajima G. Useful second-tier tests in expanded newborn screen-
    ing of isovaleric acidemia and methylmalonic aciduria. *J Inherit Metab Dis.*
    2010;33(Suppl 2):S283–S288.

212

Asch A. Prenatal diagnosis and selective abortion: a challenge to practice and policy.
    Am J Public Health. 1999;89(11):1649–1657.

Hale JE, Parad RB, Comeau AM. Newborn screening showing decreasing incidence of cystic fibrosis. *N Engl J Med*. 2008;358(9):973–974.

Massie J, Curnow L, Gaffney L, Carlin J, Francis I. Declining prevalence of cystic fibrosis since the introduction of newborn screening. *Arch Dis Child*. 2010;95(7):531–533.

Sawyer SM, Cerritelli B, Carter LS, Cooke M, Glazner JA, Massie J. Changing their minds with time: a comparison of hypothetical and actual reproductive behaviors in parents of children with cystic fibrosis. *Pediatrics*. 2006;118(3):e649–e656.

213

Atkinson K, Zuckerman B, Sharfstein JM, Levin D, Blatt RJ, Koh HK. A public health response to emerging technology: expansion of the Massachusetts newborn screening program. *Public Health Rep*. 2001;116(2):122–131.

Marshall E. Medicine. Fast technology drives new world of newborn screening. *Science*. 2001;294(5550):2272–2274.

214

Bailey DB Jr, Armstrong FD, Kemper AR, Skinner D, Warren SF. Supporting family adaptation to presymptomatic and "untreatable" conditions in an era of expanded newborn screening. *J Pediatr Psychol*. 2009;34(6):648–661.

215

Bailey DB Jr, Beskow LM, Davis AM, Skinner D. Changing perspectives on the benefits of newborn screening. *Ment Retard Dev Disabil Res Rev*. 2006;12(4):270–279.

Farrell MH, Farrell PM. Newborn screening for cystic fibrosis: ensuring more good than harm. *J Pediatr*. 2003;143(6):707–712.

Waisbren SE, Albers S, Amato S, et al. Effect of expanded newborn screening for biochemical genetic disorders on child outcomes and parental stress. *JAMA*. 2003;290(19):2564–2572.

216

Botkin JR, Anderson R, Staes C, Longo N. Developing a national registry for conditions identifiable through newborn screening. *Genet Med*. 2009;11(3):176–182.

217

Burke W, Tarini B, Press NA, Evans JP. Genetic screening. *Epidemiol Rev*. 2011;33(1):148–164.

218

Cody JD. An advocate's perspective on newborn screening policy. In: Baily MA, Murray TH, eds. *Ethics and Newborn Genetic Screening: New Technologies, New Challenges*. Baltimore: Johns Hopkins University Press; 2009:89–105.

Paul DB. Patient advocacy in newborn screening: continuities and discontinuities. *Am J Med Genet C Semin Med Genet*. 2008;148C(1):8–14.

219

Comeau AM, Larson C, Eaton RB. Integration of new genetic diseases into statewide newborn screening: New England experience. *Am J Med Genet C Semin Med Genet*. 2004;125C(1):35–41.

220

Davis PB. Therapy for cystic fibrosis—the end of the beginning? *N Engl J Med.* 2011;365(18):1734–1735.

221

Dillard JP, Shen L, Robinson JD, Farrell PM. Parental information seeking following a positive newborn screening for cystic fibrosis. *J Health Commun.* 2010;15(8):880–894.

Larsson AK, Svalenius E, Lundqvist A, Dykes AK. Parents' experiences of an abnormal ultrasound examination—vacillating between emotional confusion and sense of reality. *Reprod Health.* 2010;7(1):10.

Waisbren SE, Rones M, Read CY, Marsden D, Levy HL. Brief report: predictors of parenting stress among parents of children with biochemical genetic disorders. *J Pediatr Psychol.* 2004;29(7):565–570.

222

Downing GJ, Zuckerman AE, Coon C, Lloyd-Puryear MA. Enhancing the quality and efficiency of newborn screening programs through the use of health information technology. *Semin Perinatol.* 2010;34(2):156–162.

Downs SM, van Dyck PC, Rinaldo P, et al. Improving newborn screening laboratory test ordering and result reporting using health information exchange. *J Am Med Inform Assoc.* 2010;17(1):13–18.

223

Giusti R, Badgwell A, Iglesias AD. New York State cystic fibrosis consortium: the first 2.5 years of experience with cystic fibrosis newborn screening in an ethnically diverse population. *Pediatrics.* 2007;119(2):e460–e467.

Pass K, Green NS, Lorey F, Sherwin J, Comeau AM. Pilot programs in newborn screening. *Ment Retard Dev Disabil Res Rev.* 2006;12(4):293–300.

224

Prosser LA, Kong CY, Rusinak D, Waisbren SL. Projected costs, risks, and benefits of expanded newborn screening for MCADD. *Pediatrics.* 2010;125(2):e286–e294.

Ross LF. Minimizing risks: the ethics of predictive diabetes mellitus screening research in newborns. *Arch Pediatr Adolesc Med.* 2003;157(1):89–95.

Ross LF. Newborn screening for lysosomal storage diseases: an ethical and policy analysis. *J Inherit Metab Dis.* 2012;35(4):627–634.

Van Karnebeek C, Alfadhel M, Stockler S. Revisiting treatable forms of intellectual disability as future candidates for newborn screening. [abstract]. *J Inherit Metab Dis.* 2011;34(Suppl 1): S7.

225

National Newborn Screening and Global Resource Center. http://genes-r-us.uthscsa. edu/. Accessed July 18, 2013.

Newborn Screening Translational Research Network. https://www.nbstrn.org/. Accessed November 30, 2013.

U.S. Department of Health and Humans Services. Discretionary Advisory Committee on Heritable Disorders in Newborns and Children. http://www. hrsa.gov/advisorycommittees/mchbadvisory/heritabledisorders/. Accessed November 30, 2013.

226

Sims EJ, Clark A, McCormick J, et al. Cystic fibrosis diagnosed after 2 months of age leads to worse outcomes and requires more therapy. *Pediatrics.* 2007;119(1):19–28.

Waisbren SE, Levy HL, Noble M, et al. Short-chain acyl-CoA dehydrogenase (SCAD) deficiency: an examination of the medical and neurodevelopmental characteristics of 14 cases identified through newborn screening or clinical symptoms. *Mol Genet Metab.* 2008;95(1–2):39–45.

227

Stark AP, Lang CW, Ross LF. A pilot study to evaluate knowledge and attitudes of Illinois pediatricians toward newborn screening for sickle cell disease and cystic fibrosis. *Am J Perinatol.* 2011;28(3):169–176.

228

Tluczek A, Orland KM, Nick SW, Brown RL. Newborn screening: an appeal for improved parent education. *J Perinat Neonatal Nurs.* 2009;23(4):326–334.

229

van Maldegem BT, Wanders RJA, Wijburg FA. Clinical aspects of short-chain acyl-CoA dehydrogenase deficiency. *J Inherit Metab Dis.* 2010;33(5):507–511.

Wilcken B. Fatty acid oxidation disorders: outcome and long-term prognosis. *J Inherit Metab Dis.* 2010;33(5):501–506.

230

Forsberg JS, Hansson MG, Eriksson S. Changing perspectives in biobank research: from individual rights to concerns about public health regarding the return of results. *Eur J Hum Genet.* 2009;17(12):1544–1549.

231

Adey A, Burton JN, Kitzman JO, et al. The haplotype-resolved genome and epigenome of the aneuploid HeLa cancer cell line. *Nature.* 2013;500(7461):207–211.

Hudson KL, Collins FS. Biospecimen policy: family matters. *Nature.* 2013;500(7461):141–142.

Skloot R. *The Immortal Life of Henrietta Lacks.* New York: Crown Publishers; 2010.

232

ACOG Committee on Practice Bulletins. ACOG Practice Bulletin No. 77: screening for fetal chromosomal abnormalities. *Obstet Gynecol.* 2007;109(1):217–227.

233

American College of Obstetricians and Gynecologists. Patient choice in the maternal-fetal relationship. *Ethics in Obstetrics and Gynecology.* 2nd ed. Washington, DC: ACOG; 2004:34–36.

234

Anand G. *The Cure: How a Father Raised $100 Million—and Bucked the Medical Establishment—in a Quest to Save His Children.* New York: HarperCollins; 2009.

235

Asch A, Gostin LO, Johnson DM. Respecting persons with disabilities and preventing disability: is there a conflict? In: Herr SS, Gostin LO, Koh HH, eds.

The Human Rights of Persons with Intellectual Disabilities: Different but Equal.
New York: Oxford University Press; 2011:319–346.

236

Austin JC. Re-conceptualizing risk in genetic counseling: implications for clinical
practice. *J Genet Couns.* 2010;19(3):228–234.

237

Austin JC. Re-conceptualizing risk in genetic counseling: implications for clinical
practice. *J Genet Couns.* 2010;19(3):228–234.

238

Bell CJ, Dinwiddie DL, Miller NA, et al. Carrier testing for severe childhood recessive
diseases by next-generation sequencing. *Sci Transl Med.* 2011;3(65):65ra4.

239

Birrell J, Meares K, Wilkinson A, Freeston M. Toward a definition of intolerance
of uncertainty: a review of factor analytical studies of the Intolerance of
Uncertainty Scale. *Clin Psychol Rev.* 2011;31(7):1198–1208.

240

Botkin JR. Preimplantation and prenatal genetic testing for inherited diseases, dispositions, and traits. In: Diekema DS, Mercurio MR, Adam MB, eds. *Clinical Ethics
in Pediatrics: A Case-Based Textbook.* Cambridge, UK: Cambridge University Press;
2011:68–76.

241

Frantzen C, Links TP, Giles RH. Von Hippel-Lindau disease. *GeneReviews.* University
of Washington, Seattle. 1993–2013. http://www.ncbi.nlm.nih.gov/books/
NBK1463/. Updated June 21, 2012. Accessed July 22, 2013.

242

Jonsen AR. Casuistry and clinical ethics. In: Sugarman J, Sulmasy DP, eds. *Methods in
Medical Ethics.* Washington, DC: Georgetown University Press; 2010:109–126.

243

Mercurio MR. Pediatric ethics committees. In: Miller G, ed. *Pediatric Bioethics.*
Cambridge, UK: Cambridge University Press; 2010:87–108.

244

Kinlaw K. The healthcare ethics committee as educator. In: Hester DM, Schonfeld
T, eds. *Guidance for Healthcare Ethics Committees.* Cambridge, UK: Cambridge
University Press; 2012:155–163.

Kinlaw K. The hospital ethics committee as educator. In: Hester DM, ed. *Ethics
by Committee: A Textbook on Consultation, Organization, and Education for
Hospital Ethics Committees.* Lanham, MD: Rowman & Littlefield Publishers;
2008:203–214.

245

Largent EA, Pearson SD. Which orphans will find a home? The rule of rescue in
resource allocation for rare diseases. *Hastings Cent Rep.* 2012;42(1):27–34.

246

McGuire AL, Wang MJ, Probst FJ. Currents in contemporary bioethics. Identifying consanguinity through routine genomic analysis: reporting requirements. *J Law Med Ethics*. 2012;40(4):1040–1046.

Rehder CW, David KL, Hirsch B, Toriello HV, Wilson CM, Kearney HM. American College of Medical Genetics and Genomics: standards and guidelines for documenting suspected consanguinity as an incidental finding of genomic testing. *Genet Med*. 2013;15(2):150–152.

Schaaf CP, Scott DA, Wiszniewska J, Beaudet AL. Identification of incestuous parental relationships by SNP-based DNA microarrays. *Lancet*. 2011;377(9765):555–556.

247

Schonfeld T. Confidentiality. In: Hester DM, Schonfeld T, eds. *Guidance for Healthcare Ethics Committees*. Cambridge, UK: Cambridge University Press; 2012:71–79.

248

Selby JV, Krumholz HM. Ethical oversight: serving the best interests of patients. Commentary. *Hastings Cent Rep*. 2013;43(Suppl):S34–S36.

249

Ross LF. Disclosing misattributed paternity. *Bioethics*. 1996;10(2):114–130.

Ross LF. Disclosing misattributed paternity. In: Steinbock B, Arras J, London AJ, eds. *Ethical issues in modern medicine*. 6th ed. Boston: McGraw-Hill; 2003:120–128.

Wright L, MacRae S, Gordon D, et al. Disclosure of misattributed paternity: issues involved in the discovery of unsought information. *Semin Dial*. 2002;15(3):202–206.

250

Myring J, Beckett W, Jassi R, et al. Shock, adjust, decide: reproductive decision making in cystic fibrosis (CF) carrier couples—a qualitative study. *J Genet Couns*. 2011;20(4):404–417.

251

Ziegler A. *Photograph 51*. New York: Dramatists Play Service; 2011. Quotes from pp. 21–22, 23, 32, and 25.

252

Albee E. *Who's Afraid of Virginia Woolf? (1962)*. New York: Dramatists Play Service; 2004. Quotes from pp. 20 and 32.

253

Tolins J. *The Twilight of the Golds*. New York: Samuel French; 1994. Quotes from p. 78.

Charo RA, Rothenberg KH. The good mother: the limits of reproductive responsibility and genetic choice. In: Rothenberg KR, Thomson E, eds. *Women and Prenatal Testing: Facing the Challenges of Genetic Technology*. Columbus, OH: Ohio State University Press; 1994:105–130.

Hamer DH, Hu S, Magnuson VL, Pattatucci AM. A linkage between DNA markers on the X chromosome and male sexual orientation. *Science*. 1993;261:321–327.

Marshall E. NIH's "gay gene" study questioned. *Science*. 1995;268:1841.

Rothenberg KH. From eugenics to the 'new' genetics: "The Play's the Thing." *Fordham Law Rev.* 2010;79(2):407–434. p.426, n.113, 428 n.127 (noting studies challenging reports of a "gay" gene).

Rothenberg KH. The law's response to reproductive genetic testing: questioning assumptions about choice, causation, and control. *Fetal Diagn Ther.* 1993;8:160–163.

254

Stephenson S. *An Experiment with an Air Pump.* New York: Dramatists Play Service; 2000. Quotes from pp. 32, 33, 56, and 72.

255

Mullin P. *The Sequence.* Los Angeles, CA: Original Works Publishing; 2010. Quotes from pp. 8, 10, and 63.

256

Djerassi C. *An Immaculate Misconception: Sex in an Age of Mechanical Reproduction.* London: Imperial College Press; 2000. Quotes from pp. 16, 19, 21, and 22.

Practice Committee of the American Society for Reproductive Medicine, Practice Committee of the Society for Assisted Reproductive Technology. Genetic considerations related to intracytoplasmic sperm injection (ICSI). *Fertil Steril.* 2006;86(5 Suppl 1):S103–S105.

257

Churchill C. *A Number.* New York: Theatre Communications Group; 2002. Quotes from pp. 10–11, 18, 19, and 30–31.

Caulfield T. Human cloning laws, human dignity and the poverty of the policy making dialogue. *BMC Med Ethics.* 2003;4:E3.

Rothenberg KH. "Being human": cloning and the challenges for public policy. *Hofstra Law Rev.* 1999;27(3):639–647.

Sperling, D. Bringing life from death: is there a good justification for posthumous cloning? *J Clinic Res Bioeth* 2011;S1:001, available at http://www.omicsonline.org/bringing-life-from-death-is-there-a-good-justification-for-posthumous-cloning-2155-9627.S1-001.pdf.

258

Medley C. *Relativity.* New York: Broadway Play Publishing; 2006. Quotes from pp. 4, 5, 6, 14, and 15.

Bolnick DA, Fullwiley D, Duster T, et al. Genetics: the science and business of genetic ancestry testing. *Science.* 2007;318:399–400.

Clark AE, Shim JK, Shostak S, Nelson A. Biomedicalising genetic health, diseases and identities. In: Atkinson P, Glasner P, Lock M., eds. *Handbook of Genetics and Society: Mapping the New Genomic Era.* New York: Routledge; 2009:21–40.

Duster T. Medicine. Race and reification in science. *Science.* 2005;307(5712):1050–1051.

Kimmelman J. The post-Human Genome Project mindset: race, reliability, and health care. *Clin Genet.* 2006;70(5):427–432.

Roberts DE. Is race-based medicine good for us?: African American approaches to race, biomedicine, and equality. *J Law Med Ethics.* 2008;36(3):537–545.

259

Atkins D. *Lucy.* Toronto: Playwrights Canada Press; 2010. Quotes from pp. 55–58 and 59.

Campbell DB, Datta D, Jones ST, et al. Association of oxytocin receptor (OXTR) gene variants with multiple phenotype domains of autism spectrum disorder. *J Neurodev Disord.* 2011;3(2):101–112.

Crepel A, Steyaert J, De la Marche W, et al. Narrowing the critical deletion region for autism spectrum disorders on 16p11.2. *Am J Med Genet B Neuropsychiatr Genet.* 2011;156(2):243–245.

Godlee F, Smith J, Marcovitch H. Wakefield's article linking MMR vaccine and autism was fraudulent. *BMJ.* 2011;342:c7452.

Horev G, Ellegood J, Lerch JP, et al. Dosage-dependent phenotypes in models of 16p11.2 lesions found in autism. *Proc Natl Acad Sci U S A.* 2011;108(41):17076–17081.

Kirkland A. The legitimacy of vaccine critics: what is left after the autism hypothesis? *J Health Polit Policy Law.* 2012;37:69–97.

Vieland VJ, Hallmayer J, Huang Y, et al. Novel method for combined linkage and genome-wide association analysis finds evidence of distinct genetic architecture for two subtypes of autism. *J Neurodev Disord.* 2011;3(2):113–123.

260

Loomer L. *Distracted.* New York: Dramatists Play Service; 2009. Quotes from pp. 25, 31, 41, 45, 48, and 50.

Atkins D. *Lucy.* Toronto: Playwrights Canada Press; 2010.

Ben-Arye E, Frenkel M, Klein A, Scharf M. Attitudes toward integration of complementary and alternative medicine in primary care: perspectives of patients, physicians and complementary practitioners. *Patient Educ Couns.* 2008;70:395–402.

Kemper AR, Knapp AA, Green NS, Comeau AM, Metterville DR, Perrin JM. Weighing the evidence for newborn screening for early-infantile Krabbe disease. *Genet Med.* 2010;12(9):539–543.

Polich G, Dole C, Kaptchuk TJ. The need to act a little more 'scientific': biomedical researchers investigating complementary and alternative medicine. *Sociol Health Illn.* 2010;32:106–122.

261

Fortenberry D. *The Good Egg.* New York: Broadway Play Publishing; 2011. Quotes from pp. 14, 29, 30, 51, and 53–54.

Cahn NR, Collins JM. Eight is enough. *Northwest Univ Law Rev Colloquy.* 2009;103:501–513.

Charo RA, Rothenberg KH. The good mother: the limits of reproductive responsibility and genetic choice. In: Rothenberg KR, Thomson E, eds. *Women and Prenatal Testing: Facing the Challenges of Genetic Technology.* Columbus, OH: Ohio State University Press; 1994:105–130.

Coan AB. Is there a constitutional right to select the genes of one's offspring? *Hastings Law J.* 2011; 63:233–296.

Djerassi C. *An Immaculate Misconception: Sex in an Age of Mechanical Reproduction.* London: Imperial College Press; 2000.

Kerr A, Shakespeare T. *Genetic Politics: From Eugenics to Genome.* Cheltenham, UK: New Clarion Press; 2002.

Klitzman R, Zolovska B, Folberth W, Sauer MV, Chung W, Appelbaum P. Preimplantation genetic diagnosis on in vitro fertilization clinic websites: presentations of risks, benefits and other information. *Fertil Steril.* 2009;92:1276–1283.

262

White S. *The Other Place*. New York: Dramatists Play Service; 2011. Quotes from pp. 16 and 41–43.

Cummings JL. Alzheimer's disease clinical trials: changing the paradigm. *Curr Psychiatr Rep*. 2011;13:437–442.

Hollingworth P, Harold D, Sims R, et al. Common variants at ABCA7, MS4A6A/ MS4A4E, EPHA1, CD33 and CD2AP are associated with Alzheimer's disease. *Nat Genet*. 2011;43(5):429–435.

Illes J, Sahakian BJ, eds. *The Oxford Handbook of Neuroethics*. Oxford, UK: Oxford University Press; 2011.

Liu L, Drouet V, Wu JW, Witter MP, Small SA, Clelland C, Duff K. Trans-synaptic spread of tau pathology in vivo. *PLoS One*. 2012;7(2):E31302.

Naj AC, Jun G, Beecham GW, et al. Common variants at MS4A4/MS4A6E, CD2AP, CD33 and EPHA1 are associated with late-onset Alzheimer's disease. *Nat Genet*. 2011;43:436–441.

Specter M. Annals of science: the power of nothing. *New Yorker*. December 12, 2011, 30.

263

Kevles DJ. *In the Name of Eugenics: Genetics and the Uses of Human Heredity*. New York: Knopf; 1985.

264

Rothenberg KH. From eugenics to the 'new' genetics: "The Play's the Thing." *Fordham Law Rev*. 2010;79(2):407–434.

265

Klug A. Rosalind Franklin and the discovery of the structure of DNA. *Nature*. 1968;219(5156):808–810.

266

Jonsen AR. *The Birth of Bioethics*. Paperback ed. New York: Oxford University Press; 2003.

Lindee S. *Moments of Truth in Genetic Medicine*. Baltimore, MD: Johns Hopkins University Press; 2005.

Schwartz J. *In Pursuit of the Gene: From Darwin to DNA*. Cambridge, MA: Harvard University Press; 2008.

Watson JD, Crick FHC. Molecular structure of nucleic acids: a structure for deoxyribose nucleic acid. *Nature*. 1953;171:737–738.

267

Fins JJ, De Melo-Martin I. C.P. Snow's "Two Cultures" fifty years later: An enduring problem with an elusive solution. *Technol Soc*. 2010;32(1):1–4.

Jennings B. Enlightenment and enchantment: technology and moral limits. *Technol Soc*. 2010;32(1):25–30.

Latham SR. Law between the cultures: C.P. Snow's *The Two Cultures* and the problem of scientific illiteracy in law. *Technol Soc*. 2010;32(1):31–34.

Skorton DJ. Bridging the "Two Cultures" divide in medicine and the academy. *Technol Soc*. 2010;32(1):49–52.

Snow CP. *The Two Cultures and a Second Look: An Expanded Version of the Two Cultures and the Scientific Revolution*. London: Cambridge University Press; 1969.

268

Collins F, Galas D. A new five-year plan for the U.S. Human Genome Project. *Science*. 1993; 262:43–46.

Juengst ET. The Human Genome Project and bioethics. *Kennedy Inst Ethics J.* 1991;1:71–74.

National Human Genome Research Institute. All about the Human Genome Project (HGP). http://www.genome.gov/10001772. Updated January 24, 2013. Accessed June 21, 2013.

National Human Genome Research Institute. The Ethical, Legal and Social Implications (ELSI) Research Program. http://www.genome.gov/10001618. Updated April 10, 2013. Accessed June 21, 2013.

269

Collins FS, Green ED, Guttmacher AE, Guyer MS. US National Human Genome Research Institute. A vision for the future of genomics research. *Nature*. 2003;422(6934):835–847.

Duster T. *Backdoor to Eugenics*. 2nd ed. New York: Routledge; 2003.

National Human Genome Research Institute. ELSI research priorities and possible research projects. http://www.genome.gov/27543732. Last updated July 18, 2011. Accessed June 21, 2013.

National Human Genome Research Institute. A review and analysis of the Ethical, Legal and Social Implications (ELSI) Research Programs at the National Institutes of Health and the Department of Energy. http://www.genome. gov/10001727. Updated February 10, 2000. Accessed June 21, 2013.

Schwartz MD, Rothenberg K, Joseph L, Benkendorf J, Lerman C. Consent to the use of stored DNA for genetics research: a survey of attitudes in the Jewish population. *Am J Med Genet*. 2001;98:336–342.

270

Rothenberg KH. "Being human": cloning and the challenges for public policy. *Hofstra Law Rev*. 1999;27(3):639–647.

Rothenberg KH. From eugenics to the 'new' genetics: "The Play's the Thing." *Fordham Law Rev*. 2010;79(2):407–434.

271

Caught napping by clones. 385 *Nature*. 1997;385(6619):753.

Caulfield T, Knowles L, Meslin EM. Law and policy in the era of reproductive genetics. *J Med Ethics*. 2004;30(4):414–417.

Havstad JC. Human reproductive cloning: a conflict of liberties. *Bioethics*. 2010;24(2):71–77.

President's Council on Bioethics. Ethics of cloning-to-produce-children. *Human Cloning and Human Dignity: An Ethical Inquiry*. Washington, DC: President's Council on Bioethics; 2002:75–116.

272

Collins FS, Green ED, Guttmacher AE, Guyer MS. US National Human Genome Research Institute. A vision for the future of genomics research. *Nature*. 2003;422(6934):835–847.

273

Dicker S, Bennett E. Engulfed by the spectrum: the impact of autism spectrum disorders on law and policy. *Valparaiso Univ Law Rev*. 2011;45:415–456.

Golnik AE, Ireland M. Complementary alternative medicine for children with autism: a physician survey. *J Autism Dev Disord.* 2009;39(7):996–1005.

Levy SE, Hyman SL. Complementary and alternative medicine treatments for children with autism spectrum disorders. *Child Adolesc Psychiatr Clin N Am.* 2008;17(4):803–820.

Marchant GE, Robert JS. Genetic testing for autism predisposition: ethical, legal and social challenges. *Houston J Health Law Policy.* 2009;9(2):203–236.

Mattila ML, Kielinen M, Linna SL, et al. Autism spectrum disorders according to DSM-IV-TR and comparison with DSM-5 draft criteria: an epidemiological study. *J Am Acad Child Adolesc Psychiatry.* 2011;50(6):583–592 e511.

Sanders JL. Qualitative or quantitative differences between Asperger's disorder and autism? Historical considerations. *J Autism Dev Disord.* 2009;39(11):1560–1567.

State MW, Levitt P. The conundrums of understanding genetic risks for autism spectrum disorders. *Nat Neurosci.* 2011;14(12):1499–1506.

Timimi S. Autism is not a scientifically valid or clinically useful diagnosis. *BMJ.* 2011;343:D5105.

Wing L, Gould J, Gillberg C. Autism spectrum disorders in the DSM-V: better or worse than the DSM-IV? *Res Dev Disabil.* 2011;32(2):768–773.

274

Asch A, Gostin LO, Johnson DM. Respecting persons with disabilities and preventing disability: Is there conflict? In: Herr SS, Gostin LO, Koh HH, eds. *The Human Rights of Persons with Intellectual Disabilities: Different but Equal.* Oxford, UK: Oxford University Press; 2011:319–346.

Bickenbach JE. *Ethics, Law, and Policy.* Thousand Oaks, CA: Sage Publications; 2012.

Parens E, Asch A, eds. *Prenatal Testing and Disability Rights.* Washington, DC: Georgetown University Press; 2000.

Wasserman DT, Wachbroit RS, Bickenbach JE. *Quality of Life and Human Difference: Genetic Testing, Health Care, and Disability.* New York: Cambridge University Press; 2005.

275

Ibsen H. *Ghosts* (1881). In: Fjelde R, trans. *Four Major Plays: Ghosts; An Enemy of the People; The Lady from the Sea; John Gabriel Borkman.* Vol. 2. New York: New American Library; 1970:37–114.

MacKaye P. *To-morrow.* New York: Frederick A. Stokes Co.; 1912.

O'Neill E. *Strange Interlude* (1928). In: *Three Plays: Desire Under the Elms; Strange Interlude; Morning Becomes Electra.* New York: Vintage Books; 1995:65–256.

276

Nussbaum MC. *Love's Knowledge: Essays on Philosophy and Literature.* New York: Oxford University Press; 1990.

BIBLIOGRAPHY

Abdul-Karim R, Berkman BE, Wendler D, et al. Disclosure of incidental findings from next-generation sequencing in pediatric genomic research. *Pediatrics*. 2013;131(3):564–571.

ACMG Board of Directors. Points to consider in the clinical application of genomic sequencing. *Genet Med*. 2012;14(8):759–761.

ACOG Committee on Ethics. ACOG Committee Opinion #321: Maternal decision making, ethics, and the law. *Obstet Gynecol*. 2005;106(5 Pt 1):1127–1137.

ACOG Committee on Practice Bulletins. ACOG Practice Bulletin No. 77: Screening for fetal chromosomal abnormalities. *Obstet Gynecol*. 2007;109(1):217–227.

Affleck P. Is it ethical to deny genetic research participants individualised results? *J Med Ethics*. 2009;35(4):209–213.

Albee E. *Who's Afraid of Virginia Woolf? (1962)*. New York: Dramatists Play Service; 2004.

Albu CC, Deva DV, Severin E. Ultrasound detection of some phenotipic effects of a pericentric inversion of chromosome 9. [abstract]. *J Inherit Metab Dis*. 2011;34(Suppl 1): S10.

Alexander D, van Dyck PC. In reply: neonatal screening: old dogma or sound principle? *Pediatrics*. 2007;119(2):407.

Alexander D, van Dyck PC. A vision of the future of newborn screening. *Pediatrics*. 2006;117(5 Pt 2):S350–S354.

Ali-Khan SE, Daar AS, Shuman C, Ray PN, Scherer SW. Whole genome scanning: resolving clinical diagnosis and management amidst complex data. *Pediatr Res*. 2009;66(4):357–363.

Allyse M, Michie M. Not-so-incidental findings: the ACMG recommendations on the reporting of incidental findings in clinical whole genome and whole exome sequencing. *Trends Biotechnol*. 2013. doi: 10.1016/j.tibtech.2013.04.006.

Altshuler D, Daly MJ, Lander ES. Genetic mapping in human disease. *Science*. 2008;322(5903):881–888.

American Academy of Pediatrics, Committee on Bioethics, Committee on Genetics, American College of Medical Genetics. Ethical and policy issues in genetic testing and screening of children. *Pediatrics*. 2013;131(3):620–622.

American Academy of Pediatrics Committee on Fetus and Newborn. Screening of newborn infants for metabolic disease. *Pediatrics*. 1965;35(3):499–501.

American College of Medical Genetics and Genomics. Incidental findings in clinical genomics: a clarification. *Genet Med*. 2013;15(8):664–666.

American College of Medical Genetics and Genomics Board of Directors. Points to consider for informed consent for genome/exome sequencing. *Genet Med*. 2013;15(9):748–749.

American College of Medical Genetics Newborn Screening Expert Group. Newborn screening: toward a uniform screening panel and system. *Genet Med.* 2006;8(Suppl 1):1S–252S.

American College of Obstetricians and Gynecologists. ACOG Committee Opinion No. 393, December 2007. Newborn screening. *Obstet Gynecol.* 2007;110(6):1497–1500.

American College of Obstetricians and Gynecologists. Patient choice in the maternal-fetal relationship. *Ethics in Obstetrics and Gynecology.* 2nd ed. Washington, DC: ACOG; 2004:34–36.

American Psychiatric Association. *Diagnostic and Statistical Manual of Mental Disorders: DSM-5.* Washington, DC: American Psychiatric Publishing; 2013.

Anand G. *The Cure: How a Father Raised $100 Million—and Bucked the Medical Establishment—in a Quest to Save His Children.* New York: HarperCollins; 2009.

Anastasova V, Blasimme A, Julia S, Cambon-Thomsen A. Genomic incidental findings: reducing the burden to be fair. *Am J Bioeth.* 2013;13(2):52–54.

Andermann A, Blancquaert I, Beauchamp S, Dery V. Revisiting Wilson and Jungner in the genomic age: a review of screening criteria over the past 40 years. *Bull World Health Organ.* 2008;86(4):317–319.

Andermann A, Blancquaert I, Dery V. Genetic screening: a conceptual framework for programmes and policy-making. *J Health Serv Res Policy.* 2010;15(2):90–97.

Anderson CM, Montello M. The reader's response and why it matters in biomedical ethics. In: Charon R, Montello M, eds. *Stories Matter: The Role of Narrative in Medical Ethics.* New York: Routledge; 2002:85–94.

Anderson RR. Religious traditions and prenatal genetic counseling. *Am J Med Genet C Semin Med Genet.* 2009;151C(1):52–61.

Andresen BS, Dobrowolski SF, O'Reilly L, et al. Medium-chain acyl-CoA dehydrogenase (MCAD) mutations identified by MS/MS-based prospective screening of newborns differ from those observed in patients with clinical symptoms: identification and characterization of a new, prevalent mutation that results in mild MCAD deficiency. *Am J Hum Genet.* 2001;68(6):1408–1418.

Angell M. Respecting the autonomy of competent patients. *N Engl J Med.* 1984;310(17):1115–1116.

Angrist M. You never call, you never write: why return of 'omic' results to research participants is both a good idea and a moral imperative. *Per Med.* 2011;8(6):651–657.

Annas GJ. Mandatory PKU screening: the other side of the looking glass. *Am J Public Health.* 1982;72(12):1401–1403.

Annas GJ. Rules for research on human genetic variation—lessons from Iceland. *N Engl J Med.* 2000;342(24):1830–1833.

Anney R, Klei L, Pinto D, et al. Individual common variants exert weak effects on the risk for autism spectrum disorderspi. *Hum Mol Genet.* 2012;21(21):4781–4792.

Anthony KK, Gil KM, Schanberg LE. Brief report: Parental perceptions of child vulnerability in children with chronic illness. *J Pediatr Psychol.* 2003;28(3):185–190.

Appelbaum PS. Clarifying the ethics of clinical research: a path toward avoiding the therapeutic misconception. *Am J Bioeth.* 2002;2(2):22–23.

Appelbaum PS, Grisso T. Assessing patients' capacities to consent to treatment. *N Engl J Med.* 1988;319(25):1635–1638.

Appelbaum PS, Lidz CW. The therapeutic misconception. In: Emanuel EJ, Grady C, Crouch RA, et al., eds. *The Oxford Textbook of Clinical Research Ethics.* New York: Oxford University Press; 2008:633–644.

Appelbaum PS, Lidz CW, Grisso T. Therapeutic misconception in clinical research: frequency and risk factors. *IRB*. 2004;26(2):1–8.

Appelbaum PS, Lidz CW, Klitzman R. Voluntariness of consent to research: a conceptual model. *Hastings Cent Rep*. 2009;39(1):30–39.

Appelbaum PS, Lidz CW, Meisel A. *Informed Consent: Legal Theory and Clinical Practice*. New York: Oxford University Press; 1987.

Appelbaum PS, Roth LH, Lidz C. The therapeutic misconception: informed consent in psychiatric research. *Int J Law Psychiatry*. 1982;5(3–4):319–329.

Appelbaum PS, Roth LH, Lidz CW, Benson P, Winslade W. False hopes and best data: consent to research and the therapeutic misconception. *Hastings Cent Rep*. 1987;17(2):20–24.

Arawi T. Using medical drama to teach biomedical ethics to medical students. *Med Teach*. 2010;32(5):e205–e210.

Arnold GL, Saavedra-Matiz CA, Galvin-Parton PA, et al. Lack of genotype-phenotype correlations and outcome in MCAD deficiency diagnosed by newborn screening in New York State. *Mol Genet Metab*. 2010;99(3):263–268.

Aronson SJ, Clark EH, Varugheese M, Baxter S, Babb LJ, Rehm HL. Communicating new knowledge on previously reported genetic variants. *Genet Med*. 2012. doi: 10.1038/gim.2012.19.

Arribas-Ayllon M. The ethics of disclosing genetic diagnosis for Alzheimer's disease: do we need a new paradigm? *Br Med Bull*. 2011;100(1):7–21.

Asch A. Prenatal diagnosis and selective abortion: a challenge to practice and policy. *Am J Public Health*. 1999;89(11):1649–1657.

Asch A, Gostin LO, Johnson DM. Respecting persons with disabilities and preventing disability: is there a conflict? In: Herr SS, Gostin LO, Koh HH, eds. *The Human Rights of Persons with Intellectual Disabilities: Different but Equal*. New York: Oxford University Press; 2011:319–346.

Ashcroft R, Goodenough T, Williamson E, Kent J. Children's consent to research participation: social context and personal experience invalidate fixed cutoff rules. *Am J Bioeth*. 2003;3(4):16–18.

Ashida S, Koehly LM, Roberts JS, Chen CA, Hiraki S, Green RC. The role of disease perceptions and results sharing in psychological adaptation after genetic susceptibility testing: the REVEAL Study. *Eur J Hum Genet*. 2010;18(12):1296–1301.

Atkins D. *Lucy*. Toronto: Playwrights Canada Press; 2010.

Atkinson K, Zuckerman B, Sharfstein JM, Levin D, Blatt RJ, Koh HK. A public health response to emerging technology: expansion of the Massachusetts newborn screening program. *Public Health Rep*. 2001;116(2):122–131.

Auer-Grumbach M. The phenotypic spectrum produced by mutations in TRPV4. [abstract]. *J Inherit Metab Dis*. 2011;34(Suppl 1): S3.

Austin JC. Re-conceptualizing risk in genetic counseling: implications for clinical practice. *J Genet Couns*. 2010;19(3):228–234.

Ayuso C, Millan JM, Mancheno M, Dal-Re R. Informed consent for whole-genome sequencing studies in the clinical setting. Proposed recommendations on essential content and process. *Eur J Hum Genet*. 2013. doi: 10.1038/ejhg.2012.297.

Bailey DB Jr. The blurred distinction between treatable and untreatable conditions in newborn screening. *Health Matrix*. 2009;19(1):141–153.

Bailey DB Jr, Armstrong FD, Kemper AR, Skinner D, Warren SF. Supporting family adaptation to presymptomatic and "untreatable" conditions in an era of expanded newborn screening. *J Pediatr Psychol*. 2009;34(6):648–661.

Bailey DB Jr, Beskow LM, Davis AM, Skinner D. Changing perspectives on the benefits of newborn screening. *Ment Retard Dev Disabil Res Rev*. 2006;12(4):270–279.

Bailey DB Jr, Skinner D, Davis AM, Whitmarsh I, Powell C. Ethical, legal, and social concerns about expanded newborn screening: fragile X syndrome as a prototype for emerging issues. *Pediatrics.* 2008;121(3):e693–e704.

Baily MA, Murray TH, eds. *Ethics and Newborn Genetic Screening: New Technologies, New Challenges.* Baltimore: Johns Hopkins University Press; 2009.

Baily MA, Murray TH. Ethics, evidence, and cost in newborn screening. *Hastings Cent Rep.* 2008;38(3):23–31.

Bainbridge MN, Wiszniewski W, Murdock DR, et al. Whole-genome sequencing for optimized patient management. *Sci Transl Med.* 2011;3(87):87re3.

Bamshad MJ, Ng SB, Bigham AW, et al. Exome sequencing as a tool for Mendelian disease gene discovery. *Nat Rev Genet.* 2011;12(11):745–755.

Bamshad MJ, Shendure JA, Valle D, et al. The Centers for Mendelian Genomics: a new large-scale initiative to identify the genes underlying rare Mendelian conditions. *Am J Med* Genet A. 2012;158A(7):1523–1525.

Bard J, Mayo TW, Tovino SA. Three ways of looking at a health law and literature class. *Drexel Law Rev.* 2009;1(2):512–572.

Bayer R. Stigma and the ethics of public health: not can we but should we. *Soc Sci Med.* 2008;67(3):463–472.

Bazely R. International collaboration on genetics of Alzheimer's disease. PHG Foundation. http://www.phgfoundation.org/news/7603. Published February 10, 2011. Accessed July 22, 2013.

Bearder et al. v State of Minnesota et al., No. A10-101 (Minn. 2011).

Beauchamp TL. Methods and principles in biomedical ethics. *J Med Ethics.* 2003;29(5):269–274.

Beauchamp TL, Childress JF. *Principles of Biomedical Ethics.* 6th ed. New York: Oxford University Press; 2009.

Beaudet AL, Belmont JW. Array-based DNA diagnostics: let the revolution begin. *Annu Rev Med.* 2008;59:113–129.

Beecher HK. Ethics and clinical research. *N Engl J Med.* 1966;274(24):1354–1360.

Beleno et al. v Texas Department of State Health Services et al., Case No. 5:2009cv00188 (W.D. Tex. 2009).

Bell CJ, Dinwiddie DL, Miller NA, et al. Carrier testing for severe childhood recessive diseases by next-generation sequencing. *Sci Transl Med.* 2011;3(65):65ra4.

Bemmels HR, Wolf SM, Van Ness B. Mapping the inputs, analyses, and outputs of biobank research systems to identify sources of incidental findings and individual research results for potential return to participants. *Genet Med.* 2012;14(4):385–392.

Ben-Arye E, Frenkel M, Klein A, Scharf M. Attitudes toward integration of complementary and alternative medicine in primary care: perspectives of patients, physicians and complementary practitioners. *Patient Educ Couns.* 2008;70:395–402.

Benkendorf J, Goodspeed T, Watson MS. Newborn screening residual dried blood spot use for newborn screening quality improvement. *Genet Med.* 2010;12(12 Suppl):S269–S272.

Benkendorf JL, Reutenauer JE, Hughes CA, et al. Patients' attitudes about autonomy and confidentiality in genetic testing for breast-ovarian cancer susceptibility. *Am J Med Genet.* 1997;73(3):296–303.

Bennette CS, Trinidad SB, Fullerton SM, et al. Return of incidental findings in genomic medicine: measuring what patients value—development of an instrument to measure preferences for information from next-generation testing. *Genet Med.* 2013. doi: 10.1038/gim.2013.63.

Berg JS, Adams M, Nassar N, et al. An informatics approach to analyzing the inciden-talome. *Genet Med.* 2013;15(1):36–44.

Berg JS, Evans JP, Leigh MW, et al. Next generation massively parallel sequenc-ing of targeted exomes to identify genetic mutations in primary ciliary dyskinesia: implications for application to clinical testing. *Genet Med.* 2011;13(3):218–229.

Berg JS, Khoury MJ, Evans JP. Deploying whole genome sequencing in clinical practice and public health: meeting the challenge one bin at a time. *Genet Med.* 2011;13(6):499–504.

Bernard LE, McGillivray B, Van Allen MI, Friedman JM, Langlois S. Duty to re-contact: a study of families at risk for fragile X. *J Genet Couns.* 1999;8(1):3–15.

Berry SA, Brown C, Grant M, et al. Newborn screening 50 years later: access issues faced by adults with PKU. *Genet Med.* 2013. doi: 10.1038/gim.2013.10.

Berry SA, Lloyd-Puryear MA, Watson MS. Long-term follow-up of newborn screening patients. *Genet Med.* 2010;12(12 Suppl):S267–S268.

Beskow LM, Burke W. Offering individual genetic research results: context matters. *Sci Transl Med.* 2010;2(38):38cm20.

Beskow LM, Burke W, Merz JF, et al. Informed consent for population-based research involving genetics. *JAMA.* 2001;286(18):2315–2321.

Beskow LM, Dean E. Informed consent for biorepositories: assessing prospective participants' understanding and opinions. *Cancer Epidemiol Biomarkers Prev.* 2008;17(6):1440–1451.

Beskow LM, Smolek SJ. Prospective biorepository participants' perspectives on access to research results. *J Empir Res Hum Res Ethics.* 2009;4(3):99–111.

Betancur C. Etiological heterogeneity in autism spectrum disorders: more than 100 genetic and genomic disorders and still counting. *Brain Res.* 2011;1380:42–77.

Beucher J, Leray E, Deneuville E, et al. Psychological effects of false-positive results in cystic fibrosis newborn screening: a two-year follow-up. *J Pediatr.* 2010;156(5):771–776, 776.e1.

Bickenbach JE. *Ethics, Law, and Policy.* Thousand Oaks, CA: Sage Publications; 2012.

Biesecker LG. Exome sequencing makes medical genomics a reality. *Nat Genet.* 2010;42(1):13–14.

Biesecker LG. Incidental variants are critical for genomics. *Am J Hum Genet.* 2013;92(5):648–651.

Biesecker LG. The Nirvana fallacy and the return of results. *Am J Bioeth.* 2013;13(2):43–44.

Biesecker LG. Opportunities and challenges for the integration of massively paral-lel genomic sequencing into clinical practice: lessons from the ClinSeq project. *Genet Med.* 2012;14(4):393–398.

Biesecker LG, Mullikin JC, Facio FM, et al. The ClinSeq Project: piloting large-scale genome sequencing for research in genomic medicine. *Genome Res.* 2009;19(9):1665–1674.

Birrell J, Meares K, Wilkinson A, Freeston M. Toward a definition of intolerance of uncertainty: a review of factor analytical studies of the Intolerance of Uncertainty Scale. *Clin Psychol Rev.* 2011;31(7):1198–1208.

Black L, McClellan KA. Familial communication of research results: a need to know? *J Law Med Ethics.* 2011;39(4):605–613.

Bledsoe MJ, Clayton EW, McGuire AL, Grizzle WE, O'Rourke PP, Zeps N. Return of research results from genomic biobanks: cost matters. *Genet Med.* 2013;15(2):103–105.

Bohannon J. Genetics. Genealogy databases enable naming of anonymous DNA donors. *Science*. 2013;339(6117):262.

Bollinger JM, Scott J, Dvoskin R, Kaufman D. Public preferences regarding the return of individual genetic research results: findings from a qualitative focus group study. *Genet Med*. 2012;14(4):451–457.

Bolnick DA, Fullwiley D, Duster T, et al. Genetics: the science and business of genetic ancestry testing. *Science* 2007;318:399–400.

Bookman EB, Langehorne AA, Eckfeldt JH, et al. Comment on "Multidimensional results reporting to participants in genomic studies: getting it right." *Sci Transl Med*. 2011;3(70):70le1.

Borry P, Dierickx K. What are the limits of the duty of care? The case of clinical genetics. *Per Med*. 2008;5(2):101–104.

Bosch N, Junyent N, Gadea N, et al. What factors may influence psychological well being at three months and one year post BRCA genetic result disclosure? *Breast*. 2012;21(6):755–760.

Botkin JR. Evidence-based reviews of newborn-screening opportunities. *Pediatrics*. 2010;125(5):e1265–e1266.

Botkin JR. Newborn screening for fragile X syndrome: do we care what parents think? *Pediatrics*. 2011;127(6):e1593–e1594.

Botkin JR. Parental permission for research in newborn screening. In: Baily MA, Murray TH, eds. *Ethics and Newborn Genetic Screening: New Technologies, New Challenges*. Baltimore, MD: Johns Hopkins University Press; 2009:255–273.

Botkin JR. Preimplantation and prenatal genetic testing for inherited diseases, dispositions, and traits. In: Diekema DS, Mercurio MR, Adam MB, eds. *Clinical Ethics in Pediatrics: A Case-Based Textbook*. Cambridge, UK: Cambridge University Press; 2011:68–76.

Botkin JR. Preventing exploitation in pediatric research. *Am J Bioeth*. 2003;3(4):31–32.

Botkin JR, Anderson R, Staes C, Longo N. Developing a national registry for conditions identifiable through newborn screening. *Genet Med*. 2009;11(3):176–182.

Botkin JR, Clayton EW, Fost NC, et al. Newborn screening technology: proceed with caution. *Pediatrics*. 2006;117(5):1793–1799.

Botkin JR, Rothwell E, Anderson R, et al. Public attitudes regarding the use of residual newborn screening specimens for research. *Pediatrics*. 2012;129(2):231–238.

Boudreault P, Baldwin EE, Fox M, et al. Deaf adults' reasons for genetic testing depend on cultural affiliation: results from a prospective, longitudinal genetic counseling and testing study. *J Deaf Stud Deaf Educ*. 2010;15(3):209–227.

Bowlby J. *Attachment*. New York: Basic Books; 1969. *Attachment and Loss*; vol. 1.

Boyce WT. The vulnerable child: new evidence, new approaches. *Adv Pediatr*. 1992;39:1–33.

Bradbury AR, Patrick-Miller L, Egleston B, et al. Parent opinions regarding the genetic testing of minors for BRCA1/2. *J Clin Oncol*. 2010;28(21):3498–3505.

Bradbury AR, Patrick-Miller L, Egleston BL, et al. When parents disclose BRCA1/2 test results: their communication and perceptions of offspring response. *Cancer*. 2012;118(13):3417–3425.

Brandt AM. *No Magic Bullet: A Social History of Venereal Disease in the United States Since 1880*. New York: Oxford University Press; 1985.

Brandt DS, Shinkunas L, Hillis SL, et al. A closer look at the recommended criteria for disclosing genetic results: perspectives of medical genetic specialists, genomic researchers, and institutional review board chairs. *J Genet Couns*. 2013;22(4):544–553.

Brazelton TB, Koslowski B, Main M. The origins of reciprocity: the early mother-infant interaction. In: Lewis M, Rosenblum L, eds. *The Effect of the Infant on Its Caregiver*. New York: Wiley; 1974:49–76.

Bredenoord AL, de Vries MC, van Delden JJ. Next-generation sequencing: does the next generation still have a right to an open future? *Nat Rev Genet*. 2013;14(5):306.

Bredenoord AL, Kroes HY, Cuppen E, Parker M, van Delden JJ. Disclosure of individual genetic data to research participants: the debate reconsidered. *Trends Genet*. 2011;27(2):41–47.

Bredenoord AL, Onland-Moret NC, Van Delden JJ. Feedback of individual genetic results to research participants: in favor of a qualified disclosure policy. *Hum Mutat*. 2011;32(8):861–867.

Brehaut JC, O'Connor AM, Wood TJ, et al. Validation of a decision regret scale. *Med Decis Making*. 2003;23(4):281–292.

Brisson AR, Matsui D, Rieder MJ, Fraser DD. Translational research in pediatrics: tissue sampling and biobanking. *Pediatrics*. 2012;129(1):153–162.

Brody H. Narrative ethics and institutional impact. In: Charon R, Montello M, eds. *Stories Matter: The Role of Narrative in Medical Ethics*. New York: Routledge; 2002:153–157.

Brosco JP, Sanders LM, Dharia R, Guez G, Feudtner C. The lure of treatment: expanded newborn screening and the curious case of histidinemia. *Pediatrics*. 2010;125(3):417–419.

Brothers KB. Biobanking in pediatrics: the human nonsubjects approach. *Per Med*. 2011;8(1):79.

Brothers KB, Clayton EW. Biobanks: too long to wait for consent. *Science*. 2009;326(5954):798; author reply 799.

Buchanan AE, Brock DW. *Deciding for Others: The Ethics of Surrogate Decision Making*. New York: Cambridge University Press; 1989.

Buck v. Bell, 274 U.S. 200 (1927).

Burke W, Diekema DS. Ethical issues arising from the participation of children in genetic research. *J Pediatr*. 2006;149(1 Suppl):S34–S38.

Burke W, Matheny Antommaria AH, Bennett R, et al. Recommendations for returning genomic incidental findings? We need to talk! *Genet Med*. 2013; doi: 10.1038/gim.2013.113.

Burke W, Psaty BM. Personalized medicine in the era of genomics. *JAMA*. 2007;298(14):1682–1684.

Burke W, Tarini B, Press NA, Evans JP. Genetic screening. *Epidemiol Rev*. 2011;33(1):148–164.

Burke W, Zimmern RL, Kroese M. Defining purpose: a key step in genetic test evaluation. *Genet Med*. 2007;9(10):675–681.

Bush LW, Rothenberg KH. Dialogues, dilemmas, and disclosures: genomic research and incidental findings. *Genet Med*. 2012;14(3):293–295.

Bush LW, Rothenberg KH. It's not that simple! Genomic research & the consent process, in Rothenberg KH, Bush LW. *Genet Med*. 2012;14(2):OnlineSuppl.

Bush LW, Rothenberg KH. It's so complicated! Genomic research & incidental findings, in Bush LW, Rothenberg KH. *Genet Med*. 2012;14(3):OnlineSuppl.

Cahn NR, Collins JM. Eight is enough. *Northwest Univ Law Rev Colloquy*. 2009;103:501–513.

Calonge N, Green NS, Rinaldo P, et al. Committee report: method for evaluating conditions nominated for population-based screening of newborns and children. *Genet Med*. 2010;12(3):153–159.

Campbell DB, Datta D, Jones ST, et al. Association of oxytocin receptor (OXTR) gene variants with multiple phenotype domains of autism spectrum disorder. *J Neurodev Disord.* 2011;3(2):101–112.

Campbell E, Ross LF. Parental attitudes and beliefs regarding the genetic testing of children. *Community Genet.* 2005;8(2):94–102.

Candilis PJ, Lidz CW, Appelbaum PS, et al. The silent majority: who speaks at IRB meetings? *IRB.* 2012;34(4):15–20.

Capron AM. Human genetic engineering: Gattaca. In: Colt HG, Quadrelli S, Friedman LD, eds. *The Picture of Health: Medical Ethics and the Movies.* New York: Oxford University Press; 2011:351–356.

Capron AM. The authority of others to decide about biomedical interventions with incompetents. In: Gaylin W, Macklin R, eds. *Who Speaks for the Child: The Problems of Proxy Consent.* New York: Plenum; 1982:115–152.

Carmichael M. Newborn screening: a spot of trouble. *Nature.* 2011;475(7355):156–158.

Case GA, Brauner DJ. Perspective: the doctor as performer: a proposal for change based on a performance studies paradigm. *Acad Med.* 2010;85(1):159–163.

Caskey CT. DNA-based medicine: prevention and therapy. In: Kevles DJ, Hood L, eds. *The Code of Codes: Scientific and Social Issues in the Human Genome Project.* Cambridge, MA: Harvard University Press; 1992:112–135.

Cassa CA, Savage SK, Taylor PL, Green RC, McGuire AL, Mandl KD. Disclosing pathogenic genetic variants to research participants: quantifying an emerging ethical responsibility. *Genome Res.* 2012;22(3):421–428.

Cassa CA, Schmidt B, Kohane IS, Mandl KD. My sister's keeper?: genomic research and the identifiability of siblings. *BMC Med Genomics.* 2008;1:32.

Cassa CA, Tong MY, Jordan DM. Large numbers of genetic variants considered to be pathogenic are common in asymptomatic individuals. *Human Mutat.* 2013. doi: 10.1002/humu.22375.

Casto AM, Amid C. Beyond the genome: genomics research ten years after the human genome sequence. *Genome Biol.* 2010;11(11):309.

Caught napping by clones. 385 *Nature.* 1997;385(6619):753.

Caulfield T. Biobanks and blanket consent: the proper place of the public good and public perception rationales. *Kings Law J.* 2007;18(2):209–226.

Caulfield T. Human cloning laws, human dignity and the poverty of the policy making dialogue. *BMC Med Ethics.* 2003;4:E3.

Caulfield S, Caulfield TA. *Imagining Science: Art, Science, and Social Change.* Edmonton: University of Alberta Press; 2008.

Caulfield T, Kayet J. Broad consent in biobanking: reflections on seemingly insurmountable dilemmas. *Med Law Int.* 2009;10(2):85–100.

Caulfield T, Knowles L, Meslin EM. Law and policy in the era of reproductive genetics. *J Med Ethics.* 2004;30(4):414–417.

Caulfield T, McGuire AL, Cho M, et al. Research ethics recommendations for whole-genome research: consensus statement. *PLoS Biol.* 2008;6(3):e73.

Cavanagh L, Compton CJ, Tluczek A, Brown RL, Farrell PM. Long-term evaluation of genetic counseling following false-positive newborn screen for cystic fibrosis. *J Genet Couns.* 2010;19(2):199–210.

Chakravarti A, Kapoor A. Genetics: Mendelian puzzles. *Science.* 2012;335(6071):930–931.

Chambers T. *The Fiction of Bioethics: Cases as Literary Texts.* New York: Routledge; 1999. *Reflective Bioethics.*

Chambers T. Literature. In: Sugarman J, Sulmasy DP, eds. *Methods in Medical Ethics.* Washington, DC: Georgetown University Press; 2010:159–174.

Chambers T, Montgomery K. Plot: framing contingency and choice in bioethics. In: Charon R, Montello M, eds. *Stories Matter: The Role of Narrative in Medical Ethics.* New York: Routledge; 2002:79–87.

Chan B, Facio FM, Eidem H, et al. Genomic inheritances: disclosing individual research results from whole-exome sequencing to deceased participants' relatives. *Am J Bioeth.* 2012;12(10):1–8.

Charo RA, Rothenberg KH. The good mother: the limits of reproductive responsibility and genetic choice. In: Rothenberg KR, Thomson E, eds. *Women and Prenatal Testing: Facing the Challenges of Genetic Technology.* Columbus, OH: Ohio State University Press; 1994:105–130.

Charon R. Narrative and medicine. *N Engl J Med.* 2004;350(9):862–864.

Charon R. *Narrative Medicine: Honoring the Stories of Illness.* Oxford, UK: Oxford University Press; 2006.

Charon R. Time and ethics. In: Charon R, Montello M, eds. *Stories Matter: The Role of Narrative in Medical Ethics.* New York: Routledge; 2002:60–69.

Charon R, Montello M, eds. *Stories Matter: The Role of Narrative in Medical Ethics.* New York: Routledge; 2002. *Reflective Bioethics.*

Charon R, Trautmann Banks J, Connelly JE, et al. Literature and medicine: contributions to clinical practice. *Ann Intern Med.* 1995;122(8):599–606.

Chase M. *Harvey.* New York: Dramatists Play Service; 1971.

Chen LS, Xu L, Huang TY, Dhar SU. Autism genetic testing: a qualitative study of awareness, attitudes, and experiences among parents of children with autism spectrum disorders. *Genet Med.* 2013;15(4):274–281.

Chen LS, Zhao M, Zhou Q, Xu L. Chinese Americans' views of prenatal genetic testing in the genomic era: a qualitative study. *Clin Genet.* 2012;82(1):22–27.

Chervenak FA, McCullough LB. A comprehensive ethical framework for fetal research and its application to fetal surgery for spina bifida. *Am J Obstet Gynecol.* 2002;187(1):10–14.

Childress JF, Faden RR, Gaare RD, et al. Public health ethics: mapping the terrain. *J Law Med Ethics.* 2002;30(2):170–178.

Cho MK. Understanding incidental findings in the context of genetics and genomics. *J Law Med Ethics.* 2008;36(2):280–285, 212.

Christenhusz GM, Devriendt K, Dierickx K. To tell or not to tell? A systematic review of ethical reflections on incidental findings arising in genetics contexts. *Eur J Hum Genet.* 2013;21(3):248–255.

Church G, Heeney C, Hawkins N, et al. Public access to genome-wide data: five views on balancing research with privacy and protection. *PLoS Genet.* 2009;5(10):e1000665.

Churchill C. *A Number.* New York: Theatre Communications Group; 2002.

Churchill LR. Narrative ethics, gene stories, and the hermeneutics of consent forms. In: Charon R, Montello M, eds. *Stories Matter: The Role of Narrative in Medical Ethics.* New York: Routledge; 2002:187–199.

Clark AE, Shim JK, Shostak S, Nelson A. Biomedicalising genetic health, diseases and identities. In: Atkinson P, Glasner P, Lock M., eds. *Handbook of Genetics and Society: Mapping the New Genomic Era.* New York: Routledge; 2009:21–40.

Clayton EW. Currents in contemporary ethics. State run newborn screening in the genomic era, or how to avoid drowning when drinking from a fire hose. *J Law Med Ethics.* 2010;38(3):697–700.

Clayton EW. Incidental findings in genetics research using archived DNA. *J Law Med Ethics*. 2008;36(2):286–291, 212.

Clayton EW. Lessons to be learned from the move toward expanded newborn screening. In: Baily MA, Murray TH, eds. *Ethics and Newborn Genetic Screening: New Technologies, New Challenges*. Baltimore: Johns Hopkins University Press; 2009:125–135.

Clayton EW. Ten fingers, ten toes: newborn screening for untreatable disorders. *Health Matrix*. 2009;19(1):199–203.

Clayton EW. What should the law say about disclosure of genetic information to relatives? *J Health Care Law Policy*. 1998;1(2):373–390.

Clayton EW, Haga S, Kuszler P, Bane E, Shutske K, Burke W. Managing incidental genomic findings: legal obligations of clinicians. *Genet Med*. 2013. doi: 10.1038/gim.2013.7.

Clayton EW, Kelly SE. Let us ask better questions. *Genet Med*. 2013. doi: 10.1038/gim.2013.68.

Clayton EW, McGuire AL. The legal risks of returning results of genomics research. *Genet Med*. 2012;14(4):473–477.

Clayton EW, Ross LF. Implications of disclosing individual results of clinical research. *JAMA*. 2006;295(1):37; author reply 37–38.

Clayton EW, Smith M, Fullerton SM, et al. Confronting real time ethical, legal, and social issues in the Electronic Medical Records and Genomics (eMERGE) Consortium. *Genet Med*. 2010;12(10):616–620.

Coan AB. Is there a constitutional right to select the genes of one's offspring? *Hastings Law J*. 2011; 63:233–296.

Coates R, Williams M, Melillo S, Gudgeon J. Genetic testing for lynch syndrome in individuals newly diagnosed with colorectal cancer to reduce morbidity and mortality from colorectal cancer in their relatives. *PLoS Curr*. 2011;3:RRN1246.

Cody JD. An advocate's perspective on newborn screening policy. In: Baily MA, Murray TH, eds. *Ethics and Newborn Genetic Screening: New Technologies, New Challenges*. Baltimore: Johns Hopkins University Press; 2009:89–105.

Colaianni A, Chandrasekharan S, Cook-Deegan R. Impact of gene patents and licensing practices on access to genetic testing and carrier screening for Tay-Sachs and Canavan disease. *Genet Med*. 2010;12(4 Suppl):S5–S14.

Colgrove J, Bayer R. Manifold restraints: liberty, public health, and the legacy of Jacobson v Massachusetts. *Am J Public Health*. 2005;95(4):571–576.

Collins FS. Shattuck lecture—medical and societal consequences of the Human Genome Project. *N Engl J Med*. 1999;341(1):28–37.

Collins F, Galas D. A new five-year plan for the U.S. Human Genome Project. *Science*. 1993; 262:43–46.

Collins FS, Green ED, Guttmacher AE, Guyer MS. US National Human Genome Research Institute. A vision for the future of genomics research. *Nature*. 2003;422(6934):835–847.

Colt HG, Quadrelli S, Friedman LD, eds. *The Picture of Health: Medical Ethics and the Movies*. New York: Oxford University Press; 2011.

Comeau AM, Larson C, Eaton RB. Integration of new genetic diseases into statewide newborn screening: New England experience. *Am J Med Genet C Semin Med Genet*. 2004;125C(1):35–41.

Comeau AM, Parad RB, Dorkin HL, et al. Population-based newborn screening for genetic disorders when multiple mutation DNA testing is incorporated: a cystic fibrosis newborn screening model demonstrating increased sensitivity but more carrier detections. *Pediatrics*. 2004;113(6):1573–1581.

Connolly JJ, Hakonarson H. The impact of genomics on pediatric research and medicine. *Pediatrics*. 2012;129(6):1150–1160.

Conrad P. [book review]. Troy Duster, Backdoor to Eugenics. *J Health Politics Policy Law*. 1992;17(1):184–186.

Cooke M, Irby DM, O'Brien BC. *A Summary of Educating Physicians: A Call for Reform of Medical School and Residency*. San Francisco: Jossey Bass; 2010. http://www. carnegiefoundation.org/elibrary/summary-educating-physicians#summary. Published January 2011. Accessed July 22, 2013.

Couzin J. Genetic privacy. Whole-genome data not anonymous, challenging assumptions. *Science*. 2008;321(5894):1278.

Couzin-Frankel J. Genome sequencing. Return of unexpected DNA results urged. *Science*. 2013;339(6127):1507–1508.

Couzin-Frankel J. Human genome 10th anniversary. What would you do? *Science*. 2011;331(6018):662–665.

Couzin-Frankel J. Newborn blood collections. Science gold mine, ethical minefield. *Science*. 2009;324(5924):166–168.

Crepel A, Steyaert J, De la Marche W, et al. Narrowing the critical deletion region for autism spectrum disorders on 16p11.2. *Am J Med Genet B Neuropsychiatr Genet*. 2011;156(2):243–245.

Cross-Disorder Group of the Psychiatric Genomics Consortium. Identification of risk loci with shared effects on five major psychiatric disorders: a genome-wide analysis. *Lancet*. 2013;381(9875):1371–1379.

Cummings JL. Alzheimer's disease clinical trials: changing the paradigm. *Curr Psychiatr Rep*. 2011;13:437–442.

Czarny MJ, Faden RR, Sugarman J. Bioethics and professionalism in popular television medical dramas. *J Med Ethics*. 2010;36(4):203–206.

Daack-Hirsch S, Driessnack M, Hanish A, et al. 'Information is information': a public perspective on incidental findings in clinical and research genome-based testing. *Clin Genet*. 2013;84(1):11–18.

Daniels N, Kennedy BP, Kawachi I. Why justice is good for our health: the social determinants of health inequalities. *Daedalus*. 1999;128(4):215–251.

Danis M, Largent E, Grady C, et al. *Research Ethics Consultation: A Casebook*. Oxford, UK: Oxford University Press; 2012.

Davis DS. Child's right to an open future. *Hastings Cent Rep*. 2002;32(5):6; author reply 6.

Davis DS. Genetic dilemmas and the child's right to an open future. *Hastings Cent Rep*. 1997;27(2):7–15.

Davis DS. Groups, communities, and contested identities in genetic research. *Hastings Cent Rep*. 2000;30(6):38–45.

Davis PB. Therapy for cystic fibrosis—the end of the beginning? *N Engl J Med*. 2011;365(18):1734–1735.

Davis TC, Humiston SG, Arnold CL, et al. Recommendations for effective newborn screening communication: results of focus groups with parents, providers, and experts. *Pediatrics*. 2006;117(5 Pt 2):S326–S340.

Deloney LA, Graham CJ. Wit: using drama to teach first-year medical students about empathy and compassion. *Teach Learn Med*. 2003;15(4):247–251.

DeLuca JM, Kearney MH, Norton SA, Arnold GL. Parents' experiences of expanded newborn screening evaluations. *Pediatrics*. 2011;128(1):53–61.

de Melo-Martin I, Ho A. Beyond informed consent: the therapeutic misconception and trust. *J Med Ethics.* 2008;34(3):202–205.

Denny CC, Wilfond BS, Peters JA, Giri N, Alter BP. All in the family: disclosure of "unwanted" information to an adolescent to benefit a relative. *Am J Med Genet A.* 2008;146A(21):2719–2724.

Dhar SU, Alford RL, Nelson EA, Potocki L. Enhancing exposure to genetics and genomics through an innovative medical school curriculum. *Genet Med.* 2012;14(1):163–167.

Dicker S, Bennett E. Engulfed by the spectrum: the impact of autism spectrum disorders on law and policy. *Valparaiso Univ Law Rev.* 2011;45:415–456.

Dickert N, Sugarman J. Ethical goals of community consultation in research. *Am J Public Health.* 2005;95(7):1123–1127.

Diekema DS. Conducting ethical research in pediatrics: a brief historical overview and review of pediatric regulations. *J Pediatr.* 2006;149(1 Suppl):S3–S11.

Diekema DS. Taking children seriously: what's so important about assent? *Am J Bioeth.* 2003;3(4):25–26.

Diekema DS, Mercurio MR, Adam MB, eds. *Clinical Ethics in Pediatrics: A Case-Based Textbook.* Cambridge, UK: Cambridge University Press; 2011.

Dillard JP, Shen L, Robinson JD, Farrell PM. Parental information seeking following a positive newborn screening for cystic fibrosis. *J Health Commun.* 2010;15(8):880–894.

Djerassi C. *An Immaculate Misconception: Sex in an Age of Mechanical Reproduction.* London: Imperial College Press; 2000.

Donley G, Hull SC, Berkman BE. Prenatal whole genome sequencing: just because we can, should we? *Hastings Cent Rep.* 2012;42(4):28–40.

Doukas DJ, Berg JW. The family covenant and genetic testing. *Am J Bioeth.* 2001;1(3):3–10.

Doukas DJ, McCullough LB, Wear S. Reforming medical education in ethics and humanities by finding common ground with Abraham Flexner. *Acad Med.* 2010;85(2):318–323.

Dove ES, Avard D, Black L, Knoppers BM. Emerging issues in paediatric health research consent forms in Canada: working towards best practices. *BMC Med Ethics.* 2013;14:5.

Downie RS, Macnaughton J. *Bioethics and the Humanities: Attitudes and Perceptions.* New York: Routledge-Cavendish; 2007.

Downie RS, Randall F. Parenting and the best interests of minors. *J Med Philos.* 1997;22(3):219–231.

Downing GJ, Zuckerman AE, Coon C, Lloyd-Puryear MA. Enhancing the quality and efficiency of newborn screening programs through the use of health information technology. *Semin Perinatol.* 2010;34(2):156–162.

Downing NR, Williams JK, Daack-Hirsch S, Driessnack M, Simon CM. Genetics specialists' perspectives on disclosure of genomic incidental findings in the clinical setting. *Patient Educ Couns.* 2013;90(1):133–138.

Downs SM, van Dyck PC, Rinaldo P, et al. Improving newborn screening laboratory test ordering and result reporting using health information exchange. *J Am Med Inform Assoc.* 2010;17(1):13–18.

Dresser R. The role of patient advocates and public representatives in research. In: Emanuel EJ, Grady C, Crouch RA, et al., eds. *The Oxford Textbook of Clinical Research Ethics.* New York: Oxford University Press; 2008:231–244.

Dressler LG, Smolek S, Ponsaran R, et al. IRB perspectives on the return of individual results from genomic research. *Genet Med.* 2012;14(2):215–222.

Driessnack M, Daack-Hirsch S, Downing N, et al. The disclosure of incidental genomic findings: an "ethically important moment" in pediatric research and practice. *J Community Genet*. 2013. doi: 10.1007/s12687-013-0145-1.

Drmanac R. Medicine. The ultimate genetic test. *Science*. 2012;336(6085):1110–1112.

Dubler NN, Liebman CB. *Bioethics Mediation: A Guide to Shaping Shared Solutions*. Revised ed. Nashville, TN: Nashville University Press; 2011.

Duncan RE, Gillam L, Savulescu J, et al. "You're one of us now": young people describe their experiences of predictive genetic testing for Huntington disease (HD) and familial adenomatous polyposis (FAP). *Am J Med Genet C Semin Med Genet*. 2008;148C(1):47–55.

Dunn CT, Skrypek MM, Powers ALR, Laguna TA. The need for vigilance: the case of a false-negative newborn screen for cystic fibrosis. *Pediatrics*. 2011;128(2):e446–e449.

Duster T. *Backdoor to Eugenics*. 2nd ed. New York: Routledge; 2003.

Duster T. Lessons from history: why race and ethnicity have played a major role in biomedical research. *J Law Med Ethics*. 2006;34(3):487–496, 479.

Duster T. Medicine. Race and reification in science. *Science*. 2005;307(5712):1050–1051.

Edson M. *Wit*. New York: Dramatists Play Service; 1999.

Edvardson S, Shaag A, Zenvirt S, et al. Joubert syndrome 2 (JBTS2) in Ashkenazi Jews is associated with a TMEM216 mutation. *Am J Hum Genet*. 2010;86(1):93–97.

Edwards KL, Lemke AA, Trinidad SB, et al. Genetics researchers' and IRB professionals' attitudes toward genetic research review: a comparative analysis. *Genet Med*. 2012;14(2):236–242.

Elia J, Gai X, Hakonarson H, White PS. Structural variations in attention-deficit hyperactivity disorder. *Lancet*. 2011;377(9763):377–378; author reply 378.

Ellis TR. The materialization of ghosts in Strange Interlude. *Am Notes Queries*. March 1981:110–114.

Emanuel EJ, Grady C. Four paradigms of clinical research and research oversight. In: Emanuel EJ, Grady C, Crouch RA, et al., eds. *The Oxford Textbook of Clinical Research Ethics*. New York: Oxford University Press; 2008:222–230.

Emanuel EJ, Grady C, Crouch RA, et al., eds. *The Oxford Textbook of Clinical Research Ethics*. New York: Oxford University Press; 2008.

Emanuel EJ, Thompson DF. The concept of conflicts of interest. In: Emanuel EJ, Grady C, Crouch RA, et al., eds. *The Oxford Textbook of Clinical Research Ethics*. New York: Oxford University Press; 2008:758–766.

Emanuel EJ, Wendler D, Grady C. What makes clinical research ethical? *JAMA*. 2000;283(20):2701–2711.

Ensenauer R, Vockley J, Willard J-M, et al. A common mutation is associated with a mild, potentially asymptomatic phenotype in patients with isovaleric acidemia diagnosed by newborn screening. *Am J Hum Genet*. 2004;75(6):1136–1142.

Evans JP. Health care in the age of genetic medicine. *JAMA*. 2007;298(22):2670–2672.

Evans JP. Return of results to the families of children in genomic sequencing: tallying risks and benefits. *Genet Med*. 2013;15(6):435–436.

Evans JP. When is a medical finding "incidental"? *Genet Med*. 2013;15(7):515–516.

Evans JP, Berg JS, Olshan AF, Magnuson T, Rimer BK. We screen newborns, don't we?: realizing the promise of public health genomics. *Genet Med*. 2013;15(5):332–334.

Evans JP, Khoury MJ. The arrival of genomic medicine to the clinic is only the beginning of the journey. *Genet Med.* 2013;15(4):268–269.

Evans JP, Meslin EM, Marteau TM, Caulfield T. Genomics. Deflating the genomic bubble. *Science.* 2011;331(6019):861–862.

Evans JP, Rothschild BB. Return of results: not that complicated? *Genet Med.* 2012;14(4):358–360.

Ewart RM. Primum non nocere and the quality of evidence: rethinking the ethics of screening. *J Am Board Fam Pract.* 2000;13(3):188–196.

Fabsitz RR, McGuire A, Sharp RR, et al. Ethical and practical guidelines for reporting genetic research results to study participants: updated guidelines from a National Heart, Lung, and Blood Institute working group. *Circ Cardiovasc Genet.* 2010;3(6):574–580.

Facio FM, Brooks S, Loewenstein J, Green S, Biesecker LG, Biesecker BB. Motivators for participation in a whole-genome sequencing study: implications for translational genomics research. *Eur J Hum Genet.* 2011;19(12):1213–1217.

Facio FM, Eidem H, Fisher T, et al. Intentions to receive individual results from whole-genome sequencing among participants in the ClinSeq study. *Eur J Hum Genet.* 2013;21(3):261–265.

Faden R, Chwalow AJ, Holtzman NA, Horn SD. A survey to evaluate parental consent as public policy for neonatal screening. *Am J Public Health.* 1982;72(12):1347–1352.

Faden RR, Beauchamp TL, King NMP. *A History and Theory of Informed Consent.* New York: Oxford University Press; 1986.

Faden RR, Holtzman NA, Chwalow AJ. Parental rights, child welfare, and public health: the case of PKU screening. *Am J Public Health.* 1982;72(12):1396–1400.

Faden RR, Kass NE, Goodman SN, Pronovost P, Tunis S, Beauchamp TL. An ethics framework for a learning health care system: a departure from traditional research ethics and clinical ethics. *Hastings Cent Rep.* 2013;43(Suppl):S16–S27.

Falk MJ, Dugan RB, O'Riordan MA, Matthews AL, Robin NH. Medical geneticists' duty to warn at-risk relatives for genetic disease. *Am J Med Genet A.* 2003;120A(3):374–380.

Farrell MH, Christopher SA, Tluczek A, et al. Improving communication between doctors and parents after newborn screening. *WMJ.* 2011;110(5):221–227.

Farrell MH, Farrell PM. Newborn screening for cystic fibrosis: ensuring more good than harm. *J Pediatr.* 2003;143(6):707–712.

Farrell MH, Speiser J, Deuster L, Christopher S. Child health providers' precautionary discussion of emotions during communication about results of newborn genetic screening. *Arch Pediatr Adolesc Med.* 2012;166(1):62–67.

Fearing MK, Levy HL. Expanded newborn screening using tandem mass spectrometry. *Adv Pediatr.* 2003;50:81–111.

Feero WG, Green ED. Genomics education for health care professionals in the 21st century. *JAMA.* 2011;306(9):989–990.

Feero WG, Guttmacher AE, Collins FS. Genomic medicine—an updated primer. *N Engl J Med.* 2010;362(21):2001–2011.

Feero WG, Guttmacher AE, Collins FS. The genome gets personal—almost. *JAMA.* 2008;299(11):1351–1352.

Feinberg J. The child's right to an open future. In: Aiken W, Lafollette H, eds. *Whose Child? Children's Rights, Parental Authority, and State Power.* Totowa, NJ: Littlefield, Adams; 1980:124–153.

Fernandez CV, Gao J, Strahlendorf C, et al. Providing research results to participants: attitudes and needs of adolescents and parents of children with cancer. *J Clin Oncol.* 2009;27(6):878–883.

Fernandez CV, Strahlendorf C, Avard D, et al. Attitudes of Canadian researchers toward the return to participants of incidental and targeted genomic findings obtained in a pediatric research setting. *Genet Med.* 2013;15(7):558–564.

Fetters MD. The wizard of Osler: a brief educational intervention combining film and medical readers' theater to teach about power in medicine. *Fam Med.* 2006;38(5):323–325.

Ficicioglu C, Coughlin CR 2nd, Bennett MJ, Yudkoff M. Very long-chain acyl-CoA dehydrogenase deficiency in a patient with normal newborn screening by tandem mass spectrometry. *J Pediatr.* 2010;156(3):492–494.

Field MJ, Behrman RE, eds. Institute of Medicine. *Ethical Conduct of Clinical Research Involving Children.* Washington, DC: National Academies Press; 2004.

Fins JJ. C.P. Snow at Wesleyan: liberal learning and the origins of the "Third Culture." *Technol Soc.* 2010;32(1):10–17.

Fins JJ, De Melo-Martin I. C.P. Snow's "Two Cultures" fifty years later: An enduring problem with an elusive solution. *Technol Soc.* 2010;32(1):1–4.

Fischbach RL, Fischbach GD. Neuroethicists needed now more than ever. *Am J Bioeth.* 2008;8(1):47–48.

Fisher R. A closer look revisited: are we subjects or are we donors? *Genet Med.* 2012;14(4):458–460.

Fitzpatrick J, Hahn C, Costa T, Huggins M. The duty to recontact: attitudes of genetics service providers. *Am J Hum Genet.* 1997;61(4):A57.

Fitzpatrick JL, Hahn C, Costa T, Huggins MJ. The duty to recontact: attitudes of genetics service providers. *Am J Hum Genet.* 1999;64(3):852–860.

Flamm AL. Developing effective ethics policy. In: Hester DM, Schonfeld T, eds. *Guidance for Healthcare Ethics Committees.* Cambridge, UK: Cambridge University Press; 2012:130–138.

Fleischman AR, Collogan LK. Research with children. In: Emanuel EJ, Grady C, Crouch RA, et al., eds. *The Oxford Textbook of Clinical Research Ethics.* New York: Oxford University Press; 2008:446–460.

Fleischman AR, Howse JL. Newborn screening—the unique role of unique evidence. *Genet Med.* 2010;12(3):160–161.

Fleischman AR, Lin BK, Howse JL. A commentary on the President's Council on Bioethics report: the changing moral focus of newborn screening. *Genet Med.* 2009;11(7):507–509.

Fletcher JC. Evolution of ethical debate about human gene therapy. *Hum Gene Ther.* 1990;1(1):55–68.

Fletcher JC, Anderson WF. Germ-line gene therapy: a new stage of debate. *Law Med Health Care.* 1992;20(1–2):26–39.

Fletcher JC, Richter G. Human fetal gene therapy: moral and ethical questions. *Hum Gene Ther.* 1996;7(13):1605–1614.

Forsberg JS, Hansson MG, Eriksson S. Changing perspectives in biobank research: from individual rights to concerns about public health regarding the return of results. *Eur J Hum Genet.* 2009;17(12):1544–1549.

Fortenberry D. *The Good Egg.* New York: Broadway Play Publishing; 2011.

Foster MW, Mulvihill JJ, Sharp RR. Evaluating the utility of personal genomic information. *Genet Med.* 2009;11(8):570–574.

Foster MW, Sharp RR. Ethical issues in medical-sequencing research: implications of genotype-phenotype studies for individuals and populations. *Hum Mol Genet.* 2006;15(Spec No 1):R45–R49.

Foster MW, Sharp RR. Research with identifiable and targeted communities. In: Emanuel EJ, Grady C, Crouch RA, et al., eds. *The Oxford Textbook of Clinical Research Ethics.* New York: Oxford University Press; 2008:475–480.

Fox RC. The evolution of medical uncertainty. *Milbank Mem Fund Q.* 1980;58(1):1–49.

Frances AJ, Nardo JM. ICD-11 should not repeat the mistakes made by DSM-5. *Br J Psychiatry.* 2013;203:1–2.

Frank AW. *The Wounded Storyteller: Body, Illness, and Ethics.* Chicago, IL: University of Chicago Press; 1995.

Frantzen C, Links TP, Giles RH. Von Hippel-Lindau Disease. *GeneReviews.* University of Washington, Seattle. 1993–2013. http://www.ncbi.nlm.nih.gov/books/NBK1463/. Updated June 21, 2012. Accessed July 22, 2013.

Fritz A, Farrell P. Estimating the annual number of false negative cystic fibrosis newborn screening tests. *Pediatr Pulmonol.* 2012;47(2):207–208.

Fullerton SM, Anderson NR, Guzauskas G, Freeman D, Fryer-Edwards K. Meeting the governance challenges of next-generation biorepository research. *Sci Transl Med.* 2010;2(15):15cm3.

Fullerton SM, Wolf WA, Brothers KB, et al. Return of individual research results from genome-wide association studies: experience of the Electronic Medical Records and Genomics (eMERGE) Network. *Genet Med.* 2012;14(4):424–431.

Fyro K. Neonatal screening: life-stress scores in families given a false-positive result. *Acta Paediatr Scand.* 1988;77(2):232–238.

Gaylin W. Who speaks for the child. In: Gaylin W, Macklin R, eds. *Who Speaks for the Child: The Problems of Proxy Consent.* New York: Plenum; 1982:3–26.

Gaylin W, Macklin R, eds. *Who Speaks for the Child: The Problems of Proxy Consent.* New York: Plenum Press; 1982. *The Hastings Center Series in Ethics.*

Gemmette EV. *Law in Literature: Legal Themes in Drama.* Albany, NY: Whitston Publishing; 1995.

Gene mutations offer clues on the autistic brain. *Science Friday.* National Public Radio. June 10, 2011. http://www.npr.org/2011/06/10/137107088/gene-mutations-offer-clues-on-the-autistic-brain.

Genetic Information Nondiscrimination Act (GINA), Pub L No. 110-233, 122 Stat 881 (2008).

Gillis CM. "Seeing the difference": an interdisciplinary approach to death, dying, humanities, and medicine. *J Med Humanit.* 2006;27(2):105–115.

Girirajan S, Rosenfeld JA, Coe BP, et al. Phenotypic heterogeneity of genomic disorders and rare copy-number variants. *N Engl J Med.* 2012;367(14):1321–1331.

Giusti R, Badgwell A, Iglesias AD. New York State cystic fibrosis consortium: the first 2.5 years of experience with cystic fibrosis newborn screening in an ethnically diverse population. *Pediatrics.* 2007;119(2):e460–e467.

Gizewska M, Cabalska B, Cyrytowski L, et al. Different presentations of late-detected phenylketonuria in two brothers with the same R408W/R111X genotype in the PAH gene. *J Intellect Disabil Res.* 2003;47(Pt 2):146–152.

Gliwa C, Berkman BE. Do researchers have an obligation to actively look for genetic incidental findings? *Am J Bioeth.* 2013;13(2):32–42.

Goddard KA, Whitlock EP, Berg JS, et al. Description and pilot results from a novel method for evaluating return of incidental findings from next-generation sequencing technologies. *Genet Med.* 2013. doi: 10.1038/gim.2013.37.

Godlee F, Smith J, Marcovitch H. Wakefield's article linking MMR vaccine and autism was fraudulent. *BMJ.* 2011;342:c7452.

Goering S, Holland S, Edwards K. Making good on the promise of genetics: justice in translational science. In: Burke W, Edwards K, Goering S, Holland S, Trinidad SB, eds. *Achieving Justice in Genomic Translation: Rethinking the Pathway to Benefit.* Oxford, UK: Oxford University Press; 2011:3–21.

Goffman E. *Stigma: Notes on the Management of Spoiled Identity.* Englewood Cliffs, NJ: Prentice-Hall; 1963.

Goldenberg AJ, Dodson DS, Davis MM, Tarini BA. Parents' interest in whole-genome sequencing of newborns. *Genet Med.* 2013. doi 10.1038/gim.2013.76.

Goldenberg AJ, Hull SC, Botkin JR, Wilfond BS. Pediatric biobanks: approaching informed consent for continuing research after children grow up. *J Pediatr.* 2009;155(4):578–583.

Goldenberg AJ, Sharp RR. The ethical hazards and programmatic challenges of genomic newborn screening. *JAMA.* 2012;307(5):461–462.

Goldman MA. Perceived inheritance. *Science.* 2012;336(6079):297–298.

Goldstein J, Freud A, Solnit A. *Before the Best Interests of the Child.* New York: Free Press; 1979.

Goldstein J, Freud A, Solnit AJ. *Beyond the Best Interests of the Child.* New York: Free Press; 1973; 1979.

Goldstein J, Freud A, Solnit A, Golstein S. *In the Best Interests of the Child: Professional Boundaries.* New York: Free Press; 1986.

Golnik AE, Ireland M. Complementary alternative medicine for children with autism: a physician survey. *J Autism Dev Disord.* 2009;39(7):996–1005.

Gonzaga-Jauregui C, Lupski JR, Gibbs RA. Human genome sequencing in health and disease. *Annu Rev Med.* 2012;63:35–61.

Gonzales JL. Ethics for the pediatrician: genetic testing and newborn screening. *Pediatr Rev.* 2011;32(11):490–493.

Gooding HC, Organista K, Burack J, Biesecker BB. Genetic susceptibility testing from a stress and coping perspective. *Soc Sci Med.* 2006;62(8):1880–1890.

Goodlander EC, Berg JW. Pediatric decision-making: adolescent patients. In: Diekema DS, Mercurio MR, Adam MB, eds. *Clinical Ethics in Pediatrics: A Case-Based Textbook.* Cambridge, UK: Cambridge University Press; 2011:7–13.

Goodwin M. My sister's keeper? Law, children, and compelled donation. *West New Engl Law Rev.* 2007;29(2):357–404.

Gottesman O, Kuivaniemi H, Tromp G, et al. The Electronic Medical Records and Genomics (eMERGE) Network: past, present, and future. *Genet Med.* 2013. doi: 10.1038/gim.2013.72.

Grady C, Denny C. Research involving women. In: Emanuel EJ, ed. *The Oxford Textbook of Clinical Research Ethics.* New York: Oxford University Press; 2008:407–422.

Grady C, Wendler D. Making the transition to a learning health care system. Commentary. *Hastings Cent Rep.* 2013;43(Suppl):S32–S33.

Gray SW, Hicks-Courant K, Lathan CS, Garraway L, Park ER, Weeks JC. Attitudes of patients with cancer about personalized medicine and somatic genetic testing. *J Oncol Pract.* 2012;8(6):329–335, 2 p following 335.

Green ED, Guyer MS. Charting a course for genomic medicine from base pairs to bed-side. *Nature.* 2011;470(7333):204–213.

Green M. Vulnerable child syndrome and its variants. *Pediatr Rev.* 1986;8(3):75–80.

Green M, Solnit AJ. Reactions to the threatened loss of a child: a vulnerable child syndrome. Pediatric management of the dying child, part III. *Pediatrics.* 1964;34:58–66.

Green MJ, Botkin JR. "Genetic exceptionalism" in medicine: clarifying the differences between genetic and nongenetic tests. *Ann Intern Med.* 2003;138(7):571–575.

Green N. Every child is priceless: debating effective newborn screening policy. *Hastings Cent Rep.* 2009;39(1):6–7; author reply 7–8.

Green NS, Dolan SM, Murray TH. Newborn screening: complexities in universal genetic testing. *Am J Public Health.* 2006;96(11):1955–1959.

Green NS, Pass KA. Neonatal screening by DNA microarray: spots and chips. *Nature Rev Genet.* 2005;6(2):147–151.

Green RC, Berg JS, Berry GT, et al. Exploring concordance and discordance for return of incidental findings from clinical sequencing. *Genet Med.* 2012;14(4):405–410.

Green RC, Berg JS, Grody WW, American College of Medical Genetics and Genomics. ACMG recommendations for reporting of incidental findings in clinical exome and genome sequencing. *Genet Med.* 2013;15(7):565–574.

Green RC, Roberts JS, Cupples LA, et al. Disclosure of APOE genotype for risk of Alzheimer's disease. *N Engl J Med.* 2009;361(3):245–254.

Green RM. Research with fetuses, embryos and stem cells. In: Emanuel EJ, Grady C, Crouch RA, eds. *The Oxford Textbook of Clinical Research Ethics.* New York: Oxford University Press; 2008:488–499.

Greenbaum D, Du J, Gerstein M. Genomic anonymity: have we already lost it? *Am J Bioeth.* 2008;8(10):71–74.

Greenberg CR, Dilling LA, Thompson GR, et al. The paradox of the carnitine palmitoyltransferase type Ia P479L variant in Canadian Aboriginal populations. *Mol Genet Metab.* 2009;96(4):201–207.

Greenwood TA, Nievergelt CM, Sadovnick AD, et al. Further evidence for linkage of bipolar disorder to chromosomes 6 and 17 in a new independent pedigree series. *Bipolar Disord.* 2012;14(1):71–79.

Grisso T, Appelbaum PS. *Assessing Competence to Consent to Treatment: A Guide for Physicians and Other Health Professionals.* New York: Oxford University Press; 1998.

Grody WW, Thompson BH, Gregg AR, et al. ACMG position statement on prenatal/preconception expanded carrier screening. *Genet Med.* 2013;15(6):482–483.

Grosfeld FJ, Beemer FA, Lips CJ, Hendriks KS, ten Kroode HF. Parents' responses to disclosure of genetic test results of their children. *Am J Med Genet.* 2000;94(4):316–323.

Grosse SD, Boyle CA, Kenneson A, Khoury MJ, Wilfond BS. From public health emergency to public health service: the implications of evolving criteria for newborn screening panels. *Pediatrics.* 2006;117(3):923–929.

Grosse SD, Rogowski WH, Ross LF, Cornel MC, Dondorp WJ, Khoury MJ. Population screening for genetic disorders in the 21st century: evidence, economics, and ethics. *Public Health Genomics.* 2010;13(2):106–115.

Guiding regulatory reform in reproduction and genetics. *Harvard Law Rev.* 2006;120:574–596.

Guilmatre A, Dubourg C, Mosca AL, et al. Recurrent rearrangements in synaptic and neurodevelopmental genes and shared biologic pathways in schizophrenia, autism, and mental retardation. *Arch Gen Psychiatry.* 2009;66(9):947–956.

Gurian E, Waisbren S. The physical, emotional, and financial trauma incurred by infants and their families when an existing condition is not detected by newborn screening: in reply. *Pediatrics.* 2006;118(4):1802.

Gurian EA, Kinnamon DD, Henry JJ, Waisbren SE. Expanded newborn screening for biochemical disorders: the effect of a false-positive result. *Pediatrics.* 2006;117(6):1915–1921.

Gurrieri F. Working up autism: the practical role of medical genetics. *Am J Med Genet C Semin Med Genet.* 2012;160C(2):104–110.

Gurwitz D, Fortier I, Lunshof JE, Knoppers BM. Research ethics. Children and population biobanks. *Science.* 2009;325(5942):818–819.

Gustafson SL, Gettig EA, Watt-Morse M, Krishnamurti L. Health beliefs among African American women regarding genetic testing and counseling for sickle cell disease. *Genet Med.* 2007;9(5):303–310.

Guthrie R, Susi A. A simple phenylalanine method for detecting phenylketonuria in large populations of newborn infants. *Pediatrics.* 1963;32:338–343.

Gutmann A, Wagner JW. Found your DNA on the web: reconciling privacy and progress. *Hastings Cent Rep.* 2013;43(3):15–18.

Guttmacher AE, Collins FS. Genomic medicine—a primer. *N Engl J Med.* 2002;347(19):1512–1520.

Guttmacher AE, McGuire AL, Ponder B, Stefansson K. Personalized genomic information: preparing for the future of genetic medicine. *Nat Rev Genet.* 2010;11(2):161–165.

Guttmacher AE, Porteous ME, McInerney JD. Educating health-care professionals about genetics and genomics. *Nat Rev Genet.* 2007;8(2):151–157.

Gymrek M, McGuire AL, Golan D, Halperin E, Erlich Y. Identifying personal genomes by surname inference. *Science.* 2013;339(6117):321–324.

Hackler C, Hester DM. Introduction: what should an HEC look and act like? In: Hester DM, ed. *Ethics by Committee: A Textbook on Consultation, Organization, and Education for Hospital Ethics Committees.* Lanham, MD: Rowman & Littlefield Publishers; 2008:1–20.

Haga SB, Burke W, Agans R. Primary-care physicians' access to genetic specialists: an impediment to the routine use of genomic medicine? *Genet Med.* 2013;15(7):513–514.

Hale JE, Parad RB, Comeau AM. Newborn screening showing decreasing incidence of cystic fibrosis. *N Engl J Med.* 2008;358(9):973–974.

Hallowell N, Foster C, Eeles R, Ardern-Jones A, Murday V, Watson M. Balancing autonomy and responsibility: the ethics of generating and disclosing genetic information. *J Med Ethics.* 2003;29(2):74–79; discussion 80–83.

Halverson CM, Ross LF. Incidental findings of therapeutic misconception in biobank-based research. *Genet Med.* 2012;14(6):611–615.

Hamann HA, Croyle RT, Venne VL, Baty BJ, Smith KR, Botkin JR. Attitudes toward the genetic testing of children among adults in a Utah-based kindred tested for a BRCA1 mutation. *Am J Med Genet.* 2000;92(1):25–32.

Hamer DH, Hu S, Magnuson VL, Pattatucci AM. A linkage between DNA markers on the X chromosome and male sexual orientation. *Science* 1993;261:321–327.

Hansson MG, Maschke KJ. Biobanks: questioning distinctions. *Science.* 2009;326(5954):797; author reply 799.

Harper PS, Clarke A. Should we test children for "adult" genetic diseases? *Lancet.* 1990;335(8699):1205–1206.

Harris ED, Ziniel SI, Amatruda JG, et al. The beliefs, motivations, and expectations of parents who have enrolled their children in a genetic biorepository. *Genet Med.* 2012;14(3):330–337.

Harris J. Scientific research is a moral duty. *J Med Ethics.* 2005;31(4):242–248.

Harris R. Overview of screening: where we are and where we may be headed. *Epidemiol Rev.* 2011;33(1):1–6.

Harrison C. Fidelity and truthfulness in the pediatric setting: witholding information from children and adolescents. In: Diekema DS, Mercurio MR, Adam MB, eds.

Clinical Ethics in Pediatrics: A Case-Based Textbook. Cambridge, UK: Cambridge University Press; 2011:32–36.

Harrison C. Truth telling in pediatrics: what they don't know might hurt them. In: Miller G, ed. *Pediatric Bioethics.* New York: Cambridge University Press; 2010:73–86.

Harrison ME, Walling A. What do we know about giving bad news? A review. *Clinical Pediatr.* 2010;49(7):619–626.

Hasegawa LE, Fergus KA, Ojeda N, Au SM. Parental attitudes toward ethical and social issues surrounding the expansion of newborn screening using new technologies. *Public Health Genomics.* 2011;14(4–5):298–306.

Havasupai Tribe v Ariz. Bd. of Regents, 204 P.3d 1063 (Ariz. Ct. App. 2008).

Havstad JC. Human reproductive cloning: a conflict of liberties. *Bioethics.* 2010;24(2):71–77.

Hawkins AH. The idea of character. In: Charon R, Montello M, eds. *Stories Matter: The Role of Narrative in Medical Ethics.* New York: Routledge; 2002:70–78.

Hawkins AH, Ballard JO, eds. *Time to Go: Three Plays on Death and Dying with Commentary on End-of-Life Issues.* Philadelphia: University of Pennsylvania Press; 1995.

Hayeems RZ, Bytautas JP, Miller FA. A systematic review of the effects of disclosing carrier results generated through newborn screening. *J Genet Couns.* 2008;17(6):538–549.

Hayeems RZ, Miller FA, Li L, Bytautas JP. Not so simple: a quasi-experimental study of how researchers adjudicate genetic research results. *Eur J Hum Genet.* 2011;19(7):740–747.

Heeney C, Hawkins N, de Vries J, Boddington P, Kaye J. Assessing the privacy risks of data sharing in genomics. *Public Health Genomics.* 2010;14(1):17–25.

Helgesson G. Children, longitudinal studies, and informed consent. *Med Health Care Philos.* 2005;8(3):307–313.

Henderson GE, Juengst ET, King NM, Kuczynski K, Michie M. What research ethics should learn from genomics and society research: lessons from the ELSI Congress of 2011. *J Law Med Ethics.* 2012;40(4):1008–1024.

Henry LM. Introduction: Revising the common rule: prospects and challenges. *J Law Med Ethics.* 2013;41(2):386–389.

Hens K, Cassiman JJ, Nys H, Dierickx K. Children, biobanks and the scope of parental consent. *Eur J Hum Genet.* 2011;19(7):735–739.

Hens K, Nys H, Cassiman JJ, Dierickx K. Biological sample collections from minors for genetic research: a systematic review of guidelines and position papers. *Eur J Hum Genet.* 2009;17(8):979–990.

Hens K, Nys H, Cassiman JJ, Dierickx K. Genetic research on stored tissue samples from minors: a systematic review of the ethical literature. *Am J Med Genet A.* 2009;149A(10):2346–2358.

Hens K, Nys H, Cassiman JJ, Dierickx K. The return of individual research findings in paediatric genetic research. *J Med Ethics.* 2011;37(3):179–183.

Hens K, Nys H, Cassiman JJ, Dierickx K. Risks, benefits, solidarity: a framework for the participation of children in genetic biobank research. *J Pediatr.* 2011;158(5):842–848.

Hens K, Nys H, Cassiman JJ, Dierickx K. The storage and use of biological tissue samples from minors for research: a focus group study. *Public Health Genomics.* 2011;14(2):68–76.

Hens K, Snoeck J, Nys H, Cassiman JJ, Dierickx K. An exploratory survey of professionals on the use of stored tissue samples from minors for genetic research. *Genet Mol Res.* 2010;9(2):973–980.

Hens K, Wright J, Dierickx K. Biobanks: oversight offers protection. *Science.* 2009;326(5954):798–789; author reply 799.

Hensley Alford S, McBride CM, Reid RJ, Larson EB, Baxevanis AD, Brody LC. Participation in genetic testing research varies by social group. *Public Health Genomics.* 2011;14(2):85–93.

Hester DM. Ethical issues in pediatrics. In: Hester DM, Schonfeld T, eds. *Guidance for Healthcare Ethics Committees.* Cambridge, UK: Cambridge University Press; 2012:114–121.

Hester DM, ed. *Ethics by Committee: A Textbook on Consultation, Organization, and Education for Hospital Ethics Committees.* Lanham, MD: Rowman & Littlefield Publishers; 2008.

Hester DM, Schonfeld T. Introduction to healthcare ethics committees. In: Hester DM, Schonfeld T, eds. *Guidance for Healthcare Ethics Committees.* Cambridge, UK: Cambridge University Press; 2012:1–8.

Hester DM, Schonfeld T, eds. *Guidance for Healthcare Ethics Committees.* Cambridge, UK: Cambridge University Press; 2012.

Hewlett J, Waisbren SE. A review of the psychosocial effects of false-positive results on parents and current communication practices in newborn screening. *J Inherit Metab Dis.* 2006;29(5):677–682.

Hill MK, Archibald AD, Cohen J, Metcalfe SA. A systematic review of population screening for fragile X syndrome. *Genet Med.* 2010;12(7):396–410.

Hiraki S, Green NS. Newborn screening for treatable genetic conditions: past, present and future. *Obstet Gynecol Clin North Am.* 2010;37(1):11–21.

Hiraki S, Ormond KE, Kim K, Ross LF. Attitudes of genetic counselors towards expanding newborn screening and offering predictive genetic testing to children. *Am J Med Genet A.* 2006;140(21):2312–2319.

Hirschfeld S, Kramer B, Guttmacher A. Current status of the National Children's Study. *Epidemiology.* 2010;21(5):605–606.

Hirschhorn K, Fleisher LD, Godmilow L, et al. Duty to re-contact. *Genet Med.* 1999;1(4):171–172.

Hoff T, Hoyt A, Therrell B, Ayoob M. Exploring barriers to long-term follow-up in newborn screening programs. *Genet Med.* 2006;8(9):563–570.

Hoffmann DE, Fortenberry JD, Ravel J. Are changes to the common rule necessary to address evolving areas of research? A case study focusing on the human microbiome project. *J Law Med Ethics.* 2013;41(2):454–469.

Hoffmann DE, Rothenberg KH. Whose duty is it anyway? The Kennedy Krieger opinion and its implications for public health research. *J Health Care Law Policy.* 2002;6(1):109–147.

Hoffmann GF, Cornejo V, Pollitt RJ. Newborn screening—progress and challenges. *J Inherit Metab Dis.* 2010;33(Suppl 2):S199–S200.

Hoffmann GF, Fang-Hoffmann J, Lindner M, Burgard P. Clinical advances and challenges of extended newborn screening. [abstract]. *J Inherit Metab Dis.* 2011;34(Suppl 1): S1.

Hollingworth P, Harold D, Sims R, et al. Common variants at ABCA7, MS4A6A/MS4A4E, EPHA1, CD33 and CD2AP are associated with Alzheimer's disease. *Nat Genet.* 2011;43(5):429–435.

Holm IA, Taylor PL. The Informed Cohort Oversight Board: from values to architecture. *Minn J Law Sci Technol.* 2012;13:669–690.

Holm S. Informed consent and the bio-banking of material from children. *Genomics Soc Policy.* 2005;1(1):16–26.

Holmes C, McDonald F, Jones M, Ozdemir V, Graham JE. Standardization and omics science: technical and social dimensions are inseparable and demand symmetrical study. *OMICS*. 2010;14(3):327–332.

Holtzman NA. Expanding newborn screening: how good is the evidence? *JAMA*. 2003;290(19):2606–2608.

Holtzman NA, Faden R, Chwalow AJ, Horn SD. Effect of informed parental consent on mothers' knowledge of newborn screening. *Pediatrics*. 1983;72(6):807–812.

Horev G, Ellegood J, Lerch JP, et al. Dosage-dependent phenotypes in models of 16p11.2 lesions found in autism. *Proc Natl Acad Sci USA*. 2011;108(41):17076–17081.

Horton R, Brody H. Informed consent, shared decision-making, and the ethics committee. In: Hester DM, Schonfeld T, eds. *Guidance for Healthcare Ethics Committees*. Cambridge, UK: Cambridge University Press; 2012:48–54.

Howell RR. Every child is priceless: debating effective newborn screening policy. *Hastings Cent Rep*. 2009;39(1):4–6; author reply 7–8.

Howell RR. The high price of false positives. *Mol Genet Metab*. 2006;87(3):180–183.

Howell RR, Lloyd-Puryear MA. From developing guidelines to implementing legislation: actions of the US Advisory Committee on Heritable Disorders in Newborns and Children toward advancing and improving newborn screening. *Semin Perinatol*. 2010;34(2):121–124.

Hudson KL. Genomics, health care, and society. *N Engl J Med*. 2011;365(11):1033–1041.

Hudson KL, Collins FS. Biospecimen policy: family matters. *Nature*. 2013;500(7461):141–142.

Hull SC, Colloca L, Avins A, et al. Patients' attitudes about the use of placebo treatments: telephone survey. *BMJ*. 2013;347:f3757.

Hull SC, Gooding H, Klein AP, Warshauer-Baker E, Metosky S, Wilfond BS. Genetic research involving human biological materials: a need to tailor current consent forms. *IRB*. 2004;26(3):1–7.

Hull SC, Sharp RR, Botkin JR, et al. Patients' views on identifiability of samples and informed consent for genetic research. *Am J Bioeth*. 2008;8(10):62–70.

Hunter AG, Sharpe N, Mullen M, Meschino WS. Ethical, legal, and practical concerns about recontacting patients to inform them of new information: the case in medical genetics. *Am J Med Genet*. 2001;103(4):265–276.

Hunter KM, Charon R, Coulehan JL. The study of literature in medical education. *Acad Med*. 1995;70(9):787–794.

Hurle B, Citrin T, Jenkins JF, et al. What does it mean to be genomically literate?: National Human Genome Research Institute Meeting Report. *Genet Med*. 2013. doi: 10.1038/gim.2013.14.

Ibsen H. *Ghosts* (1881). In: Fjelde R, trans. *Four Major Plays: Ghosts; An Enemy of the People; The Lady from the Sea; John Gabriel Borkman*. Vol. 2. New York: Signet Classics; 1970.

Illes J, Sahakian BJ, eds. *The Oxford Handbook of Neuroethics*. Oxford, UK: Oxford University Press; 2011.

Im HK, Gamazon ER, Nicolae DL, Cox NJ. On sharing quantitative trait GWAS results in an era of multiple-omics data and the limits of genomic privacy. *Am J Hum Genet*. 2012;90(4):591–598.

International Congress on Prevention of Congenital Diseases. Screening newborns: current state and future challenges. Abstracts of the International Congress on Prevention of Congenital Diseases. Vienna, Austria. May 13–14, 2011. *J Inherit Metab Dis*. 2011;34(Suppl 1):S1–S16.

International HapMap Consortium. Integrating ethics and science in the International HapMap Project. *Nat Rev Genet.* 2004;5(6):467–475.

International HapMap 3 Consortium, Altshuler DM, Gibbs RA, et al. Integrating common and rare genetic variation in diverse human populations. *Nature.* 2010;467(7311):52–58.

Ioannidis JP. Expectations, validity, and reality in omics. *J Clin Epidemiol.* 2010;63(9):945–949.

Jackson L, Pyeritz RE. Molecular technologies open new clinical genetic vistas. *Sci Transl Med.* 2011;3(65):65ps2.

James PM, Levy HL. The clinical aspects of newborn screening: importance of newborn screening follow-up. *Ment Retard Dev Disabil Res Rev.* 2006;12(4):246–254.

Javitt GH. Take another little piece of my heart(1): regulating the research use of human biospecimens. *J Law Med Ethics.* 2013;41(2):424–439.

Jennings B. Enlightenment and enchantment: technology and moral limits. *Technol Soc.* 2010;32(1):25–30.

Jennings B. Frameworks for ethics in public health. *Acta Bioethica.* 2003;9(2):165–176.

Johnson AD, Bhimavarapu A, Benjamin EJ, et al. CLIA-tested genetic variants on commercial SNP arrays: potential for incidental findings in genome-wide association studies. *Genet Med.* 2010;12(6):355–363.

Johnson G, Lawrenz F, Thao M. An empirical examination of the management of return of individual research results and incidental findings in genomic biobanks. *Genet Med.* 2012;14(4):444–450.

Johnson JO, Mandrioli J, Benatar M, et al. Exome sequencing reveals VCP mutations as a cause of familial ALS. *Neuron.* 2010;68(5):857–864.

Johnston JJ, Rubinstein WS, Facio FM, et al. Secondary variants in individuals undergoing exome sequencing: screening of 572 individuals identifies high-penetrance mutations in cancer-susceptibility genes. *Am J Hum Genet.* 2012;91(1):97–108.

Jonsen AR. Casuistry and clinical ethics. In: Sugarman J, Sulmasy DP, eds. *Methods in Medical Ethics.* Washington, DC: Georgetown University Press; 2010:109–126.

Jonsen AR. *The Birth of Bioethics.* New York: Oxford University Press; 1998. Paperback ed. New York: Oxford University Press; 2003.

Jonsen AR, Siegler M, Winslade WJ. *Clinical Ethics: A Practical Approach to Ethical Decisions in Clinical Medicine.* 6th ed. New York: McGraw-Hill; 2006.

Jordan BR, Tsai DF. Whole-genome association studies for multigenic diseases: ethical dilemmas arising from commercialization—the case of genetic testing for autism. *J Med Ethics.* 2010;36(7):440–444.

Juengst ET. FACE facts: why human genetics will always provoke bioethics. *J Law Med Ethics.* 2004;32(2):267–275, 191.

Juengst ET. Group identity and human diversity: keeping biology straight from culture. *Am J Hum Genet.* 1998;63(3):673–677.

Juengst ET. The Human Genome Project and bioethics. *Kennedy Inst Ethics J.* 1991;1:71–74.

Juengst ET. Self-critical federal science? The ethics experiment within the U.S. Human Genome Project. *Soc Philos Policy.* 1996; 13(2):63–95.

Juengst ET, Goldenberg A. Genetic diagnostic, pedigree, and screening research. In: Emanuel EJ, Grady C, Crouch RA, et al., eds. *The Oxford Textbook of Clinical Research Ethics.* New York: Oxford University Press; 2008:298–314.

Kaiser J. Human genetics. Genetic influences on disease remain hidden. *Science.* 2012;338(6110):1016–1017.

Kaltman JR, Thompson PD, Lantos J, et al. Screening for sudden cardiac death in the young: report from a national heart, lung, and blood institute working group. *Circulation.* 2011;123(17):1911–1918.

Kandaswamy R, McQuillin A, Curtis D, Gurling H. Tests of linkage and allelic association between markers in the 1p36 PRKCZ (Protein Kinase C Zeta) gene region and bipolar affective disorder. *Am J Med Genet B Neuropsychiatr Genet.* 2012;159:201–209.

Karp DR, Carlin S, Cook-Deegan R, et al. Ethical and practical issues associated with aggregating databases. *PLoS Med.* 2008;5(9):e190.

Kass NE, Faden RR, Goodman SN, Pronovost P, Tunis S, Beauchamp TL. The research-treatment distinction: a problematic approach for determining which activities should have ethical oversight. *Hastings Cent Rep.* 2013;43(Suppl):S4–S15.

Katz J. *The Silent World of Doctor and Patient.* New York: Free Press; 1984.

Katz J, Capron AM. *The Silent World of Doctor and Patient:* Baltimore, MD: Johns Hopkins University Press; 2002.

Kaufman D, Geller G, Leroy L, Murphy J, Scott J, Hudson K. Ethical implications of including children in a large biobank for genetic-epidemiologic research: a qualitative study of public opinion. *Am J Med Genet C Semin Med Genet.* 2008;148C(1):31–39.

Kaufman D, Murphy J, Scott J, Hudson K. Subjects matter: a survey of public opinions about a large genetic cohort study. *Genet Med.* 2008;10(11):831–839.

Kaye J, Boddington P, de Vries J, Hawkins N, Melham K. Ethical implications of the use of whole genome methods in medical research. *Eur J Hum Genet.* 2010;18(4):398–403.

Kaye J, Curren L, Anderson N, et al. From patients to partners: participant-centric initiatives in biomedical research. *Nat Rev Genet.* 2012;13(5):371–376.

Kaye J, Heeney C, Hawkins N, de Vries J, Boddington P. Data sharing in genomics—re-shaping scientific practice. *Nat Rev Genet.* 2009;10(5):331–335.

Kaye J, Meslin EM, Knoppers BM, et al. Research priorities. ELSI 2.0 for genomics and society. *Science.* 2012;336(6082):673–674.

Kaye J, Wilbanks J. Privacy II—control, access, and human genome sequence data. *Presentation to the Presidential Commission for the Study of Bioethical Issues.* http://bioethics.gov/cms/node/659. Presented February 2, 2013. Accessed July 26, 2013.

Kemper AR, Knapp AA, Green NS, Comeau AM, Metterville DR, Perrin JM. Weighing the evidence for newborn screening for early-infantile Krabbe disease. *Genet Med.* 2010;12(9):539–543.

Kemper KJ, Vohra S, Walls R, Task Force on Complementary and Alternative Medicine, Provisional Section on Complementary, Holistic, and Integrative Medicine. American Academy of Pediatrics: the use of complementary and alternative medicine in pediatrics. *Pediatrics.* 2008;122:1374–1386.

Kerr A, Shakespeare T. *Genetic Politics: From Eugenics to Genome.* Cheltenham, UK: New Clarion Press; 2002.

Kevles DJ. *In the Name of Eugenics: Genetics and the Uses of Human Heredity.* New York: Knopf; 1985.

Khoury MJ. Public health genomics: the end of the beginning. *Genet Med.* 2011;13(3):206–209.

Khoury MJ, Coates RJ, Evans JP. Evidence-based classification of recommendations on use of genomic tests in clinical practice: dealing with insufficient evidence. *Genet Med.* 2010;12(11):680–683.

Khoury MJ, Feero WG, Reyes M, et al. The genomic applications in practice and prevention network. *Genet Med.* 2009;11(7):488–494.

Khoury MJ, Feero WG, Valdez R. Family history and personal genomics as tools for improving health in an era of evidence-based medicine. *Am J Prev Med.* 2010;39(2):184–188.

Khoury MJ, Gwinn M, Yoon PW, Dowling N, Moore CA, Bradley L. The continuum of translation research in genomic medicine: how can we accelerate the appropriate integration of human genome discoveries into health care and disease prevention? *Genet Med.* 2007;9(10):665–674.

Kim SJ, Silva RM, Flores CG, et al. A quantitative association study of SLC25A12 and restricted repetitive behavior traits in autism spectrum disorders. *Mol Autism.* 2011;2(1):8.

Kimmelman J. The post-Human Genome Project mindset: race, reliability, and health care. *Clin Genet.* 2006;70(5):427–432.

King N, Robeson R. Dramatic arts casuistry in bioethics education and outreach. Paper presented at: ELSI Congress; 2011; Chapel Hill, NC.

King NM, Henderson GE, Churchill LR, et al. Consent forms and the therapeutic misconception: the example of gene transfer research. *IRB.* 2005;27(1):1–8.

King NMP, Churchill LR. Assessing and comparing potential benefits and risks of harm. In: Emanuel EJ, Grady C, Crouch RA, et al., eds. *The Oxford Textbook of Clinical Research Ethics.* New York: Oxford University Press; 2008:514–526.

Kinlaw K. The healthcare ethics committee as educator. In: Hester DM, Schonfeld T, eds. *Guidance for Healthcare Ethics Committees.* Cambridge, UK: Cambridge University Press; 2012:155–163.

Kinlaw K. The hospital ethics committee as educator. In: Hester DM, ed. *Ethics by Committee: A Textbook on Consultation, Organization, and Education for Hospital Ethics Committees.* Lanham, MD: Rowman & Littlefield Publishers; 2008:203–214.

Kirkland A. The legitimacy of vaccine critics: what is left after the autism hypothesis? *J Health Polit Policy Law.* 2012;37:69–97.

Kitzman JO, Snyder MW, Ventura M, et al. Noninvasive whole-genome sequencing of a human fetus. *Sci Transl Med.* 2012;4(137):137ra176.

Kladny B, Williams A, Gupta A, Gettig EA, Krishnamurti L. Genetic counseling following the detection of hemoglobinopathy trait on the newborn screen is well received, improves knowledge, and relieves anxiety. *Genet Med.* 2011;13(7):658–661.

Kleinman A. *The Illness Narratives: Suffering, Healing, and the Human Condition.* New York: Basic Books; 1988.

Klima J, Fitzgerald-Butt SM, Kelleher KJ, et al. Understanding of informed consent by parents of children enrolled in a genetic biobank. *Genet Med.* 2013. doi: 10.1038/gim.2013.86.

Kline W. *Building a Better Race.* Berkeley: University of California Press; 2001.

Klitzman R. "Am I my genes?": Questions of identity among individuals confronting genetic disease. *Genet Med.* 2009;11(12):880–889.

Klitzman R. Questions, complexities, and limitations in disclosing individual genetic results. *Am J Bioeth.* 2006;6(6):34–36; author reply W10–W12.

Klitzman R, Appelbaum PS. Research ethics. To protect human subjects, review what was done, not proposed. *Science.* 2012;335(6076):1576–1577.

Klitzman R, Appelbaum PS, Fyer A, et al. Researchers' views on return of incidental genomic research results: qualitative and quantitative findings. *Genet Med.* 2013. doi: 10.1038/gim.2013.87.

Klitzman R, Chung W, Marder K, et al. Attitudes and practices among internists concerning genetic testing. *J Genet Couns.* 2013;22(1):90–100.

Klitzman R, Zolovska B, Folberth W, Sauer MV, Chung W, Appelbaum P. Preimplantation genetic diagnosis on in vitro fertilization clinic websites: presentations of risks, benefits and other information. *Fertil Steril.* 2009;92:1276–1283.

Klug A. Rosalind Franklin and the discovery of the structure of DNA. *Nature.* 1968;219(5156):808–810.

Knoppers BM. Paediatric research and the communication of not-so incidental findings. *Paediatr Child Health.* 2012;17(4):190–192.

Knoppers BM, Avard D, Cardinal G, Glass KC. Science and society: children and incompetent adults in genetic research: consent and safeguards. *Nat Rev Genet.* 2002;3(3):221–225.

Knoppers BM, Chadwick R. Human genetic research: emerging trends in ethics. *Nat Rev Genet.* 2005;6(1):75–79.

Knoppers BM, Dove ES, Litton JE, Nietfeld JJ. Questioning the limits of genomic privacy. *Am J Hum Genet.* 2012;91(3):577–578; author reply 579.

Knoppers BM, Joly Y, Simard J, Durocher F. The emergence of an ethical duty to disclose genetic research results: international perspectives. *Eur J Hum Genet.* 2006;14(11):1170–1178.

Kodish E. Ethics and research with children: an introduction. In: Kodish E, ed. *Ethics and Research with Children: A Case-Based Approach.* Oxford; New York: Oxford University Press; 2005:3–25.

Kohane IS. No small matter: qualitatively distinct challenges of pediatric genomic studies. *Genome Med.* 2011;3(9):62.

Kohane IS. Using electronic health records to drive discovery in disease genomics. *Nat Rev Genet.* 2011;12(6):417–428.

Kohane IS, Hsing M, Kong SW. Taxonomizing, sizing, and overcoming the incidentalome. *Genet Med.* 2012;14(4):399–404.

Kohane IS, Mandl KD, Taylor PL, Holm IA, Nigrin DJ, Kunkel LM. Medicine. Reestablishing the researcher-patient compact. *Science.* 2007;316(5826):836–837.

Kohane IS, Masys DR, Altman RB. The incidentalome: a threat to genomic medicine. *JAMA.* 2006;296(2):212–215.

Kohane IS, Taylor PL. Multidimensional results reporting to participants in genomic studies: getting it right. *Sci Transl Med.* 2010;2(37):37cm19.

Konrad M. *Narrating the New Predictive Genetics: Ethics, Ethnography, and Science.* Cambridge, UK: Cambridge University Press; 2005.

Kopelman L. Genetic screening in newborns: voluntary or compulsory? *Perspect Biol Med.* 1978;21:83–89.

Kopelman LM. On the evaluative nature of competency and capacity judgments. *Int J Law Psychiatry.* 1990;13(4):309–329.

Kopelman LM. Using the best-interests standard in treatment decisions for young children. In: Miller G, ed. *Pediatric Bioethics.* New York: Cambridge University Press; 2010:22–37.

Kopelman LM. Using the best interests standard to decide whether to test children for untreatable, late-onset genetic diseases. *J Med Philos.* 2007;32(4):375–394.

Korf BR. Genetics and genomics education: the next generation. *Genet Med.* 2011;13(3):201–202.

Krauss LM. An update on C.P. Snow's "Two Cultures." *Scientific American.* September 2009. http://www.scientificamerican.com/article.cfm?id=an-update-on-cp-snows-two-cultures. Published August 31, 2009. Accessed July 25, 2013.

Krier JB, Green RC. Management of incidental findings in clinical genomic sequencing. *Curr Protoc Hum Genet.* 2013;Chapter 9:Unit 9.23.

Kronenthal C, Delaney SK, Christman MF. Broadening research consent in the era of genome-informed medicine. *Genet Med.* 2012;14(4):432–436.

Kuehn BM. 1000 Genomes Project finds substantial genetic variation among populations. *JAMA.* 2012;308(22):2322, 2325.

Kullo IJ, Jarvik GP, Manolio TA, et al. Leveraging the electronic health record to implement genomic medicine. *Genet Med.* 2013;15(4):270–271.

Kupersmith J. Advances in the research enterprise. Commentary. *Hastings Cent Rep.* 2013;43(Suppl):S43–S44.

Kwon C, Farrell PM. The magnitude and challenge of false-positive newborn screening test results. *Arch Pediatr Adolesc Med.* 2000;154(7):714–718.

Kwon JM, Steiner RD. "I'm fine; I'm just waiting for my disease": the new and growing class of presymptomatic patients. *Neurology.* 2011;77(6):522–523.

LaCombe MA, Elpern DJ, eds. *Osler's Bedside Library: Great Writers Who Inspired a Great Physician.* Philadelphia, PA: American College of Physicians; 2010.

La Pean A, Collins JL, Christopher SA, et al. A qualitative secondary evaluation of statewide follow-up interviews for abnormal newborn screening results for cystic fibrosis and sickle cell hemoglobinopathy. *Genet Med.* 2012;14(2):207–214.

La Pean A, Farrell MH. Initially misleading communication of carrier results after newborn genetic screening. *Pediatrics.* 2005;116(6):1499–1505.

Lakes KD, Vaughan E, Jones M, Burke W, Baker D, Swanson JM. Diverse perceptions of the informed consent process: implications for the recruitment and participation of diverse communities in the National Children's Study. *Am J Community Psychol.* 2012;49(1–2):215–232.

Lander ES. Initial impact of the sequencing of the human genome. *Nature.* 2011;470(7333):187–197.

Lander ES, Linton LM, Birren B, et al. Initial sequencing and analysis of the human genome. *Nature.* 2001;409(6822):860–921.

Lang CW, McColley SA, Lester LA, Ross LF. Parental understanding of newborn screening for cystic fibrosis after a negative sweat-test. *Pediatrics.* 2011;127(2):276–283.

Lang CW, Stark AP, Acharya K, Ross LF. Maternal knowledge and attitudes about newborn screening for sickle cell disease and cystic fibrosis. *Am J Med Genet A.* 2009;149A(11):2424–2429.

Lantos J. Reconsidering action: day-to-day ethics in the work of medicine. In: Charon R, Montello M, eds. *Stories Matter: The Role of Narrative in Medical Ethics.* New York: Routledge; 2002:158–163.

Lantos JD. Dangerous and expensive screening and treatment for rare childhood diseases: the case of Krabbe disease. *Dev Disabil Res Rev.* 2011;17(1):15–18.

Lantos JD. Maybe we are getting better at counseling. [eLetter]. *Pediatrics.* http://pediatrics.aappublications.org/content/128/4/715.abstract/reply#pediatrics_el_51684. Published September 26, 2011. Accessed July 18, 2013.

Lantos JD. Reconsidering action: day-to-day ethics in the work of medicine. In: Charon R, Montello M, eds. *Stories Matter: The Role of Narrative in Medical Ethics.* New York: Routledge; 2002:158–163.

Lantos JD. Should we always tell children the truth? *Perspect Biol Med.* 1996;40(1):78–92.

Lapointe J, Bouchard K, Patenaude AF, Maunsell E, Simard J, Dorval M. Incidence and predictors of positive and negative effects of BRCA1/2 genetic testing on familial relationships: a 3-year follow-up study. *Genet Med.* 2012;14(1):60–68.

Largent EA, Joffe S, Miller FG. Can research and care be ethically integrated? Commentary. *Hastings Cent Rep.* 2011;41(4):37–46.

Largent EA, Miller FG, Joffe S. A prescription for ethical learning. Commentary. *Hastings Cent Rep.* 2013;43(Suppl):S28–S29.

Largent EA, Pearson SD. Which orphans will find a home? The rule of rescue in resource allocation for rare diseases. *Hastings Cent Rep.* 2012;42(1):27–34.

Larsson AK, Svalenius E, Lundqvist A, Dykes AK. Parents' experiences of an abnormal ultrasound examination—vacillating between emotional confusion and sense of reality. *Reprod Health.* 2010;7(1):10.

Latham S. Healthcare ethics committees and the law. In: Hester DM, Schonfeld T, eds. *Guidance for Healthcare Ethics Committees.* Cambridge, UK: Cambridge University Press; 2012:17–24.

Latham SR. Law between the cultures: C.P. Snow's *The Two Cultures* and the problem of scientific illiteracy in law. *Technol Soc.* 2010;32(1):31–34.

Latham S. Reproductive cloning: Multiplicity. In: Colt HG, Quadrelli S, Friedman LD, eds. *The Picture of Health: Medical Ethics and the Movies.* New York: Oxford University Press; 2011:357–361.

Lemke A, Bick D, Dimmock D, Simpson P, Veith R. Perspectives of clinical genetics professionals toward genome sequencing and incidental findings: a survey study. *Clin Genet.* 2012. doi: 10.1111/cge.12060.

Lemke AA, Halverson C, Ross LF. Biobank participation and returning research results: perspectives from a deliberative engagement in South Side Chicago. *Am J Med Genet A.* 2012;158A(5):1029–1037.

Letendre M, Godard B. Expanding the physician's duty of care: a duty to recontact? *Med Law.* 2004;23(3):531–539.

Levenson D. A majority of parents accept newborn screening for fragile X. *Am J Med Genet A.* 2011;155A(9):viii–ix.

Levin BW, Fleischman AR. Public health and bioethics: the benefits of collaboration. *Am J Public Health.* 2002;92(2):165–167.

Levine C, Faden R, Grady C, Hammerschmidt D, Eckenwiler L, Sugarman J. The limitations of "vulnerability" as a protection for human research participants. *Am J Bioeth.* 2004;4(3):44–49.

Levine RJ. The nature, scope, and justification of clinical research: what is research? Who is a Subject? In: Emanuel EJ, Grady C, Crouch RA, et al., eds. *The Oxford Textbook of Clinical Research Ethics.* New York: Oxford University Press; 2008:211–221.

Levy DE, Byfield SD, Comstock CB, et al. Underutilization of BRCA1/2 testing to guide breast cancer treatment: black and Hispanic women particularly at risk. *Genet Med.* 2011;13(4):349–355.

Levy HL. Lessons from the past—looking to the future. Newborn screening. *Pediatric Annals.* 2003;32(8):505–508.

Levy HL. Newborn screening by tandem mass spectrometry: a new era. *Clin Chem.* 1998;44(12):2401–2402.

Levy HL. Newborn screening conditions: what we know, what we do not know, and how we will know it. *Genet Med.* 2010;12(12 Suppl):S213–S214.

Levy SE, Hyman SL. Complementary and alternative medicine treatments for children with autism spectrum disorders. *Child Adolesc Psychiatr Clin N Am.* 2008;17(4):803–820.

Lewis C, Skirton H, Jones R. Can we make assumptions about the psychosocial impact of living as a carrier, based on studies assessing the effects of carrier testing? *J Genet Couns.* 2011;20(1):80–97.

Lewis MH. Laboratory specimens and genetic privacy: evolution of legal theory. *J Law Med Ethics.* 2013;41(Suppl 1):65–68.

Lewis MH, Goldenberg A, Anderson R, Rothwell E, Botkin JR. State laws regarding the retention and use of residual newborn screening blood samples. *Pediatrics.* 2011;127(4):703–712.

Liberati A, Mosconi P, Meyerowitz B. Truth telling: a cultural or individual choice? *JAMA.* 1993;269(8):989.

Lidz CW, Appelbaum PS. The therapeutic misconception: problems and solutions. *Med Care.* 2002;40(9 Suppl):V55–V63.

Lidz CW, Appelbaum PS, Grisso T, Renaud M. Therapeutic misconception and the appreciation of risks in clinical trials. *Soc Sci Med.* 2004;58(9):1689–1697.

Lidz CW, Garverich S. What the ANPRM missed: additional needs for IRB reform. *J Law Med Ethics.* 2013;41(2):390–396.

Lidz CW, Simon LJ, Seligowski AV, et al. The participation of community members on medical institutional review boards. *J Empir Res Hum Res Ethics.* 2012;7(1):1–6.

Lieve KV, Williams L, Daly A, et al. Results of genetic testing in 855 consecutive unrelated patients referred for long QT syndrome in a clinical laboratory. *Genet Test Mol Biomarkers.* 2013;17(7):553–561.

Lin Z, Owen AB, Altman RB. Genetics. Genomic research and human subject privacy. *Science.* 2004;305(5681):183.

Lindee S. *Moments of Truth in Genetic Medicine.* Baltimore, MD: Johns Hopkins University Press; 2005.

Lindor NM, Johnson KJ, McCormick JB, Klee EW, Ferber MJ, Farrugia G. Preserving personal autonomy in a genomic testing era. *Genet Med.* 2013;15(5):408–409.

Lionel AC, Vaags AK, Sato D, et al. Rare exonic deletions implicate the synaptic organizer Gephyrin (GPHN) in risk for autism, schizophrenia and seizures. *Hum Mol Genet.* 2013;22(10):2055–2066.

Lipinski SE, Lipinski MJ, Biesecker LG, Biesecker BB. Uncertainty and perceived personal control among parents of children with rare chromosome conditions: the role of genetic counseling. *Am J Med Genet C Semin Med Genet.* 2006;142C(4):232–240.

Lipstein EA, Brinkman WB, Britto MT. What is known about parents' treatment decisions? A narrative review of pediatric decision making. *Med Decis Making.* 2012;32(2):246–258.

Lipstein EA, Nabi E, Perrin JM, Luff D, Browning MF, Kuhlthau KA. Parents' decision-making in newborn screening: opinions, choices, and information needs. *Pediatrics.* 2010;126(4):696–704.

Lipstein EA, Perrin JM, Waisbren SE, Prosser LA. Impact of false-positive newborn metabolic screening results on early health care utilization. *Genet Med.* 2009;11(10):716–721.

Lipstein EA, Vorono S, Browning MF, et al. Systematic evidence review of newborn screening and treatment of severe combined immunodeficiency. *Pediatrics.* 2010;125(5):e1226–e1235.

Liu L, Drouet V, Wu JW, Witter MP, Small SA, Clelland C, Duff K. Trans-synaptic spread of tau pathology in vivo. *PLoS One.* 2012;7(2):E31302.

Lloyd-Puryear MA, Brower A. Long-term follow-up in newborn screening: A systems approach for improving health outcomes. *Genet Med.* 2010;12(12 Suppl):S256–S260.

Lockhart NC, Yassin R, Weil CJ, Compton CC. Intersection of biobanking and clinical care: should discrepant diagnoses and pathological findings be returned to research participants? *Genet Med.* 2012;14(4):417–423.

Lohn Z, Adam S, Birch P, Townsend A, Friedman J. Genetics professionals' perspectives on reporting incidental findings from clinical genome-wide sequencing. *Am J Med Genet A.* 2013;161(3):542–549.

Lohn Z, Adam S, Birch PH, Friedman JM. Incidental findings from clinical genome-wide sequencing: a review. *J Genet Couns.* 2013. doi: 10.1007/s10897-013-9604-4.

Loo KK. Procedural challenges in international collaborative research. *Acad Psychiatry.* 2009;33(3):229–233.

Loomer L. *Distracted.* New York: Dramatists Play Service; 2009.

Lord C, Petkova E, Hus V, et al. A multisite study of the clinical diagnosis of different autism spectrum disorders. *Arch Gen Psychiatry.* 2012;69(3):306–313.

Lorenz KA, Steckart MJ, Rosenfeld KE. End-of-life education using the dramatic arts: the Wit educational initiative. *Acad Med.* 2004;79(5):481–486.

Loukides G, Denny JC, Malin B. The disclosure of diagnosis codes can breach research participants' privacy. *J Am Med Inform Assoc.* 2010;17(3):322–327.

Lowrance WW, Collins FS. Ethics. Identifiability in genomic research. *Science.* 2007;317(5838):600–602.

Lunshof JE, Chadwick R, Vorhaus DB, Church GM. From genetic privacy to open consent. *Nat Rev Genet.* 2008;9(5):406–411.

Lupski JR, Belmont JW, Boerwinkle E, Gibbs RA. Clan genomics and the complex architecture of human disease. *Cell.* 2011;147(1):32–43.

Lupski JR, de Oca-Luna RM, Slaugenhaupt S, et al. DNA duplication associated with Charcot-Marie-Tooth disease type 1A. *Cell.* 1991;66(2):219–232.

Lupski JR, Reid JG, Gonzaga-Jauregui C, et al. Whole-genome sequencing in a patient with Charcot-Marie-Tooth neuropathy. *N Engl J Med.* 2010;362(13):1181–1191.

Lurie N. Health disparities—less talk, more action. *N Engl J Med.* 2005;353(7):727–729.

Lyon GJ, Jiang T, Van Wijk R, et al. Exome sequencing and unrelated findings in the context of complex disease research: ethical and clinical implications. *Discov Med.* 2011;12(62):41–55.

MacKaye P. *To-morrow.* New York: Frederick A. Stokes Co.; 1912.

Macklin R. Bioethics, vulnerability, and protection. *Bioethics.* 2003;17(5–6):472–486.

Macklin R. Return to the best interests of the child. In: Gaylin W, Macklin R, eds. *Who Speaks for the Child: The Problems of Proxy Consent.* New York: Plenum; 1982:265–301.

Maddox B. *Rosalind Franklin: The Dark Lady of DNA.* New York: HarperCollins; 2002.

Malm HM. Medical screening and the value of early detection. When unwarranted faith leads to unethical recommendations. *Hastings Cent Rep.* 1999;29(1):26–37.

Malpas PJ. Predictive genetic testing of children for adult-onset diseases and psychological harm. *J Med Ethics.* 2008;34(4):275–278.

Mand C, Duncan RE, Gillam L, Collins V, Delatycki MB. Genetic selection for deafness: the views of hearing children of deaf adults. *J Med Ethics.* 2009;35(12):722–728.

Manolio TA, Chisholm RL, Ozenberger B, et al. Implementing genomic medicine in the clinic: the future is here. *Genet Med.* 2013;15(4):258–267.

Manolio TA, Collins FS, Cox NJ, et al. Finding the missing heritability of complex diseases. *Nature.* 2009;461(7265):747–753.

Marchant GE, Robert JS. Genetic testing for autism predisposition: ethical, legal and social challenges. *Houston J Health Law Policy.* 2009;9:203–236.

Mardis ER. A decade's perspective on DNA sequencing technology. *Nature.* 2011;470(7333):198–203.

Marion R. *Genetics Rounds: A Doctor's Encounters in the Field That Revolutionized Medicine.* New York: Kaplan Publishing; 2009.

Marsden D, Levy H. Newborn screening of lysosomal storage disorders. *Clin Chem.* 2010;56(7):1071–1079.

Marshall E. Medicine. Fast technology drives new world of newborn screening. *Science.* 2001;294(5550):2272–2274.

Marshall E. NIH's "gay gene" study questioned. *Science* 1995;268:1841.

Marteau TM, French DP, Griffin SJ, et al. Effects of communicating DNA-based disease risk estimates on risk-reducing behaviours. *Cochrane Database Syst Rev.* 2010(10):CD007275.

Mascalzoni D, Hicks A, Pramstaller P, Wjst M. Informed consent in the genomics era. *PLoS Med.* 2008;5(9):e192.

Maschke KE. Ethical and policy issues involving research with newborn screening blood samples. In: Baily MA, Murray TH, eds. *Ethics and Newborn Genetic Screening: New Technologies, New Challenges.* Baltimore, MD: Johns Hopkins University Press; 2009:237–254.

Maschke KJ. Wanted: human biospecimens. *Hastings Cent Rep.* 2010;40(5):21–23.

Massie J, Curnow L, Gaffney L, Carlin J, Francis I. Declining prevalence of cystic fibrosis since the introduction of newborn screening. *Arch Dis Child.* 2010;95(7):531–533.

Master Z, Claudio JO, Rachul C, Wang JC, Minden MD, Caulfield T. Cancer patient perceptions on the ethical and legal issues related to biobanking. *BMC Med Genomics.* 2013;6:8.

Mastroianni AC, Kahn JP. Risk and responsibility: ethics, Grimes v Kennedy Krieger, and public health research involving children. *Am J Public Health.* 2002;92(7):1073–1076.

Matern D, Tortorelli S, Oglesbee D, Gavrilov D, Rinaldo P. Reduction of the false-positive rate in newborn screening by implementation of MS/MS-based second-tier tests: the Mayo Clinic experience (2004–2007). *J Inherit Metab Dis.* 2007;30(4):585–592.

Matsunami N, Hadley D, Hensel CH, et al. Identification of rare recurrent copy number variants in high-risk autism families and their prevalence in a large ASD population. *PLoS One.* 2013;8(1):e52239.

Matteson S, Paulauskis J, Foisy S, Hall S, Duval M. Opening the gate for genomics data into clinical research: a use case in managing patients' DNA samples from the bench to drug development. *Pharmacogenomics.* 2010;11(11):1603–1612.

Mattila ML, Kielinen M, Linna SL, et al. Autism spectrum disorders according to DSM-IV-TR and comparison with DSM-5 draft criteria: an epidemiological study. *J Am Acad Child Adolesc Psychiatry.* 2011;50(6):583–592.e511.

May T. Rethinking clinical risk for DNA sequencing. *Am J Bioeth.* 2012;12(10):24–26.

Mayer AN, Dimmock DP, Arca MJ, et al. A timely arrival for genomic medicine. *Genet Med.* 2011;13(3):195–196.

Mazzocco MMM, Ross JL, eds. *Neurogenetic Developmental Disorders: Variation of Manifestation in Childhood.* Cambridge, MA: MIT Press; 2007. *Issues in Clinical and Cognitive Neuropsychology.*

McBride CM, Guttmacher AE. Commentary: trailblazing a research agenda at the interface of pediatrics and genomic discovery—a commentary on the psychological aspects of genomics and child health. *J Pediatr Psychol.* 2009;34(6):662–664.

McCabe LL, Therrell BL Jr, McCabe ERB. Newborn screening: rationale for a comprehensive, fully integrated public health system. *Mol Genet Metab.* 2002;77(4):267–273

McCandless SE, Chandrasekar R, Linard S, Kikano S, Rice L. Sequencing from dried blood spots in infants with "false positive" newborn screen for MCAD deficiency. *Mol Genet Metab.* 2013;108(1):51–55.

McCarty CA, Chisholm RL, Chute CG, et al. The eMERGE Network: a consortium of biorepositories linked to electronic medical records data for conducting genomic studies. *BMC Med Genomics.* 2011;4:13.

McClaren BJ, Aitken M, Massie J, Amor D, Ukoumunne OC, Metcalfe SA. Cascade carrier testing after a child is diagnosed with cystic fibrosis through newborn screening: investigating why most relatives do not have testing. *Genet Med.* 2013;15(7):533–540.

McCullough LB. Contributions of ethical theory to pediatric ethics: pediatricians and parents as co-fiduciaries of pediatric patients. In: Miller G, ed. *Pediatric Bioethics.* Cambridge, UK: Cambridge University Press; 2010:11–21.

McCullough M. Bringing drama into medical education. *Lancet.* 2012;379(9815):512–513.

McEwen JE, Boyer JT, Sun KY. Evolving approaches to the ethical management of genomic data. *Trends Genet.* 2013;29(6):375–382.

McGuire AL, Achenbaum LS, Whitney SN, et al. Perspectives on human microbiome research ethics. *J Empir Res Hum Res Ethics.* 2012;7(3):1–14.

McGuire AL, Basford M, Dressler LG, et al. Ethical and practical challenges of sharing data from genome-wide association studies: the eMERGE Consortium experience. *Genome Res.* 2011;21(7):1001–1007.

McGuire AL, Beskow LM. Informed consent in genomics and genetic research. *Annu Rev Genomics Hum Genet.* 2010;11:361–381.

McGuire AL, Caulfield T, Cho MK. Research ethics and the challenge of whole-genome sequencing. *Nat Rev Genet.* 2008;9(2):152–156.

McGuire AL, Fisher R, Cusenza P, et al. Confidentiality, privacy, and security of genetic and genomic test information in electronic health records: points to consider. *Genet Med.* 2008;10(7):495–499.

McGuire AL, Hamilton JA, Lunstroth R, McCullough LB, Goldman A. DNA data sharing: research participants' perspectives. *Genet Med.* 2008;10(1):46–53.

McGuire AL, Joffe S, Koenig BA, et al. Point-counterpoint. Ethics and genomic incidental findings. *Science.* 2013;340(6136):1047–1048.

McGuire AL, Lupski JR. Personal genome research: what should the participant be told? *Trends Genet.* 2010;26(5):199–201.

McGuire AL, Majumder MA. Two cheers for GINA? *Genome Med.* 2009;1(1):6.

McGuire AL, McCullough LB, Evans JP. The indispensable role of professional judgment in genomic medicine. *JAMA.* 2013;309(14):1465–1466.

McGuire AL, Oliver JM, Slashinski MJ, et al. To share or not to share: a randomized trial of consent for data sharing in genome research. *Genet Med.* 2011;13(11):948–955.

McGuire AL, Robinson JO, Ramoni RB, Morley DS, Joffe S, Plon SE. Returning genetic research results: study type matters. *Per Med*. 2013;10(1):27–34.

McGuire AL, Wang MJ, Probst FJ. Currents in contemporary bioethics. Identifying consanguinity through routine genomic analysis: reporting requirements. *J Law Med Ethics*. 2012;40(4):1040–1046.

McHugh DMS, Cameron CA, Abdenur JE, et al. Clinical validation of cutoff target ranges in newborn screening of metabolic disorders by tandem mass spectrometry: a worldwide collaborative project. *Genet Med*. 2011;13(3):230–254.

Meacham MC, Starks H, Burke W, Edwards K. Researcher perspectives on disclosure of incidental findings in genetic research. *J Empir Res Hum Res Ethics*. 2010;5(3):31–41.

Medley C. *Relativity*. New York: Broadway Play Publishing; 2006.

Mefford HC, Batshaw ML, Hoffman EP. Genomics, intellectual disability, and autism. *N Engl J Med*. 2012;366(8):733–743.

Mercurio MR. Pediatric ethics committees. In: Miller G, ed. *Pediatric Bioethics*. Cambridge, UK: Cambridge University Press; 2010:87–108.

Merelle ME, Huisman J, Alderden-van der Vecht A, et al. Early versus late diagnosis: psychological impact on parents of children with cystic fibrosis. *Pediatrics*. 2003;111(2):346–350.

Meslin EM, Thomson EJ, Boyer JT. The ethical, legal, and social implications research program at the National Human Genome Research Institute. *Kennedy Inst Ethics J*. 1997;7:291–298.

Metcalfe A, Coad J, Plumridge GM, Gill P, Farndon P. Family communication between children and their parents about inherited genetic conditions: a meta-synthesis of the research. *Eur J Hum Genet*. 2008;16(10):1193–1200.

Miller BM, Moore DE Jr., Stead WW, Balser JR. Beyond Flexner: a new model for continuous learning in the health professions. *Acad Med*. 2010;85(2):266–272.

Miller FA, Christensen R, Giacomini M, Robert JS. Duty to disclose what? Querying the putative obligation to return research results to participants. *J Med Ethics*. 2008;34(3):210–213.

Miller FA, Giacomini M, Ahern C, Robert JS, de Laat S. When research seems like clinical care: a qualitative study of the communication of individual cancer genetic research results. *BMC Med Ethics*. 2008;9:4.

Miller FA, Hayeems RZ, Bombard Y, et al. Clinical obligations and public health programmes: healthcare provider reasoning about managing the incidental results of newborn screening. *J Med Ethics*. 2009;35(10):626–634.

Miller FA, Hayeems RZ, Bytautas JP. What is a meaningful result? Disclosing the results of genomic research in autism to research participants. *Eur J Hum Genet*. 2010;18(8):867–871.

Miller FA, Hayeems RZ, Carroll JC, et al. Consent for newborn screening: the attitudes of health care providers. *Public Health Genomics*. 2010;13(3):181–190.

Miller FA, Hayeems RZ, Li L, Bytautas JP. One thing leads to another: the cascade of obligations when researchers report genetic research results to study participants. *Eur J Hum Genet*. 2012;20(8):837–843.

Miller FA, Paynter M, Hayeems RZ, et al. Understanding sickle cell carrier status identified through newborn screening: a qualitative study. *Eur J Hum Genet*. 2010;18(3):303–308.

Miller FA, Robert JS, Hayeems RZ. Questioning the consensus: managing carrier status results generated by newborn screening. *Am J Public Health*. 2009;99(2):210–215.

Miller FG, Mello MM, Joffe S. Incidental findings in human subjects research: what do investigators owe research participants? *J Law Med Ethics.* 2008;36(2):271–279.

Miller G, ed. *Pediatric Bioethics.* Cambridge, UK: Cambridge University Press; 2010.

Miller VA, Drotar D, Kodish E. Children's competence for assent and consent: a review of empirical findings. *Ethics Behav.* 2004;14(3):255–295.

Millington DS, Kodo N, Norwood DL, Roe CR. Tandem mass spectrometry: a new method for acylcarnitine profiling with potential for neonatal screening for inborn errors of metabolism. *J Inherit Metab Dis.* 1990;13(3):321–324.

Mitchell GJ, Jonas-Simpson C, Ivonoffski V. Research-based theatre: the making of *I'm Still Here! Nurs Sci Q.* 2006;19(3):198–206.

Moore CA, Khoury MJ, Bradley LA. From genetics to genomics: using gene-based medicine to prevent disease and promote health in children. *Semin Perinatol.* 2005;29(3):135–143.

Moreno JD, Kravitt A. The ethics of pediatric research. In: Miller G, ed. *Pediatric Bioethics.* Cambridge, UK: Cambridge University Press; 2010:54–72.

Morrison DR, Clayton EW. False positive newborn screening results are not always benign. *Public Health Genomics.* 2011;14(3):173–177.

Moyer VA, Calonge N, Teutsch SM, Botkin JR. Expanding newborn screening: process, policy, and priorities. *Hastings Cent Rep.* 2008;38(3):32–39.

Mullin P. *The Sequence.* Los Angeles, CA: Original Works Publishing; 2010.

Munger KM, Gill CJ, Ormond KE, Kirschner KL. The next exclusion debate: assessing technology, ethics, and intellectual disability after the Human Genome Project. *Ment Retard Dev Disabil Res Rev.* 2007;13(2):121–128.

Muntoni F, Torelli S, Ferlini A. Dystrophin and mutations: one gene, several proteins, multiple phenotypes. *Lancet Neurol.* 2003;2(12):731–740.

Murphy J, Scott J, Kaufman D, Geller G, LeRoy L, Hudson K. Public expectations for return of results from large-cohort genetic research. *Am J Bioeth.* 2008;8(11):36–43.

Murphy J, Scott J, Kaufman D, Geller G, LeRoy L, Hudson K. Public perspectives on informed consent for biobanking. *Am J Public Health.* 2009;99(12):2128–2134.

Murphy TF. Hospital ethics committees and research with human beings. In: Hester DM, ed. *Ethics by Committee: A Textbook on Consultation, Organization, and Education for Hospital Ethics Committees.* Lanham, MD: Rowman & Littlefield Publishers; 2008:215–230.

Murray TH. Moral obligations to the not-yet born: the fetus as patient. *Clin Perinatol.* 1987;14(2):329–343.

Murray TH. *The Worth of a Child.* Berkeley, CA: University of California Press; 1996.

Myring J, Beckett W, Jassi R, et al. Shock, adjust, decide: reproductive decision making in cystic fibrosis (CF) carrier couples—a qualitative study. *J Genet Couns.* 2011;20(4):404–417.

Naj AC, Jun G, Beecham GW, et al. Common variants at MS4A4/MS4A6E, CD2AP, CD33 and EPHA1 are associated with late-onset Alzheimer's disease. *Nat Genet.* 2011;43:436–441.

Najafzadeh M, Lynd LD, Davis JC, et al. Barriers to integrating personalized medicine into clinical practice: a best-worst scaling choice experiment. *Genet Med.* 2012;14(5):520–526.

National Commission for the Protection of Human Subjects of Biomedical and Behavioral Research. *The Belmont Report: Ethical Principles and Guidelines for the Protection of Human Subjects of Research.* Bethesda, MD: National

Commission for the Protection of Human Subjects of Biomedical and Behavioral Research; 1978.

National Human Genome Research Institute. All about the Human Genome Project (HGP). http://www.genome.gov/10001772. Updated January 24, 2013. Accessed June 21, 2013.

National Human Genome Research Institute. ELSI research priorities and possible research projects. http://www.genome.gov/27543732. Last updated July 18, 2011. Accessed June 21, 2013.

National Human Genome Research Institute. The Ethical, Legal and Social Implications (ELSI) Research Program. http://www.genome.gov/10001618. Updated April 10, 2013. Accessed June 21, 2013.

National Human Genome Research Institute. *International consortium completes Human Genome Project [news release]*. Bethesda, MD: National Human Genome Research Institute and Department of Energy, April 14, 2003. http://web.ornl. gov/sci/techresources/Human_Genome/project/press4_2003.shtml. Accessed July 26, 2013.

National Human Genome Research Institute, ELSI Research Planning and Evaluation Group. *A Review and Analysis of the Ethical, Legal and Social Implications (ELSI) Research Programs at the National Institutes of Health and the Department of Energy*. http://www.genome.gov/10001727. Updated February 10, 2000. Accessed June 21, 2013.

National Human Genome Research Institute. *Summary of population-based carrier screening for single gene disorders: lessons learned and new opportunities*. Rockville, MD: NIH, February 6–7, 2008. http://www.genome.gov/27026048. Accessed July 25, 2013.

National Institutes of Health Recombinant DNA Advisory Committee. Prenatal gene transfer: Scientific, medical, and ethical issues. *Hum Gene Ther*. 2000;11(8):1211–1229.

National Newborn Screening and Global Resource Center. http://genes-r-us.uthscsa. edu/. Accessed July 18, 2013.

Neale BM, Medland SE, Ripke S, et al. Meta-analysis of genome-wide association studies of attention-deficit/hyperactivity disorder. *J Am Acad Child Adolesc Psychiatry*. 2010;49(9):884–897.

Nelkin D, Lindee MS. *The DNA Mystique: The Gene as a Cultural Icon*. 2nd ed. Ann Arbor, MI: University of Michigan Press; 2004.

Nelkin D, Tancredi LR. *Dangerous Diagnostics: The Social Power of Biological Information*. New York: Basic Books; 1989.

Nelson HL. Context: backward, sideways, and forward. In: Charon R, Montello M, eds. *Stories Matter: The Role of Narrative in Medical Ethics*. New York: Routledge; 2002:39–47.

Nelson HL. *Stories and Their Limits: Narrative Approaches to Bioethics*. New York: Routledge; 1997. *Reflective Bioethics*.

Netzer C, Klein C, Kohlhase J, Kubisch C. New challenges for informed consent through whole genome array testing. *J Med Genet*. 2009;46(7):495–496.

Newborn Screening Translational Research Network. https://www.nbstrn.org/. Accessed November 30, 2013.

Newson A. Should parental refusals of newborn screening be respected? *Camb Q Healthc Ethics*. 2006;15(2):135–146.

Ng SB, Turner EH, Robertson PD, et al. Targeted capture and massively parallel sequencing of 12 human exomes. *Nature*. 2009;461(7261):272–276.

Nijsingh N. Blurring boundaries. *Am J Bioeth.* 2012;12(10):26–27.

Nobile H, Vermeulen E, Thys K, Bergmann MM, Borry P. Why do participants enroll in population biobank studies? A systematic literature review. *Expert Rev Mol Diagn.* 2013;13(1):35–47.

Nowaczyk, MJM. Narrative medicine in clinical genetics practice. *Am J Med Genet A.* 2012; 158A:1941–1947.

Nuland SB. *The Soul of Medicine: Tales from the Bedside.* New York: Kaplan Publishing; 2009.

Nussbaum MC. *Love's Knowledge: Essays on Philosophy and Literature.* New York: Oxford University Press; 1990.

Nyholt DR, Yu CE, Visscher PM. On Jim Watson's APOE status: genetic information is hard to hide. *Eur J Hum Genet.* 2009;17(2):147–149.

O'Daniel J, Haga SB. Public perspectives on returning genetics and genomics research results. *Public Health Genomics.* 2011;14(6):346–355.

Offit K. Personalized medicine: new genomics, old lessons. *Hum Genet.* 2011;130(1):3–14.

Oliver JM, McGuire AL. Exploring the ELSI universe: critical issues in the evolution of human genomic research. *Genome Med.* 2011;3(6):38.

Oliver JM, Slashinski MJ, Wang T, Kelly PA, Hilsenbeck SG, McGuire AL. Balancing the risks and benefits of genomic data sharing: genome research participants' perspectives. *Public Health Genomics.* 2012;15(2):106–114.

Olney RS, Moore CA, Ojodu JA, Lindegren ML, Hannon WH. Storage and use of residual dried blood spots from state newborn screening programs. *J Pediatr.* 2006;148(5):618–622.

O'Neill E. *Strange Interlude* (1928). In: *Three Plays: Desire Under the Elms; Strange Interlude; Morning Becomes Electra.* New York:Vintage Books; 1995:65–256.

1000 Genomes Project Consortium, Abecasis GR, Altshuler D, et al. A map of human genome variation from population-scale sequencing. *Nature.* 2010;467(7319):1061–1073.

Opel DJ, Diekema DS, Marcuse EK. Assuring research integrity in the wake of Wakefield. *BMJ.* 2011;342:d2.

Ormond KE, Cirino AL, Helenowski IB, Chisholm RL, Wolf WA. Assessing the understanding of biobank participants. *Am J Med Genet A.* 2009;149A(2):188–198.

Ormond KE, Wheeler MT, Hudgins L, et al. Challenges in the clinical application of whole-genome sequencing. *Lancet.* 2010;375(9727):1749–1751.

O'Roak BJ, Deriziotis P, Lee C, et al. Exome sequencing in sporadic autism spectrum disorders identifies severe de novo mutations. *Nat Genet.* 2011;43(6):585–589.

Ossorio P. Taking aims seriously: repository research and limits on the duty to return individual research findings. *Genet Med.* 2012;14(4):461–466.

Ossorio P, Duster T. Race and genetics: controversies in biomedical, behavioral, and forensic sciences. *Am Psychol.* 2005;60(1):115–128.

Otto EA, Hurd TW, Airik R, et al. Candidate exome capture identifies mutation of SDCCAG8 as the cause of a retinal-renal ciliopathy. *Nat Genet.* 2010;42(10):840–850.

Ozonoff S, Young GS, Carter A, et al. Recurrence risk for autism spectrum disorders: a Baby Siblings Research Consortium study. *Pediatrics.* 2011;128(3):e488–e495.

Paasche-Orlow M. The ethics of cultural competence. *Acad Med.* 2004;79(4):347–350.

Palermo G, Joris H, Devroey P, Van Steirteghem AC. Pregnancies after intra-cytoplasmic injection of single spermatozoon into an oocyte. *Lancet.* 1992;340(8810):17–18.

Parens E. Should we hold the (germ) line? *J Law Med Ethics.* 1995;23(2):173–176.

Parens E, Appelbaum P, Chung W. Incidental findings in the era of whole genome sequencing? *Hastings Cent Rep.* 2013;43(4):16–19.

Parens E, Asch A. Disability rights critique of prenatal genetic testing: reflections and recommendations. *Ment Retard Dev Disabil Res Rev.* 2003;9(1):40–47.

Parens E, Asch A. The disability rights critique of prenatal genetic testing. Reflections and recommendations. *Hastings Cent Rep.* 1999;29(5):S1–S22.

Parens E, Asch A, eds. *Prenatal Testing and Disability Rights.* Washington, DC: Georgetown University Press; 2000.

Parker LS. Best laid plans for offering results go awry. *Am J Bioeth.* 2006;6(6):22–23; author reply W10–W12.

Parker LS. The future of incidental findings: should they be viewed as benefits? *J Law Med Ethics.* 2008;36(2):341–351.

Parker LS. Returning individual research results: what role should people's preferences play? *Minn JL Sci & Tech.* 2012;13(2):449–484.

Parker M. *Ethical Problems and Genetics Practice.* New York: Cambridge University Press; 2012.

Pass K, Green NS, Lorey F, Sherwin J, Comeau AM. Pilot programs in newborn screening. *Ment Retard Dev Disabil Res Rev.* 2006;12(4):293–300.

Patenaude AF. The genetic testing of children for cancer susceptibility: ethical, legal, and social issues. *Behav Sci Law.* 1996;14(4):393–410.

Patenaude AF, Basili L, Fairclough DL, Li FP. Attitudes of 47 mothers of pediatric oncology patients toward genetic testing for cancer predisposition. *J Clin Oncol.* 1996;14(2):415–421.

Paul D. Contesting consent: the challenge to compulsory neonatal screening for PKU. *Perspect Biol Med.* 1999;42(2):207–219.

Paul DB. A double-edged sword. *Nature.* 2000;405(6786):515.

Paul DB. Patient advocacy in newborn screening: continuities and discontinuities. *Am J Med Genet C Semin Med Genet.* 2008;148C(1):8–14.

Pelias MK. Genetic testing of children for adult-onset diseases: is testing in the child's best interests? *Mt Sinai J Med.* 2006;73(3):605–608.

Pelias MZ, Blanton SH. Genetic testing in children and adolescents: parental authority, the rights of children, and duties of geneticists. *Univ Chicago Law School Roundtable.* 1996;3(2):525–544.

Pennings G, Schots R, Liebaers I. Ethical considerations on preimplantation genetic diagnosis for HLA typing to match a future child as a donor of haematopoietic stem cells to a sibling. *Hum Reprod.* 2002;17(3):534–538.

Pennisi E. Genomics. ENCODE project writes eulogy for junk DNA. *Science.* 2012;337(6099):1159, 1161.

Perrin EC, West PD, Culley BS. Is my child normal yet? Correlates of vulnerability. *Pediatrics.* 1989;83(3):355–363.

Perrin JM, Knapp AA, Browning MF, et al. An evidence development process for newborn screening. *Genet Med.* 2010;12(3):131–134.

Petros M. Revisiting the Wilson-Jungner criteria: how can supplemental criteria guide public health in the era of genetic screening? *Genet Med.* 2012;14(1):129–134.

Plass AMC, van El CG, Pieters T, Cornel MC. Neonatal screening for treatable and untreatable disorders: prospective parents' opinions. *Pediatrics.* 2010;125(1):e99–e106.

Platt J, Bollinger J, Dvoskin R, Kardia SL, Kaufman D. Public preferences regarding informed consent models for participation in population-based genomic research. *Genet Med.* 2013. doi: 10.1038/gim.2013.59.

Platt R, Grossmann C, Selker HP. Evaluation as part of operations: reconciling the common rule and continuous improvement. Commentary. *Hastings Cent Rep.* 2013;43(Suppl):S37–S39.

Poirier S. Voice in the medical narrative. In: Charon R, Montello M, eds. *Stories Matter: The Role of Narrative in Medical Ethics.* New York: Routledge; 2002:48–59.

Polich G, Dole C, Kaptchuk TJ. The need to act a little more 'scientific': biomedical researchers investigating complementary and alternative medicine. *Sociol Health Illn.* 2010;32:106–122.

Pollitt RJ. Introducing new screens: why are we all doing different things? *J Inherit Metab Dis.* 2007;30(4):423–429.

Potter BK, Avard D, Entwistle V, et al. Ethical, legal, and social issues in health technology assessment for prenatal/preconceptional and newborn screening: a workshop report. *Public Health Genomics.* 2009;12(1):4–10.

Potter BK, O'Reilly N, Etchegary H, et al. Exploring informed choice in the context of prenatal testing: findings from a qualitative study. *Health Expect.* 2008;11(4):355–365.

Powers M, Faden RR. *Social Justice: The Moral Foundations of Public Health and Health Policy.* Oxford, UK: Oxford University Press; 2006. *Issues in Biomedical Ethics.*

Practice Committee of the American Society for Reproductive Medicine, Practice Committee of the Society for Assisted Reproductive Technology. Genetic considerations related to intracytoplasmic sperm injection (ICSI). *Fertil Steril.* 2006;86(5 Suppl 1):S103–S105.

Presidential Commission for the Study of Bioethical Issues. *Moral Science: Protecting Participants in Human Subjects Research.* http://bioethics.gov/sites/default/files/Moral%20Science%20June%202012.pdf. Published December 2011. Accessed July 9, 2013.

Presidential Commission for the Study of Bioethical Issues. *Privacy and Progress in Whole Genome Sequencing.* http://bioethics.gov/sites/default/files/PrivacyProgress508_1.pdf. Published October 2012. Accessed July 23, 2013.

President's Commission for the Study of Ethical Problems in Medicine and Biomedical and Behavioral Research. *Screening and Counseling for Genetic Conditions: A Report on the Ethical, Social, and Legal Implications of Genetic Screening, Counseling, and Education Programs.* Washington, DC: President's Commission for the Study of Ethical Problems in Medicine and Biomedical and Behavioral Research; 1983.

President's Commission for the Study of Ethical Problems in Medicine and Biomedical and Behavioral Research. *Summing Up: The Ethical and Legal Problems in Medicine and Biomedical and Behavioral Research.* Washington, DC: President's Commission for the Study of Ethical Problems in Medicine and Biomedical Research; 1983.

President's Council on Bioethics. *The Changing Moral Focus of Newborn Screening: An Ethical Analysis by the President's Council on Bioethics.* Washington, DC: President's Council on Bioethics; 2008.

President's Council on Bioethics. Ethics of cloning-to-produce-children. *Human Cloning and Human Dignity: An Ethical Inquiry.* Washington, DC: President's Council on Bioethics; 2002:75–116.

President's Council on Bioethics. *Human Cloning and Human Dignity: An Ethical Inquiry.* Washington, DC: President's Council on Bioethics; 2002.

President's Panel on Mental Retardation. *A Proposed Program for National Action to Combat Mental Retardation.* Washington, DC: The President's Panel on Mental Retardation; 1962.

Press N, Browner CH. Why women say yes to prenatal diagnosis. *Soc Sci Med.* 1997;45(7):979–989.

Press N, Clayton EW. Genetics and public health: informed consent beyond the clinical encounter. In: Khoury MJ, Burke W, Thomson EJ, eds. *Genetics and Public Health in the 21st Century: Using Genetic Information to Improve Health and Prevent Disease*. New York: Oxford University Press; 2000:505–526.

Prince AE, Berkman BE. When does an illness begin: genetic discrimination and disease manifestation. *J Law Med Ethics*. 2012;40(3):655–664.

Prosser LA, Kong CY, Rusinak D, Waisbren SL. Projected costs, risks, and benefits of expanded newborn screening for MCADD. *Pediatrics*. 2010;125(2):e286–e294.

Prosser LA, Ladapo JA, Rusinak D, Waisbren SE. Parental tolerance of false-positive newborn screening results. *Arch Pediatr Adolesc Med*. 2008;162(9):870–876.

Puckett RL, Lorey F, Rinaldo P, et al. Maple syrup urine disease: further evidence that newborn screening may fail to identify variant forms. *Mol Genet Metab*. 2010;100(2):136–142.

Puglisi T. Reform within the common rule? Commentary. *Hastings Cent Rep*. 2013;43(Suppl):S40–S42.

Pulley J, Clayton E, Bernard GR, Roden DM, Masys DR. Principles of human subjects protections applied in an opt-out, de-identified biobank. *Clin Transl Sci*. 2010;3(1):42–48.

Pullman D, Hodgkinson K. Genetic knowledge and moral responsibility: ambiguity at the interface of genetic research and clinical practice. *Clin Genet*. 2006;69(3):199–203.

Pyeritz RE. The coming explosion in genetic testing—is there a duty to recontact? *N Engl J Med*. 2011;365(15):1367–1369.

Quaid KA. Presymptomatic genetic testing in children. In: Miller G, ed. *Pediatric Bioethics*. New York: Cambridge University Press; 2010:125–140.

Rabkin J. American exceptionalism and the healthcare reform debate. *Harvard J Law Public Policy*. 2012;35(1):153–170.

Ramoni RB, McGuire AL, Robinson JO, Morley DS, Plon SE, Joffe S. Experiences and attitudes of genome investigators regarding return of individual genetic test results. *Genet Med*. 2013;15(11):882–887.

Ramos EM, Din-Lovinescu C, Bookman EB, et al. A mechanism for controlled access to GWAS data: experience of the GAIN Data Access Committee. *Am J Hum Genet*. 2013;92(4):479–488.

Raspberry K, Skinner D. Experiencing the genetic body: parents' encounters with pediatric clinical genetics. *Med Anthropol*. 2007;26(4):355–391.

Ravitsky V, Wilfond BS. Disclosing individual genetic results to research participants. *Am J Bioeth*. 2006;6(6):8–17.

Reeves S, Zwarenstein M, Goldman J, et al. Interprofessional education: effects on professional practice and health care outcomes. *Cochrane Database Syst Rev*. 2008(1):CD002213.

Refsgaard L, Holst AG, Sadjadieh G, Haunsø S, Nielsen JB, Olesen MS. High prevalence of genetic variants previously associated with LQT syndrome in new exome data. *Eur J Hum Genet*. 2012;20(8):905–908.

Rehder CW, David KL, Hirsch B, Toriello HV, Wilson CM, Kearney HM. American College of Medical Genetics and Genomics: standards and guidelines for documenting suspected consanguinity as an incidental finding of genomic testing. *Genet Med*. 2013;15(2):150–152.

Reverby SM. Invoking "Tuskegee": problems in health disparities, genetic assumptions, and history. *J Health Care Poor Underserved*. 2010;21(3 Suppl):26–34.

Reverby SM. Listening to narratives from the Tuskegee syphilis study. *Lancet*. 2011;377(9778):1646–1647.

Reynolds RC, Stone J, eds. *On Doctoring: Stories, Poems, Essays*. 3rd ed. New York: Simon & Schuster; 2001.

Rhodes R. Genetic links, family ties, and social bonds: rights and responsibilities in the face of genetic knowledge. *J Med Philos*. 1998;23(1):10–30.

Richardson HS. Incidental findings and ancillary-care obligations. *J Law Med Ethics*. 2008;36(2):256–270.

Richardson HS, Belsky L. The ancillary-care responsibilities of medical researchers. An ethical framework for thinking about the clinical care that researchers owe their subjects. *Hastings Cent Rep*. 2004;34(1):25–33.

Richardson HS, Cho MK. Secondary researchers' duties to return incidental findings and individual research results: a partial-entrustment account. *Genet Med*. 2012;14(4):467–472.

Ries NM, LeGrandeur J, Caulfield T. Handling ethical, legal and social issues in birth cohort studies involving genetic research: responses from studies in six countries. *BMC Med Ethics*. 2010;11(1):4.

Rinaldo P, Cowan TM, Matern D. Acylcarnitine profile analysis. *Genet Med*. 2008;10(2):151–156.

Rinaldo P, Matern D. Newborn screening for inherited metabolic disease. In: Hoffman GF, Zschocke J, Nyhan WL, eds. *Inherited Metabolic Diseases: A Clinical Approach*. Berlin: Springer-Verlag; 2010:251–261.

Rinaldo P, Zafari S, Tortorelli S, Matern D. Making the case for objective performance metrics in newborn screening by tandem mass spectrometry. *Ment Retard Dev Disabil Res Rev*. 2006;12(4):255–261.

Rini C, O'Neill SC, Valdimarsdottir H, et al. Cognitive and emotional factors predicting decisional conflict among high-risk breast cancer survivors who receive uninformative BRCA1/2 results. *Health Psychol*. 2009;28(5):569–578.

Roach JC, Glusman G, Smit AFA, et al. Analysis of genetic inheritance in a family quartet by whole-genome sequencing. *Science*. 2010;328(5978):636–639.

Roberts DE. Is race-based medicine good for us?: African American approaches to race, biomedicine, and equality. *J Law Med Ethics*. 2008;36(3):537–545.

Roberts DE. Legal constraints on the use of race in biomedical research: toward a social justice framework. *J Law Med Ethics*. 2006;34(3):526–534.

Robertson S, Savulescu J. Is there a case in favour of predictive genetic testing in young children? *Bioethics*. 2001;15(1):26–49.

Robinson WM. The narrative of rescue in pediatric practice. In: Charon R, Montello M, eds. *Stories Matter: The Role of Narrative in Medical Ethics*. New York: Routledge; 2002:100–111.

Roche MI. A case of genetic counselling for Dr Watson. *Nature*. 2008;453(7193):281.

Roche MI, Skinner D. How parents search, interpret, and evaluate genetic information obtained from the internet. *J Genet Couns*. 2009;18(2):119–129.

Rodriguez LL, Brooks LD, Greenberg JH, Green ED. Research ethics. The complexities of genomic identifiability. *Science*. 2013;339(6117):275–276.

Roe AM, Shur N. From new screens to discovered genes: the successful past and promising present of single gene disorders. *Am J Med Genet C Semin Med Genet*. 2007;145C(1):77–86.

Rorty MV. Ethics in and for the organization. In: Hester DM, Schonfeld T, eds. *Guidance for Healthcare Ethics Committees*. Cambridge, UK: Cambridge University Press; 2012:147–154.

Rosenberg LE. Legacies of Garrod's brilliance: one hundred years—and counting. *J Inherit Metab Dis*. 2008;31(5):574–579.

Rosenberg RN, DiMauro S, Paulson HL, Ptacek L, Nestler E, eds. *The Molecular and Genetic Basis of Neurologic and Psychiatric Disease*. 4th ed. Philadelphia: Wolters Kluwer Health/Lippincott Williams & Wilkins; 2008.

Rosenfeld JA, Ballif BC, Torchia BS, et al. Copy number variations associated with autism spectrum disorders contribute to a spectrum of neurodevelopmental disorders. *Genet Med*. 2010;12(11):694–702.

Ross LF. *Children, Families, and Health Care Decision-Making*. Oxford, UK: Oxford University Press; 1998.

Ross LF. Disclosing misattributed paternity. *Bioethics*. 1996;10(2):114–130.

Ross LF. Disclosing misattributed paternity. In: Steinbock B, Arras J, London AJ, eds. *Ethical issues in modern medicine*. 6th ed. Boston: McGraw-Hill; 2003:120–128.

Ross LF. Ethical and policy issues in pediatric genetics. *Am J Med Genet C Semin Med Genet*. 2008;148C(1):1–7.

Ross LF. Genetic testing of children: who should consent? In: Burley J, Harris J, eds. *A Companion to Genethics*. Oxford: Blackwell; 2002:114–126.

Ross LF. Informed consent in pediatric research. *Camb Q Healthc Ethics*. 2004;13(4):346–358.

Ross LF. Mandatory versus voluntary consent for newborn screening? *Kennedy Inst Ethics J*. 2010;20(4):299–328.

Ross LF. Minimizing risks: the ethics of predictive diabetes mellitus screening research in newborns. *Arch Pediatr Adolesc Med*. 2003;157(1):89–95.

Ross LF. Newborn screening. In: Miller G, ed. *Pediatric Bioethics*. Cambridge, UK: Cambridge University Press; 2010:111–124.

Ross LF. Newborn screening for conditions that do not meet the Wilson and Jungner criteria: the case of Duchenne muscular dystrophy. In: Baily MA, Murray TH, eds. *Ethics and Newborn Genetic Screening: New Technologies, New Challenges*. Baltimore: Johns Hopkins University Press; 2009:106–124.

Ross LF. Newborn screening for cystic fibrosis: a lesson in public health disparities. *J Pediatr*. 2008;153(3):308–313.

Ross LF. Newborn screening for lysosomal storage diseases: an ethical and policy analysis. *J Inherit Metab Dis*. 2012;35(4):627–634.

Ross LF. Predictive genetic testing for conditions that present in childhood. *Kennedy Inst Ethics J*. 2002;12(3):225–244.

Ross LF, Moon MR. Ethical issues in genetic testing of children. *Arch Pediatr Adolesc Med*. 2000;154(9):873–879.

Ross LF, Saal HM, David KL, Anderson RR. Technical report: ethical and policy issues in genetic testing and screening of children. *Genet Med*. 2013;15(3):234–245.

Rothenberg K. Eugenics, genetics and gender: theatre and the role of women. In: Caulfield ST, Gillespie C, Caulfield TA, eds. *Perceptions of Promise: Biotechnology, Society and Art*. Edmonton: University of Alberta; 2011:73–78.

Rothenberg K, Bush L. Manipulating fate: medical innovations, ethical implications, theatrical illuminations. *Houston J Health Law Policy*. 2012;13(1):1–77.

Rothenberg KH. "Being human": cloning and the challenges for public policy. *Hofstra Law Rev*. 1999;27(3):639–647.

Rothenberg KH. From eugenics to the 'new' genetics: "The Play's the Thing." *Fordham Law Rev*. 2010;79(2):407–434.

Rothenberg KH. The law's response to reproductive genetic testing: questioning assumptions about choice, causation, and control. *Fetal Diagn Ther*. 1993;8:160–163.

Rothenberg KH, Bush LW. Genes and plays: bringing ELSI issues to life. *Genet Med.* 2012;14(2):274–277.

Rothenberg MB, Sills EM. Iatrogenesis: the PKU anxiety syndrome. *J Am Acad Child Psychiatry.* 1968;7(4):689–692.

Rothman DJ. Ethics and human experimentation. Henry Beecher revisited. *New Engl J Med.* 1987;317(19):1195–1199.

Rothman DJ. *Strangers at the Bedside: A History of How Law and Bioethics Transformed Medical Decision Making.* New York: BasicBooks; 1991.

Rothstein M, Siegal G. Health Information Technology and physicians' duty to notify patients of new medical developments. *Houston J Health Law Policy.* 2012;12(1):93–136.

Rothstein MA. Currents in contemporary bioethics: physicians' duty to inform patients of new medical discoveries: the effect of health information technology. *J Law Med Ethics.* 2011;39(4):690–693.

Rothstein MA. Disclosing decedents' research results to relatives violates the HIPAA Privacy Rule. *Am J Bioeth.* 2012;12(10):16–17.

Rothstein MA. Tiered disclosure options promote the autonomy and well-being of research subjects. *Am J Bioeth.* 2006;6(6):20–21; author reply W10–W12.

Rothwell E, Anderson R, Goldenberg A, et al. Assessing public attitudes on the retention and use of residual newborn screening blood samples: a focus group study. *Soc Sci Med.* 2012;74(8):1305–1309.

Rothwell EW, Anderson RA, Burbank MJ, et al. Concerns of newborn blood screening advisory committee members regarding storage and use of residual newborn screening blood spots. *Am J Public Health.* 2011;101(11):2111–2116.

Rubinstein YR, Groft SC, Bartek R, et al. Creating a global rare disease patient registry linked to a rare diseases biorepository database: Rare Disease-HUB (RD-HUB). *Contemp Clin Trials.* 2010;31(5):394–404.

Russo AJ, Devito R. Analysis of copper and zinc plasma concentration and the efficacy of zinc therapy in individuals with Asperger's syndrome, pervasive developmental disorder not otherwise specified (PDD-NOS) and autism. *Biomark Insights.* 2011;6:127–133.

Saha K, Hurlbut JB. Research ethics: treat donors as partners in biobank research. *Nature.* 2011;478(7369):312–313.

Saleem T, Khalid U. Institutional review boards—a mixed blessing. *Int Arch Med.* 2011;4:19.

Samuel J, Knoppers BM, Avard D. Paediatric biobanks: what makes them so unique? *J Paediatr Child Health.* 2012;48(2):E1–E3.

Sandel MJ. *The Case Against Perfection: Ethics in the Age of Genetic Engineering.* Cambridge, MA: Belknap Harvard University Press; 2007.

Sandel MJ. The ethical implications of human cloning. *Perspect Biol Med.* 2005;48(2):241–247.

Sanders JL. Qualitative or quantitative differences between Asperger's disorder and autism? Historical considerations. *J Autism Dev Disord.* 2009;39(11):1560–1567.

Sanders SJ, Ercan-Sencicek AG, Hus V, et al. Multiple recurrent de novo CNVs, including duplications of the 7q11.23 Williams syndrome region, are strongly associated with autism. *Neuron.* 2011;70(5):863–885.

Sankar P. Communication and miscommunication in informed consent to research. *Med Anthropol Q.* 2004;18(4):429–446.

Saunders CJ, Miller NA, Soden SE, et al. Rapid whole-genome sequencing for genetic disease diagnosis in neonatal intensive care units. *Sci Transl Med.* 2012;4(154):154ra135.

Savitt TL. *Medical Readers' Theater: A Guide and Scripts*. Iowa City, IA: University of Iowa Press; 2002.

Sawyer SM, Cerritelli B, Carter LS, Cooke M, Glazner JA, Massie J. Changing their minds with time: a comparison of hypothetical and actual reproductive behaviors in parents of children with cystic fibrosis. *Pediatrics*. 2006;118(3):e649–e656.

Sayeed SA. The moral and legal status of children and parents. In: Miller G, ed. *Pediatric Bioethics*. Cambridge, UK: Cambridge University Press; 2010:38–53.

Sayre A. *Rosalind Franklin and DNA*. New York: Norton; 1975.

Schaaf CP, Scott DA, Wiszniewska J, Beaudet AL. Identification of incestuous parental relationships by SNP-based DNA microarrays. *Lancet*. 2011;377(9765):555–556.

Schaefer GB, Mendelsohn NJ. Clinical genetics evaluation in identifying the etiology of autism spectrum disorders: 2013 guideline revisions. *Genet Med*. 2013;15(5):399–407.

Scheuner MT, Edelen MO, Hilborne LH, Lubin IM. Effective communication of molecular genetic test results to primary care providers. *Genet Med*. 2013;15(6):444–449.

Schmidt JL, Castellanos-Brown K, Childress S, et al. The impact of false-positive newborn screening results on families: a qualitative study. *Genet Med*. 2012;14(1):76–80.

Schonfeld T. Confidentiality. In: Hester DM, Schonfeld T, eds. *Guidance for healthcare ethics committees*. Cambridge, UK: Cambridge University Press; 2012:71–79.

Schrijver I, Aziz N, Farkas DH, et al. Opportunities and challenges associated with clinical diagnostic genome sequencing: a report of the Association for Molecular Pathology. *J Mol Diagn*. 2012;14(6):525–540.

Schwartz J. *In Pursuit of the Gene: From Darwin to DNA*. Cambridge, MA: Harvard University Press; 2008.

Schwartz MD, Rothenberg K, Joseph L, Benkendorf J, Lerman C. Consent to the use of stored DNA for genetics research: a survey of attitudes in the Jewish population. *Am J Med Genet*. 2001;98:336–342.

Schwarzbraun T, Obenauf AC, Langmann A, et al. Predictive diagnosis of the cancer prone Li-Fraumeni syndrome by accident: new challenges through whole genome array testing. *J Med Genet*. 2009;46(5):341–344.

Selby JV, Krumholz HM. Ethical oversight: serving the best interests of patients. Commentary. *Hastings Cent Rep*. 2013;43(Suppl):S34–S36.

Sermet-Gaudelus I, Mayell SJ, Southern KW. Guidelines on the early management of infants diagnosed with cystic fibrosis following newborn screening. *J Cyst Fibros*. 2010;9(5):323–329.

Sevick MA, Nativio DG, McConnell T. Genetic testing of children for late onset disease. *Camb Q Healthc Ethics*. 2005;14(1):47–56.

Shah S, Wendler D. Interpretation of the subjects' condition requirement: a legal perspective. *J Law Med Ethics*. 2010;38(2):365–373.

Shah S, Whittle A, Wilfond B, Gensler G, Wendler D. How do institutional review boards apply the federal risk and benefit standards for pediatric research? *JAMA*. 2004;291(4):476–482.

Shah S, Wolitz R, Emanuel E. Refocusing the responsiveness requirement. *Bioethics*. 2013;27(3):151–159.

Shah SK. Outsourcing ethical obligations: should the revised common rule address the responsibilities of investigators and sponsors? *J Law Med Ethics*. 2013;41(2):397–410.

Shalowitz DI, Miller FG. Communicating the results of clinical research to participants: attitudes, practices, and future directions. *PLoS Med.* 2008;5(5):e91.

Shalowitz DI, Miller FG. Disclosing individual results of clinical research: implications of respect for participants. *JAMA.* 2005;294(6):737–740.

Shapiro J. Walking a mile in their patients' shoes: empathy and othering in medical students' education. *Philos Ethics Humanit Med.* 2008;3:10.

Shapiro J, Hunt L. All the world's a stage: the use of theatrical performance in medical education. *Med Educ.* 2003;37(10):922–927.

Shapiro J, Kasman D, Shafer A. Words and wards: a model of reflective writing and its uses in medical education. *J Med Humanit.* 2006;27(4):231–244.

Sharp RR. Downsizing genomic medicine: approaching the ethical complexity of whole-genome sequencing by starting small. *Genet Med.* 2011;13(3):191–194.

Sharp RR, Foster MW. Clinical utility and full disclosure of genetic results to research participants. *Am J Bioeth.* 2006;6(6):42–44; author reply W10–W12.

Shelton W, Bjarnadottir D. Ethics consultation and the committee. In: Hester DM, ed. *Ethics by Committee: A Textbook on Consultation, Organization, and Education for Hospital Ethics Committees.* Lanham, MD: Rowman & Littlefield Publishers; 2008:49–78.

Shen Y, Chen X, Wang L, et al. Intra-family phenotypic heterogeneity of 16p11.2 deletion carriers in a three-generation Chinese family. *Am J Med Genet B Neuropsychiatr Genet.* 2011;156(2):225–232.

Shen Y, Dies KA, Holm IA, et al. Clinical genetic testing for patients with autism spectrum disorders. *Pediatrics.* 2010;125(4):e727–e735.

Shepherd-Barr K. *Science on Stage: From Doctor Faustus to Copenhagen.* Princeton, NJ: Princeton University Press; 2006.

Shigematsu Y, Hata I, Tajima G. Useful second-tier tests in expanded newborn screening of isovaleric acidemia and methylmalonic aciduria. *J Inherit Metab Dis.* 2010;33(Suppl 2):S283–S288.

Shonkoff CJ. Reactions to the threatened loss of a child: a vulnerable child syndrome, by Morris Green, MD, and Albert A. Solnit, MD, Pediatrics, 1964;34:58–66. *Pediatrics.* 1998;102(1 Pt 2):239–241.

Sibley A, Sheehan M, Pollard AJ. Assent is not consent. *J Med Ethics.* 2012;38(1):3.

Siegler M. A legacy of Osler. Teaching clinical ethics at the bedside. *JAMA.* 1978;239(10):951–956.

Simon C, Shinkunas LA, Brandt D, Williams JK. Individual genetic and genomic research results and the tradition of informed consent: exploring US review board guidance. *J Med Ethics.* 2012;38(7):417–422.

Simon CM, Williams JK, Shinkunas L, Brandt D, Daack-Hirsch S, Driessnack M. Informed consent and genomic incidental findings: IRB chair perspectives. *J Empir Res Hum Res Ethics.* 2011;6(4):53–67.

Sims EJ, Clark A, McCormick J, et al. Cystic fibrosis diagnosed after 2 months of age leads to worse outcomes and requires more therapy. *Pediatrics.* 2007;119(1):19–28.

Sivell S, Elwyn G, Gaff CL, et al. How risk is perceived, constructed and interpreted by clients in clinical genetics, and the effects on decision making: systematic review. *J Genet Couns.* 2008;17(1):30–63.

Skinner D, Choudhury S, Sideris J, et al. Parents' decisions to screen newborns for FMR1 gene expansions in a pilot research project. *Pediatrics.* 2011;127(6):e1455–e1463.

Skinner D, Schaffer R. Families and genetic diagnoses in the genomic and internet age. *Infants Young Child.* 2006;19(1):16–24.

Skinner D, Sparkman KL, Bailey DB Jr. Screening for fragile X syndrome: parent attitudes and perspectives. *Genet Med.* 2003;5(5):378–384.

Skloot R. *The Immortal Life of Henrietta Lacks.* New York: Crown Publishers; 2010.

Skorton DJ. Bridging the "Two Cultures" divide in medicine and the academy. *Technol Soc.* 2010;32(1):49–52.

Smith EH, Thomas C, McHugh D, et al. Allelic diversity in MCAD deficiency: the biochemical classification of 54 variants identified during 5 years of ACADM sequencing. *Mol Genet Metab.* 2010;100(3):241–250.

Smith ML. Mission, vision, goals: defining the parameters of ethics consultation. In: Hester DM, Schonfeld T, eds. *Guidance for Healthcare Ethics Committees.* Cambridge, UK: Cambridge University Press; 2012:32–40.

Snow CP. *The Two Cultures and a Second Look: An Expanded Version of the Two Cultures and the Scientific Revolution.* London: Cambridge University Press; 1969.

Solomon BD, Hadley DW, Pineda-Alvarez DE, et al. Incidental medical information in whole-exome sequencing. *Pediatrics.* 2012;129(6):e1605–e1611.

Solomon MZ, Bonham AC. Ethical oversight of research on patient care. *Hastings Cent Rep.* 2013;43(Suppl):S2–S3.

Sousa I, Clark TG, Holt R, et al. Polymorphisms in leucine-rich repeat genes are associated with autism spectrum disorder susceptibility in populations of European ancestry. *Mol Autism.* 2010;1(1):7.

Specter M. Annals of science: the power of nothing. *New Yorker.* December 12, 2011, 30.

Sperling, D. Bringing life from death: is there a good justification for posthumous cloning? *J Clinic Res Bioeth* 2011;S1:001, available at http://www.omicsonline.org/2155-9627/2155-9627-S1-001.pdf.

Spike J. Ethics consultation process. In: Hester DM, Schonfeld T, eds. *Guidance for Healthcare Ethics Committees.* Cambridge, UK: Cambridge University Press; 2012:41–47.

Stack CB, Gharani N, Gordon ES, Schmidlen T, Christman MF, Keller MA. Genetic risk estimation in the Coriell Personalized Medicine Collaborative. *Genet Med.* 2011;13(2):131–139.

Stark AP, Lang CW, Ross LF. A pilot study to evaluate knowledge and attitudes of Illinois pediatricians toward newborn screening for sickle cell disease and cystic fibrosis. *Am J Perinatol.* 2011;28(3):169–176.

State MW, Levitt P. The conundrums of understanding genetic risks for autism spectrum disorders. *Nat Neurosci.* 2011;14(12):1499–1506.

Stephenson S. *An Experiment with an Air Pump.* New York: Dramatists Play Service; 2000.

Stockdale A, Terry S. Advocacy groups and the new genetics. In: Alper JS, Ard C, Asch A, eds. *The Double-Edged Helix: Social Implications of Genetics in a Diverse Society.* Baltimore, MD: Johns Hopkins University Press; 2002:80–101.

Stripling MY. *Bioethics and Medical Issues in Literature.* Westport, CT: Greenwood Press; 2005. *Exploring Social Issues Through Literature.*

Strong C. Abortion decisions as inclusion and exclusion criteria in research involving pregnant women and fetuses. *J Med Ethics.* 2012;38(1):43–47.

Subbaraman N. Alzheimer's genetic map. *Nat Biotech.* 2011;29(3):179–179.

Sugarman J, Sulmasy DP, eds. *Methods in Medical Ethics.* 2nd ed. Washington, DC: Georgetown University Press; 2010.

Suther S, Kiros GE. Barriers to the use of genetic testing: a study of racial and ethnic disparities. *Genet Med.* 2009;11(9):655–662.

Tabor HK, Berkman BE, Hull SC, Bamshad MJ. Genomics really gets personal: how exome and whole genome sequencing challenge the ethical framework of human genetics research. *Am J Med Genet A.* 2011;155A(12):2916–2924.

Tabor HK, Cho MK. Ethical implications of array comparative genomic hybridization in complex phenotypes: points to consider in research. *Genet Med.* 2007;9(9):626–631.

Tabor HK, Stock J, Brazg T, et al. Informed consent for whole genome sequencing: a qualitative analysis of participant expectations and perceptions of risks, benefits, and harms. *Am J Med Genet A.* 2012;158A(6):1310–1319.

Tarini BA. Communicating with parents about newborn screening: the skill of eliciting unspoken emotions. *Arch Pediatr Adolesc Med.* 2012;166(1):95–96.

Tarini BA. The current revolution in newborn screening: new technology, old controversies. *Arch Pediatr Adolesc Med.* 2007;161(8):767–772.

Tarini BA. Storage and use of residual newborn screening blood spots: a public policy emergency. *Genet Med.* 2011;13(7):619–620.

Tarini BA, Burke W, Scott CR, Wilfond BS. Waiving informed consent in newborn screening research: balancing social value and respect. *Am J Med Genet C Semin Med Genet.* 2008;148C(1):23–30.

Tarini BA, Christakis DA, Welch HG. State newborn screening in the tandem mass spectrometry era: more tests, more false-positive results. *Pediatrics.* 2006;118(2):448–456.

Tarini BA, Clark SJ, Pilli S, et al. False-positive newborn screening result and future health care use in a state Medicaid cohort. *Pediatrics.* 2011;128(4):715–722.

Tarini BA, Goldenberg A, Singer D, Clark SJ, Butchart A, Davis MM. Not without my permission: parents' willingness to permit use of newborn screening samples for research. *Public Health Genomics.* 2010;13(3):125–130.

Tarini BA, Singer D, Clark SJ, Davis MM. Parents' interest in predictive genetic testing for their children when a disease has no treatment. *Pediatrics.* 2009;124(3):e432–e438.

Tarini BA, Tercyak KP, Wilfond BS. Commentary: Children and predictive genomic testing: disease prevention, research protection, and our future. *J Pediatr Psychol.* 2011;36(10):1113–1121.

Tercyak KP, Hensley Alford S, Emmons KM, Lipkus IM, Wilfond BS, McBride CM. Parents' attitudes toward pediatric genetic testing for common disease risk. *Pediatrics.* 2011;127(5):e1288–e1295.

Terry SF. The tension between policy and practice in returning research results and incidental findings in genomic biobank research. *Minn J Law Sci & Tech.* 2012;13(2):691–736.

Therrell BL Jr. U.S. newborn screening policy dilemmas for the twenty-first century. *Mol Genet Metab.* 2001;74(1–2):64–74.

Therrell BL Jr., Hannon WH, Bailey DB Jr., et al. Committee report: considerations and recommendations for national guidance regarding the retention and use of residual dried blood spot specimens after newborn screening. *Genet Med.* 2011;13(7):621–624.

Therrell BL, Johnson A, Williams D. Status of newborn screening programs in the United States. *Pediatrics.* 2006;117(5 Pt 2):S212–S252.

Timimi S. Autism is not a scientifically valid or clinically useful diagnosis. *BMJ.* 2011;343:D5105.

Timmermans S, Buchbinder M. Patients-in-waiting: living between sickness and health in the genomics era. *J Health Soc Behav.* 2010;51(4):408–423.

Tluczek A, Chevalier McKechnie A, Lynam PA. When the cystic fibrosis label does not fit: a modified uncertainty theory. *Qual Health Res.* 2010;20(2):209–223.

Tluczek A, McKechnie AC, Brown RL. Factors associated with parental perception of child vulnerability 12 months after abnormal newborn screening results. *Res Nurs Health.* 2011;34(5):389–400.

Tluczek A, Orland KM, Cavanagh L. Psychosocial consequences of false-positive newborn screens for cystic fibrosis. *Qual Health Res.* 2011;21(2):174–186.

Tluczek A, Orland KM, Nick SW, Brown RL. Newborn screening: an appeal for improved parent education. *J Perinat Neonatal Nurs.* 2009;23(4):326–334.

Tluczek A, Zaleski C, Stachiw-Hietpas D, et al. A tailored approach to family-centered genetic counseling for cystic fibrosis newborn screening: the Wisconsin model. *J Genet Couns.* 2011;20(2):115–128.

Tolins J. *The Twilight of the Golds.* New York: Samuel French; 1994.

Townsend A, Adam S, Birch PH, Lohn Z, Rousseau F, Friedman JM. "I want to know what's in Pandora's box": comparing stakeholder perspectives on incidental findings in clinical whole genomic sequencing. *Am J Med Genet A.* 2012;158A(10):2519–2525.

Trillin AS. Of dragons and garden peas: a cancer patient talks to doctors. *N Engl J Med.* 1981;304(12):699–701.

Trinidad SB, Fullerton SM, Bares JM, Jarvik GP, Larson EB, Burke W. Genomic research and wide data sharing: views of prospective participants. *Genet Med.* 2010;12(8):486–495.

Trinidad SB, Fullerton SM, Ludman EJ, Jarvik GP, Larson EB, Burke W. Research ethics. Research practice and participant preferences: the growing gulf. *Science.* 2011;331(6015):287–288.

Trotter TL, Fleischman AR, Howell RR, Lloyd-Puryear M. Secretary's Advisory Committee on Heritable Disorders in Newborns and Children response to the President's Council on Bioethics report: the changing moral focus of newborn screening. *Genet Med.* 2011;13(4):301–304.

Tsai LY, Ghaziuddin M. DSM-5 ASD moves forward into the past. *J Autism Dev Disord.* 2013. doi: 10.1007/s10803-013-1870-3.

Turner CG, Tworetzky W, Wilkins-Haug LE, Jennings RW. Cardiac anomalies in the fetus. *Clin Perinatol.* 2009;36(2):439–449.

Uhlmann W, Schuette J, Yashar B, eds. *A Guide to Genetic Counseling.* 2nd ed. Hoboken, NJ: Wiley-Blackwell; 2011.

Ulrich M. The duty to rescue in genomic research. *Am J Bioeth.* 2013;13(2):50–51.

Unalan PC, Uzuner A, Cifcili S, Akman M, Hancioglu S, Thulesius HO. Using theatre in education in a traditional lecture oriented medical curriculum. *BMC Med Educ.* 2009;9:73.

Ungar D, Joffe S, Kodish E. Children are not small adults: documentation of assent for research involving children. *J Pediatr.* 2006;149(1 Suppl):S31–S33.

Unguru Y. Pediatric decision-making: informed consent, parental permission, and child assent. In: Diekema DS, Mercurio MR, Adam MB, eds. *Clinical Ethics in Pediatrics: A Case-Based Textbook.* Cambridge, UK: Cambridge University Press; 2011:1–6.

Unguru Y, Coppes MJ, Kamani N. Rethinking pediatric assent: from requirement to ideal. *Pediatr Clin North Am.* 2008;55(1):211–222.

United Nations. United Nations Convention on the Rights of the Child, GA Res 44/736. Art. 18.01, 1989.

U.S. Department of Health and Humans Services. Discretionary Advisory Committee on Heritable Disorders in Newborns and Children. http://www.hrsa.gov/advisorycommittees/mchbadvisory/heritabledisorders/. Accessed November 30, 2013.

U.S. Department of Health and Human Services. *Institutional Review Board Guidebook*, Chapter VI: Special Classes of Subjects. Updated 1993. http://www.hhs.gov/ohrp/archive/irb/irb_chapter6.htm. Accessed August 15, 2013.

U.S. Department of Health and Human Services Office of the Secretary. Human subjects research protections: enhancing protections for research subjects and reducing burden, delay, and ambiguity for investigators—advance notice of proposed rulemaking. *Fed Regist.* 2011;76(143):44512–44531.

U.S. Department of Health and Human Services. Protection of human subjects. 45 CFR Pt. 46. Updated October 1, 2012.

U.S. Department of Health and Human Services. Protection of human subjects: subpart d—additional protections for children involved as subjects in research. 45 CFR 46.401–46.409 (2012).

U.S. Department of Health and Human Services, Secretary's Advisory Committee on Heritable Disorders and Genetic Diseases in Newborns and Children. Briefing paper—considerations and recommendations for a national policy regarding the retention and use of dried blood spot specimens after newborn screening. http://www.hrsa.gov/advisorycommittees/mchbadvisory/heritabledisorders/recommendations/correspondence/briefingdriedblood.pdf. Published September 2010. Accessed July 17, 2013.

U.S. National Commission for the Protection of Human Subjects of Biomedical and Behavioral Research. *Research Involving Children: Report and Recommendations*. Bethesda, MD: National Commission for the Protection of Human Subjects of Biomedical and Behavioral Research; 1977.

van Calcar SC, Gleason LA, Lindh H, et al. 2-methylbutyryl-CoA dehydrogenase deficiency in Hmong infants identified by expanded newborn screen. *WMJ.* 2007;106(1):12–15.

van den Berg M, Timmermans DRM, Ten Kate LP, van Vugt JMG, van der Wal G. Are pregnant women making informed choices about prenatal screening? *Genet Med.* 2005;7(5):332–338.

van Dijck J. *Imagenation: Popular Images of Genetics*. Basingstoke, UK: Palgrave Macmillan Limited; 1998.

Van Karnebeek C, Alfadhel M, Stockler S. Revisiting treatable forms of intellectual disability as future candidates for newborn screening. [abstract]. *J Inherit Metab Dis.* 2011;34(Suppl 1): S7.

van Maldegem BT, Wanders RJA, Wijburg FA. Clinical aspects of short-chain acyl-CoA dehydrogenase deficiency. *J Inherit Metab Dis.* 2010;33(5):507–511.

Van Ness B. Genomic research and incidental findings. *J Law Med Ethics.* 2008;36(2):292–297.

Vansenne F, Bossuyt PM, de Borgie CA. Evaluating the psychological effects of genetic testing in symptomatic patients: a systematic review. *Genet Test Mol Biomarkers.* 2009;13(5):555–563.

Varma S, Wendler D. Risk-benefit assessment in pediatric research. In: Emanuel EJ, Grady C, Crouch RA, et al., eds. *The Oxford Textbook of Clinical Research Ethics.* New York: Oxford University Press; 2008:527–540.

Varmus H. Ten years on—the human genome and medicine. *N Engl J Med.* 2010;362(21):2028–2029.

Veenstra DL, Roth JA, Garrison LP Jr., Ramsey SD, Burke W. A formal risk-benefit framework for genomic tests: facilitating the appropriate translation of genomics into clinical practice. *Genet Med.* 2010;12(11):686–693.

Vermeulen E, Schmidt MK, Aaronson NK, et al. Opt-out plus, the patients' choice: preferences of cancer patients concerning information and consent regimen for future research with biological samples archived in the context of treatment. *J Clin Pathol.* 2009;62(3):275–278.

Vieland VJ, Hallmayer J, Huang Y, et al. Novel method for combined linkage and genome-wide association analysis finds evidence of distinct genetic architecture for two subtypes of autism. *J Neurodev Disord.* 2011;3(2):113–123.

Viera AJ. Predisease: when does it make sense? *Epidemiol Rev.* 2011;33(1):122–134.

Vockley J. Newborn screening: after the thrill is gone. *Mol Genet Metab.* 2007;92(1–2):6–12.

Volandes A. Medical ethics on film: towards a reconstruction of the teaching of healthcare professionals. *J Med Ethics.* 2007;33(11):678–680.

von Bubnoff A. Next-generation sequencing: the race is on. *Cell.* 2008;132(5):721–723.

von Heijne G. A Day in the Life of Dr K. or How I Learned to Stop Worrying and Love Lysozyme: a tragedy in six acts. *J Mol Biol.* 1999;293(2):367–379.

Waddell L, Wiley V, Carpenter K, et al. Medium-chain acyl-CoA dehydrogenase deficiency: genotype-biochemical phenotype correlations. *Mol Genet Metab.* 2006;87(1):32–39.

Wade CH, Wilfond BS, McBride CM. Effects of genetic risk information on children's psychosocial wellbeing: a systematic review of the literature. *Genet Med.* 2010;12(6):317–326.

Wailoo K, Pemberton SG. *The Troubled Dream of Genetic Medicine: Ethnicity and Innovation in Tay-Sachs, Cystic Fibrosis, and Sickle Cell Disease*. Baltimore, MD: Johns Hopkins University Press; 2006.

Waisbren SE, Albers S, Amato S, et al. Effect of expanded newborn screening for biochemical genetic disorders on child outcomes and parental stress. *JAMA.* 2003;290(19):2564–2572.

Waisbren SE, Levy HL, Noble M, et al. Short-chain acyl-CoA dehydrogenase (SCAD) deficiency: an examination of the medical and neurodevelopmental characteristics of 14 cases identified through newborn screening or clinical symptoms. *Mol Genet Metab.* 2008;95(1–2):39–45.

Waisbren SE, Rones M, Read CY, Marsden D, Levy HL. Brief report: predictors of parenting stress among parents of children with biochemical genetic disorders. *J Pediatr Psychol.* 2004;29(7):565–570.

Wakefield AJ. MMR vaccination and autism. *Lancet.* 1999;354(9182):949–950.

Wald N. Neonatal screening: old dogma or sound principle? *Pediatrics.* 2007;119(2):406–407; author reply 407.

Walters L. Ethical and public policy issues in fetal resarch. *Research on the Fetus: Appendix. National Commission for the Protection of Human Subjects of Biomedical and Behavioral Research*, DHEW Publication No. (OS) 76–128. Bethesda, MD: Department of Health, Education and Welfare; 1975:8-1 to 8-18.

Walters L. Genetics and bioethics: how our thinking has changed since 1969. *Theor Med Bioeth.* 2012;33(1):83–95.

Walters L. Human gene therapy: ethics and public policy. *Hum Gene Ther.* 1991;2(2):115–122.

Walters L, Palmer JG. *The Ethics of Human Gene Therapy*. New York: Oxford University Press; 1997.

Wang K, Zhang H, Ma D, et al. Common genetic variants on 5p14.1 associate with autism spectrum disorders. *Nature*. 2009;459(7246):528–533.

Warren S, Brandeis LD. The right to privacy. *Harvard Law Rev*. 1890;15(4):193–220.

Warren ZE, Stone WL. Clinical best practices: diagnosis and assessment of young children. In: Amaral D, Dawson G, Geschwind DH, eds. *Autism Spectrum Disorders*. New York: Oxford University Press; 2011:1269–1280.

Wasserman DT, Wachbroit RS, Bickenbach JE. *Quality of Life and Human Difference: Genetic Testing, Health Care, and Disability*. New York: Cambridge University Press; 2005.

Watson JD, Crick FHC. Molecular structure of nucleic acids: a structure for deoxyribose nucleic acid. *Nature* 1953;171:737–738.

Watson MS. Current status of newborn screening: decision-making about the conditions to include in screening programs. *Ment Retard Dev Disabil Res Rev*. 2006;12(4):230–235.

Weijer C, Emanuel EJ. Ethics. Protecting communities in biomedical research. *Science*. 2000;289(5482):1142–1144.

Weil CJ, Mechanic LE, Green T, et al. NCI think tank concerning the identifiability of biospecimens and "omic" data. *Genet Med*. 2013. doi: 10.1038/gim.2013.40.

Weinstein AL. *A Scream Goes Through the House: What Literature Teaches Us About Life*. New York: Random House; 2003.

Welch HG, Schwartz L, Woloshin S. *Overdiagnosed: Making People Sick in the Pursuit of Health*. Boston, MA: Beacon Press; 2011.

Wendler D. The assent requirement in pediatric research. In: Emanuel EJ, Grady C, Crouch RA, et al., eds. *The Oxford Textbook of Clinical Research Ethics*. New York: Oxford University Press; 2008:661–672.

Wendler D. One-time general consent for research on biological samples. *BMJ*. 2006;332(7540):544–547.

Wendler D, Emanuel E. The debate over research on stored biological samples: what do sources think? *Arch Intern Med*. 2002;162(13):1457–1462.

Wendler D, Shah S. Should children decide whether they are enrolled in nonbeneficial research? *Am J Bioeth*. 2003;3(4):1–7.

Wendler D, Varma S. Minimal risk in pediatric research. *J Pediatr*. 2006;149(6):855–861.

Wendler DS. Assent in paediatric research: theoretical and practical considerations. *J Med Ethics*. 2006;32(4):229–234.

Wertz DC. Testing children and adolescents. In: Burley J, Harris J, eds. *A Companion to Genethics*. Malden, MA: Blackwell Publishers; 2002:92–113.

Wertz DC, Fanos JH, Reilly PR. Genetic testing for children and adolescents. Who decides? *JAMA*. 1994;272(11):875–881.

Wertz DC, Fletcher JC, Berg K, Boulyjenkov V. *Guidelines on Ethical Issues in Medical Genetics and the Provision of Genetics Services*. Geneva: WHO; 1995.

Westbrook MJ, Wright MF, Van Driest SL, et al. Mapping the incidentalome: estimating incidental findings generated through clinical pharmacogenomics testing. *Genet Med*. 2013;15(5):325–331.

Wexler A. *Mapping Fate: A Memoir of Family, Risk, and Genetic Research*. New York: Times Books: Random House; 1995.

Wheeler DA, Srinivasan M, Egholm M, et al. The complete genome of an individual by massively parallel DNA sequencing. *Nature*. 2008;452(7189):872–876.

Wheeler PG, Smith R, Dorkin HL, Parad RB, Comeau AM, Bianchi DW. Genetic counseling after implementation of statewide cystic fibrosis newborn screening: Two years' experience in one medical center. *Genet Med*. 2001;3(6):411–415.

White S. *The Other Place*. New York: Dramatists Play Service; 2011.

Whitehead NS, Brown DS, Layton CM. *Survey of Parental Attitudes Regarding Voluntary Newborn Screening. [pamphlet]*. Research Triangle Park, NC: RTI Press; 2010.

Whitmarsh I, Davis AM, Skinner D, Bailey DB Jr. A place for genetic uncertainty: parents valuing an unknown in the meaning of disease. *Soc Sci Med.* 2007;65(6):1082–1093.

Wilcken B. The consequences of extended newborn screening programmes: do we know who needs treatment? *J Inherit Metab Dis.* 2008;31(2):173–177.

Wilcken B. Expanded newborn screening: reducing harm, assessing benefit. *J Inherit Metab Dis.* 2010;33(Suppl 2):S205–S210.

Wilcken B. Fatty acid oxidation disorders: outcome and long-term prognosis. *J Inherit Metab Dis.* 2010;33(5):501–506.

Wilcken B. Rare diseases and the assessment of intervention: what sorts of clinical trials can we use? *J Inherit Metab Dis.* 2001;24(2):291–298.

Wilfond B. Predicting our future: lessons from Winnie-the-Pooh. *Hastings Cent Rep.* 2012;42(4):3.

Wilfond B, Ross LF. From genetics to genomics: ethics, policy, and parental decision-making. *J Pediatr Psychol.* 2009;34(6):639–647.

Wilfond BS. Ethical and policy implications of conducting carrier testing and newborn screening for the same condition. In: Baily MA, Murray TH, eds. *Ethics and Newborn Genetic Screening: New Technologies, New Challenges*. Baltimore, MD: Johns Hopkins University Press; 2009:292–311.

Wilfond BS, Carpenter KJ. Incidental findings in pediatric research. *J Law Med Ethics.* 2008;36(2):332–340, 213.

Wilfond BS, Diekema DS. Engaging children in genomics research: decoding the meaning of assent in research. *Genet Med.* 2012;14(4):437–443.

Wilfond BS, Gollust SE. Policy issues for expanding newborn screening programs: the cystic fibrosis newborn screening experience in the United States. *J Pediatr.* 2005;146(5):668–674.

Wilfond BS, Parad RB, Fost N. Balancing benefits and risks for cystic fibrosis newborn screening: implications for policy decisions. *J Pediatr.* 2005;147(3 Suppl):S109–S113.

Wilfond BS, Thomson EJ. Models of public health genetic policy development. In: Khoury MJ, Burke W, Thomson EJ, eds. *Genetics and Public Health in the 21st Century: Using Genetic Information to Improve Health and Prevent Disease*. New York: Oxford University Press; 2000:61–81.

Wilkinson D. Dissent about assent in paediatric research. *J Med Ethics.* 2012;38(1):2.

Wilkinson S. "Eugenics talk" and the language of bioethics. *J Med Ethics.* 2008;34(6):467–471.

Williams BA, Wolf LE. Biobanking, consent, and certificates of confidentiality: does the ANPRM muddy the water? *J Law Med Ethics.* 2013;41(2):440–453.

Williams JK, Daack-Hirsch S, Driessnack M, et al. Researcher and institutional review board chair perspectives on incidental findings in genomic research. *Genet Test Mol Biomarkers.* 2012;16(6):508–513.

Wilson JMG. Current trends and problems in health screening. *J Clin Pathol.* 1973;26(8):555–563.

Wilson JMG, Jungner G. *Principles and Practice of Screening for Disease*. Public Health Papers No. 34. Geneva: WHO; 1968. http://whqlibdoc.who.int/php/WHO_PHP_34.pdf. Accessed July 26, 2013.

Wing L, Gould J, Gillberg C. Autism spectrum disorders in the DSM-V: better or worse than the DSM-IV? *Res Dev Disabil.* 2011;32(2):768–773.

Wivel NA, Walters L. Germ-line gene modification and disease prevention: some medical and ethical perspectives. *Science*. 1993;262(5133):533–538.

Wjst M. Caught you: threats to confidentiality due to the public release of large-scale genetic data sets. *BMC Med Ethics*. 2010;11:21.

Wolf LE. Advancing research on stored biological materials: reconciling law, ethics, and practice. *Minn J Law Sci & Tech*. 2010;11(1):99–156.

Wolf LE, Bouley TA, McCulloch CE. Genetic research with stored biological materials: ethics and practice. *IRB*. 2010;32(2):7–18.

Wolf LE, Catania JA, Dolcini MM, Pollack LM, Lo B. IRB chairs' perspectives on genomics research involving stored biological materials: ethical concerns and proposed solutions. *J Empir Res Hum Res Ethics*. 2008;3(4):99–111.

Wolf SM. The past, present, and future of the debate over return of research results and incidental findings. *Genet Med*. 2012;14(4):355–357.

Wolf SM, Annas GJ, Elias S. Point-counterpoint. Patient autonomy and incidental findings in clinical genomics. *Science*. 2013;340(6136):1049–1050.

Wolf SM, Crock BN, Van Ness B, et al. Managing incidental findings and research results in genomic research involving biobanks and archived data sets. *Genet Med*. 2012;14(4):361–384.

Wolf SM, et al. Symposium: incidental findings in human subjects research: from imaging to genomics. *J Law Med Ethics*. 2008;36(2):211–435.

Wolf SM, Lawrenz FP, Nelson CA, et al. Managing incidental findings in human subjects research: analysis and recommendations. *J Law Med Ethics*. 2008;36(2):219–248.

Wolf SM, Paradise J, Caga-anan C. The law of incidental findings in human subjects research: establishing researchers' duties. *J Law Med Ethics*. 2008;36(2):361–383.

Wolff T. *Mendel's Theatre: Heredity, Eugenics, and Early Twentieth-Century American Drama*. 1st ed. New York: Palgrave Macmillan; 2009. *Palgrave Studies in Theatre and Performance History*.

World Health Organization Scientific Group on Screening for Inborn Errors of Metabolism. *Screening for Inborn Errors of Metabolism*. World Health Organization Technical Report Series. Geneva: World Health Organization; 1968.

World Health Organization. *Genomics and World Health: Report of the Advisory Committee on Health Research*. Geneva: World Health Organization; 2002.

World Medical Association. WMA Declaration of Helsinki: Ethical Principles for Medical Research Involving Human Subjects. *JAMA*. 2013;310(20):2191–2194.

World Medical Association. *WMA Declaration of Helsinki—Ethical Principles for Medical Research Involving Human Subjects*. WMA. http://www.wma.net/en/30publications/10policies/b3/. Amended October 2008. Accessed July 26, 2013.

Worthey EA, Mayer AN, Syverson GD, et al. Making a definitive diagnosis: successful clinical application of whole exome sequencing in a child with intractable inflammatory bowel disease. *Genet Med*. 2011;13(3):255–262.

Wright L, MacRae S, Gordon D, et al. Disclosure of misattributed paternity: issues involved in the discovery of unsought information. *Semin Dial*. 2002;15(3):202–206.

Yu JH, Jamal SM, Tabor HK, Bamshad MJ. Self-guided management of exome and whole-genome sequencing results: changing the results return model. *Genet Med*. 2013. doi: 10.1038/gim.2013.35.

Zawati MH, Knoppers BM. International normative perspectives on the return of individual research results and incidental findings in genomic biobanks. *Genet Med.* 2012;14(4):484–489.

Zelkowitz P, Papageorgiou A, Bardin C, Wang T. Persistent maternal anxiety affects the interaction between mothers and their very low birthweight children at 24 months. *Early Hum Dev* 2009;85(1):51–58.

Ziegler A. *Photograph 51.* New York: Dramatists Play Service; 2011.

Zusevics K. Ancillary care, genomics, and the need and opportunity for community-based participatory research. *Am J Bioeth.* 2013;13(2):54–56.